AGE ERASERS

for

MEN

HUNDREDS
OF FAST
AND
EASY WAYS
TO BEAT
THE YEARS

By Doug Dollemore, Mark Giuliucci
and the Editors of Men'sHealth Magazine

 Rodale Press, Emmaus, Pennsylvania

Copyright © 1994 by Rodale Press, Inc.
Cover photograph copyright © 1994 by James McLoughlin
Illustrations copyright © 1994 by Susan Rosenberger

Printed in the United States of America on acid-free ∞, recycled paper containing a minimum of 20% post-consumer waste ♲

Library of Congress Cataloging-in-Publication Data

Dollemore, Doug.
    Age erasers for men : hundreds of fast and easy ways to beat the years / by Doug
 Dollemore, Mark Giuliucci, and the editors of Men's health magazine.
        p.   cm.
    Includes index.
    ISBN 0–87596–213–0 hardcover
      1. Middle aged men—Health and hygiene.   2. Aged men—Health and hygiene.
  3. Middle aged men—Mental health.   4. Aged men—Mental health.   5. Longevity.
  I. Giuliucci, Mark.   II. Men's health (Magazine).   III. Title.
  RA777.8.D65   1994
  613′.04234—dc20   94–26444
                                                                            CIP

Distributed in the book trade by St. Martin's Press

2   4   6   8   10   9   7   5   3   1   hardcover

OUR MISSION
We publish books that empower people's lives.
RODALE ❧ BOOKS

Age Erasers for Men Editorial and Design Staff

SENIOR MANAGING EDITOR: PATRICIA FISHER

SENIOR EDITOR: RUSSELL WILD

STAFF WRITERS: DOUG DOLLEMORE AND MARK GIULIUCCI
WITH SID KIRCHHEIMER, ELLEN MICHAUD, ELISABETH TORG,
LAURA WALLACE-SMITH, MARK D. WISNIEWSKI

CONTRIBUTING WRITERS: STEFAN BECHTEL, JEFF CSATARI,
LISA DELANEY, TIM FRIEND, MARK GOLIN, MARCIA HOLMAN,
CLAIRE KOWALCHIK, RICHARD LALIBERTE, JEFF MEADE,
MELISSA MEYERS, RICHARD TRUBO, JOSEPH M. WARGO,
STEPHEN WILLIAMS

ART DIRECTOR: STAN GREEN
INTERIOR AND COVER DESIGNER: ACEY LEE
STUDIO MANAGER: JOE GOLDEN
LAYOUT DESIGNERS: DEBORAH KRIGER, RICHARD SNYDER
TECHNICAL ARTISTS: KRISTEN PAGE MORGAN, DAVID Q. PRYOR,
COLIN SHERMAN
COVER PHOTOGRAPHER: JAMES MCLOUGHLIN
ILLUSTRATOR: SUSAN ROSENBERGER

RESEARCHERS AND FACT-CHECKERS: SUSAN E. BURDICK, HILTON CASTON,
CHRISTINE DREISBACH, VALERIE EDWARDS-PAULIK, JAN EICKMEIER,
THERESA FOGARTY, CAROL J. GILMORE, DEBORAH PEDRON,
SALLY A. REITH, SANDRA SALERA-LLOYD, ANITA SMALL, CAROL SVEC,
MICHELLE M. SZULBORSKI, JOHN WALDRON

COPY EDITORS: SUSAN G. BERG, KATHY DIEHL

OFFICE STAFF: ROBERTA MULLINER, MARY LOU STEPHEN, JULIE KEHS

Men's Health Books

EDITOR-IN-CHIEF, RODALE BOOKS: BILL GOTTLIEB
EXECUTIVE EDITOR: DEBORA A. TKAC
ART DIRECTOR: JANE COLBY KNUTILA
RESEARCH MANAGER: ANN GOSSY YERMISH
COPY MANAGER: LISA D. ANDRUSCAVAGE
EDITOR, _MEN'S HEALTH_ MAGAZINE: MICHAEL LAFAVORE

CONTENTS

Part III: Boost Your Youthfulness

INTRODUCTION

This, Bud, Is for You

There's an old saying that goes something like "Getting old is tough, but it sure beats the alternative." Well, yes, it does, but I would argue that getting older doesn't have to be so tough, nor should we accept a gradual physical and mental decline as inevitable.

There's no such thing as an "aging process." There aren't any rules that say you'll have trouble walking at this age or lose your memory skills at that age. Sure, we all know men who seem to begin a rapid slide downhill in their fifties, but if you think about it, you probably also know guys in their seventies and eighties who have tremendous energy and enthusiasm, men who are in great shape not just "for their age" but for any age.

Theories about aging are changing rapidly as scientists learn more about human potential. One thing is already quite clear from their studies: Aging is inevitable—there's no way to stop the clock—but a gradual decline in good health and good looks isn't. "Many of the things we blame on aging really have nothing to do with getting older," says Ben Douglas, Ph.D., professor of anatomy at the University of Mississippi Medical Center in Jackson and author of *AgeLess: Living Younger Longer*. Things such as diminished vitality, strength and sexual vigor, mental fogginess, even premature wrinkling—none of these is a natural side effect of aging at 40, 50, 60 or 70 years old, and each of them can be controlled.

You can lead the pack, staying strong and active well past middle age, or you can fall into line with those who accept the notion that aging and decline are inseparable. But make no mistake, you have a choice: You can take an active role and hold on to your looks, your strength and your sexuality, or you can let a little bit of each slip away with each birthday.

The earlier you start thumb wrestling with the hands of time, the better. The problems that lead to aging are cumulative, and the sooner you start correcting them, the better off you'll be in the long run.

But neither is it ever too late to start. A study at Tufts University, in Medford, Massachusetts, showed that people in their nineties were able to increase their leg strength by as much as 200 percent when they started lifting weights.

We created *Age Erasers for Men* to help you redefine your personal agenda for the coming years and to change your thinking about what it means to age in the 1990s. Within its pages, you'll find all you need to know about how to combat the forces that can make you look and feel older than you are—not just facts but practical, simple steps you can take right now to start turning back the clock. And because males and females age differently, we've created this book for men only. It deals specifically with your strengths, problems and challenges. We did a companion book for women called *Age Erasers for Women*.

If you're ready to take an active role in your future health, read on. And if you need a quote to live by, forget that stuff about aging being tough. Here's a better thought, from noted anthropologist Ashley Montagu: "The goal of life is to die young—as late as possible."

Michael Lafavore
Executive Editor
Men's Health Magazine

Part I

How a Man Ages

Moving Through the Decades

Plot Your Own Course

You've noticed the changes.

Maybe it's as subtle as aches and pains from a weekend pickup game that last well into Tuesday, maybe as obvious as thinning hair or a thickening gut. It could be that you're squinting a little more or hearing a little less, panting too hard from exercise or not hard enough over sex.

Whatever it is, it means you're putting on a few years. But that doesn't mean that you have to get old.

Scientists who study the aging process readily acknowledge that there's little you can do about some aspects of aging. The fact is, as men age, certain changes tend to occur—what those in the aging biz call biomarkers of aging.

Some of these changes are obvious: Hair gets thinner and grayer, skin gets looser and more wrinkled, vision gets more fuzzy, and hearing begins to fade. Muscles get weaker. Lungs wind more easily. And of course, the gut tends to expand as metabolism slows down, making you more likely to gain weight even if you eat the same amount of calories.

Some changes are less noticeable but can be even more significant to overall health: Cholesterol levels start increasing steadily, raising your risk of heart disease. Immunity weakens, so you're more susceptible to illness and you take longer to bounce back. Even brain cells start dying off by the thousands each day starting around age 30.

To further add insult to injury, the part of us that for so long did a lot of our thinking, our libido, also begins to wane, thanks to lower levels of testosterone that decrease our sexual appetite.

But none of these changes is inevitable.

Outpacing Aging

You may not be able to outrun Father Time, but more and more, research seems to indicate that you can keep one step ahead of him.

"How you age is more of a reflection of how you live, a lifetime's accumulation of the things you do every day," says William Evans, Ph.D., director of the Noell Laboratory for Human Performance Research at Pennsylvania State University in University Park and co-author of *Biomarkers: The Ten Determinants of Aging You Can Control.* "And to a very great degree, those things are under your control."

And it's never too late to change. "There is a lot of research showing that this wonderful body of ours is almost indefinitely renewable if we give it a chance," says Walter Bortz, M.D., clinical associate professor of medicine at Stanford University in Stanford, California, and author of *We Live Too Short and Die Too Long.* In fact, researchers at Duke University in Durham, North Carolina, have calculated that simply by taking charge of certain key actions in your life—like eating right and exercising regularly—you can boost your life expectancy by up to 15 years.

Decades of Change

The typical guy starts to show the first signs of aging soon after reaching full maturity—around age 22. In other words, just as we reach our peak, many of us begin our decline.

"But there's no reason for it. The human body is designed to last 110 years," says Ben Douglas, Ph.D., professor of anatomy at the University of Mississippi Medical Center in Jackson and author of *AgeLess: Living Younger Longer.* "Just like other members of the animal kingdom, our bodies are designed to last roughly five times the age of when we reach our sexual maturity. And with proper care, we should."

Here's a decade-by-decade breakdown of the likely aging process—and what you can do to beat the odds.

In your twenties, the first faint signs of aging usually begin. Metabolism, the rate at which your body burns calories at rest, slows by about 2 percent per decade from this point on. This means that every extra dessert or helping of chips could mean a tighter belt. Lung capacity and muscle strength also start to diminish, an ongoing trend that can result in one-third of current capacity by age 70. So now is no time to rest on your laurels—or anything else.

"Most of these changes result from inactivity, and you can minimize all these adverse effects just by staying active," says Dr. Douglas. "That's not to say that you won't notice any change. But something as simple as taking deep breaths religiously several times a day—anything that helps you breathe in and out as deeply as possible—can minimize the lung damage dramatically: Instead of the 60 percent reduction you'll get in later years, you'll get only a 20 percent reduction."

Why Do We Die Younger?

In the United States, and in virtually every other society, males typically die seven years earlier than females—and we're not just talking about humans. From apes to canaries to leopard frogs, "studies disclose that greater female longevity is virtually universal in zoology," says William R. Hazzard, M.D., chairman of the Department of Internal Medicine at the Bowman Gray School of Medicine of Wake Forest University in Winston-Salem, North Carolina.

Sorry, we can't explain the whys for the critters, but researchers have some theories on why women typically die at age 79, while men pass on at 72.

While smoking and violence play some role—men are more fond of both, although men now smoke less and women smoke more than they used to—the main reason is that we get diseases sooner. Guys under 50 are twice as likely to die from heart disease as women of the same age, largely because of our testosterone, which doesn't offer the same protection against cholesterol levels as estrogen. We're also more likely to get strokes, cancer or other life-threatening diseases at an earlier age.

Some of this, of course, is fate, but a lot of it is up to you. With the right lifestyle, you can minimize the damage prompted by your genes or even avoid illness altogether—for a longer, healthier and happier life decades beyond what's written in the statistics.

Meanwhile, he advocates a regular exercise program that emphasizes fun over anything else to keep muscles strong and metabolism high, so calories are burned more efficiently. "Do it daily, in moderation, and pick something you enjoy so you stick with it."

In your thirties, skin starts to lose its tightness, and crow's-feet may start to appear. "Limiting sun exposure—or wearing a hat that shields your face—can help offset that," says Dr. Douglas. And keep skin moisturized, since there's a tendency toward dryness.

Meanwhile, hearing worsens—the result of continued exposure to loud noise. So turn down the music and wear ear protection when working with tools or guns. "People assume that you have to lose your hearing, but I have studied people in their nineties who had no hearing loss whatsoever because they protected themselves from continued exposure to loud noise," he adds. "Meanwhile, you take anyone in the army who is right-handed, and by his thirties, his

(continued on page 8)

Before the Looking Glass

Most of us keep track of the aging process with mirrors. Here's what a man can and can't see as he watches his face and body through the years.

Twenties. He's probably starting a career, maybe a family. But unfortunately, he's also starting to show the first subtle signs of aging—probably in the form of thinning hair. Muscles weaken, and he gets winded easier during exercise. But it's no time to hang up the sneakers, as the rate at which his body burns calories begins to slow. So now it's especially important to pay attention to diet and exercise.

Thirties. Laugh lines and fine furrows appear around his eyes and mouth as the skin starts to lose its elasticity. Hearing starts to fade, especially if he likes to pump up the volume on the stereo. Cholesterol control becomes important as levels of LDL (low-density lipoprotein, the dangerous kind) continue to climb, along with hairlines. Meanwhile, the good HDL (high-density lipoprotein) cholesterol starts to drop. After around age 35, gray hair starts to show, especially at the temples, along with a potbelly.

Forties. Uh-oh! Middle age kicks into high gear. Male pattern baldness rears its ugly head in full force (at least in guys prone to baldness). Wrin-

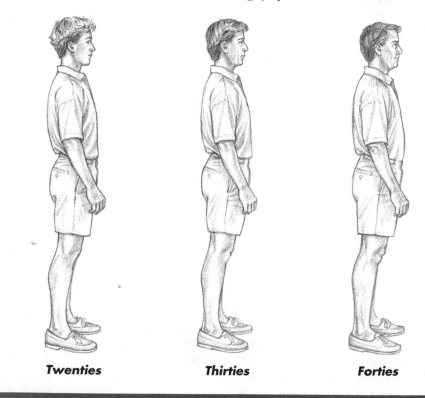

Twenties   **Thirties**   **Forties**

kles show up on his eyelids, and crow's-feet and other facial lines begin to appear. He may need glasses or bifocals as the eye lens starts to stiffen. But he can now concentrate on things other than sex—the libido starts to wane as testosterone levels start to taper off.

Fifties. Some good news: After decades of climbing, cholesterol finally levels off. The bad news: Immunity weakens, making him more prone to illness and infection. Gums start to recede noticeably, and early signs of prostate problems may start, such as weak or dribbling urine flow. Jowls and a double chin may become noticeable.

Sixties. He loses weight as muscle mass decreases, resulting in sagging skin, especially around the arms and shoulders; bags under eyes are also noticeable. Shoulders are narrower, and hair color fades. Mentally, he's every bit the man he was 30 years ago; problem-solving skills are strong.

Seventies. His skin is rougher and loses its uniform color, resulting in more splotches and age spots. The nose becomes longer and wider; earlobes are fatter. He needs less sleep, which may mean more illness, since the body repairs itself during slumber. His memory also suffers.

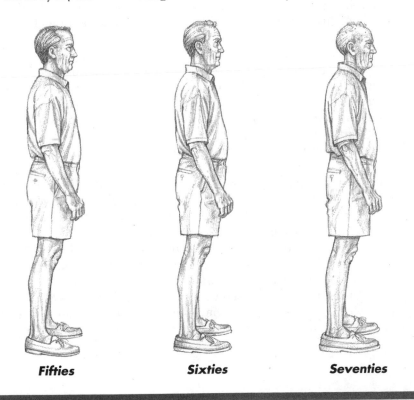

| **Fifties** | **Sixties** | **Seventies** |

left ear has less hearing because of the way he shoots his weapons. But his right ear doesn't suffer as much damage, so it doesn't lose as much hearing."

Levels of LDL (low-density lipoprotein) cholesterol, the dangerous kind, continue a steady rise that begins around puberty, while artery-scouring HDL (high-density lipoprotein) cholesterol, the good kind, drops in this decade. So it's essential to eat low-fat (to lower LDLs) and exercise (to raise HDLs). Kidneys begin working less efficiently, dropping off by around 1 percent a year after age 30; so drink eight to ten glasses of water a day to keep them in top shape.

In your forties, your eye lens begins to stiffen, making it difficult to focus on close objects. But you can minimize this with a series of eye exercises, such as holding your thumb at arm's length and slowly moving it in circles and figures eights while following it with your eyes. Your optometrist can give you a series of such exercises, which take about 15 minutes a day, to delay or avoid the need for glasses or bifocals.

A little lower, you might find that your sexual urges have waned as testosterone levels begin slowly tapering off. The good news is that you can concentrate on something other than sex; the other good news is there's no reason why you still can't be a horizontal dynamo. "Frequency of sexual activity may change, but for the most part, sexual ability doesn't," says Dr. Douglas. In other words, focus on quality rather than quantity. Staying aerobically fit will maintain killer erections as well as do wonders for that ever-slowing metabolism.

In your fifties, cholesterol levels—which had been climbing steadily since your teens—finally plateau, so you'll notice a welcome steadying trend. But it's no time to hit the doughnuts. Since immunity is likely to weaken, making you more susceptible to infections and disease, diet remains very important—especially one rich in immune-building antioxidant vitamins like vitamin C, vitamin E and beta-carotene.

In your sixties, you may be amazed to discover that you're actually beginning to lose weight; it's likely caused by a loss in muscle mass (which weighs more than fat). You also begin to shrink in another way, losing about a half-inch in height over the next 20 years. Skin is noticeably sagging, especially around your arms and shoulders. "Some of this can be minimized with regular exercise to keep muscles toned and skin tight," says Dr. Douglas.

Mentally, though, you're every bit the man you've always been: Problem-solving abilities are still strong and won't begin to fade until your mid seventies—especially if you stay sharp with crossword puzzles and other brainteasers.

In your seventies, there's no reason why you shouldn't be fit as a fiddle, says Dr. Douglas. "Most of what we blame on aging has nothing to do with getting older," he says. "Instead, it's a question of staying active in mind and body."

AGING: IT'S A STATE OF MIND

You're as Young as You Think

Forget about the birthday candles on your cake or gray hairs on your head. Age isn't a number, say researchers. It's an attitude. Some guys are barely past puberty and already worried about midlife crisis. Other men are pushing 75—and feeling great.

"It's absolutely true that you're as young as you think," says Ben Douglas, Ph.D., professor of anatomy at the University of Mississippi Medical Center in Jackson and author of *AgeLess: Living Younger Longer*. "By having the right attitude, not only will you live longer, but you'll remain younger longer."

He ought to know. Part of his job is to research why old people remain young in heart, mind and body despite reaching ages usually achieved only by tortoises. And after studying scores of centenarians—including one man who was still enjoying a vibrant and disease-free life at age 110—he concludes that there's no reason why we all can't live through that triple figure . . . as long as the healthiest part of you is between your ears.

"Regardless of race, religion, socioeconomic background, even their diet, in my research the people who age the best all seem to share similar characteristics," says Dr. Douglas. "They all have a good sense of humor; they don't take life too seriously. They tend to be active, having worked hard every day of their lives. And they also tend to be forward-looking people. Rather than looking back at what they have done or didn't do, they focus on what's ahead, whether it's the election or a baseball game or seeing their grandchildren."

Those findings seem to go along with what other scientists have been saying for years: How you think about aging may be the most crucial point in how you actually age.

How Many More Years Have You Got?

The long and the short of longevity is this: You're born with a genetic wiring diagram imprinted on your cells, and that affects your life span. But beyond that, it's really up to you. To get a clearer idea of what your life expectancy may be, try the following quiz. It's based on the work of experts on aging, primarily Robert F. Allen, Ph.D., author of *Lifegain*. Keep a running tally of your score as you answer the following questions.

Family History

1. Did your grandparents live to be at least 80? _____ (+1 for each instance)
2. Did your mother or father live that long? _____ (+3 for each)
3. Did your mother or father die of a heart attack or stroke before age 50? _____ (–4 for each)
4. Do any immediate family members (parent, sibling, grandparent) have now or did have cancer, a heart condition or diabetes since childhood? _____ (–3 for each)
5. Did any die of the above problems before age 60? _____ (–2 for each)
6. Did any immediate family member die of prostate cancer, colon cancer or any other natural cause before age 60? _____ (–1 for each)

Exercise

7. Do you exercise aerobically for at least 30 minutes three or more times a week? _____ (+2)
8. Do you play sports or do light physical activities like yard work once or twice a week? _____ (+1)
9. Do you almost never exercise? _____ (–2)

Diet

10. Do you get five or more helpings of fruits and vegetables daily? _____ (+5)
11. Do you eat a lot of high-fat foods but rarely, if ever, eat fruits and vegetables? _____ (–4)
12. Do you eat a lot of high-fat foods but try to balance these with plenty of fruits and vegetables? _____ (+1)

Cholesterol

13. Has your total cholesterol always been 200 or less? _____ (+4)

14. Is your total cholesterol now 200 or less but once was between 240 and 299? _____ (+3)

15. Is your total cholesterol now 200 or less but once was 300 or more? _____ (+2)

16. Is your total cholesterol now between 240 and 299? _____ (–1)

17. Is your total cholesterol now above 300? _____ (–2)

Blood Pressure

The following questions all pertain to your diastolic blood pressure (the 80 in a reading of 120/80), considered the more important number.

18. Has your diastolic pressure always been 88 or lower? _____ (+3)

19. Is it 88 or lower but once was 90 or higher? _____ (+2)

20. Is 88 or lower but once was 105 or higher? _____ (+1)

21. Is it 90 to 104? _____ (–1)

22. Is it above 104? _____ (–2)

Smoking

23. Did you ever smoke? _____ (If no, +2)

24. Did you quit five or more years ago? _____ (+1)

25. Do you smoke less than a pack a day? _____ (–1)

26. Do you smoke one-half to one pack a day? _____ (–2)

27. Do you smoke one to two packs a day? _____ (–6)

28. Do you smoke more than two packs a day? _____ (–10)

29. Do you smoke marijuana once a week or more? _____ (–1)

Stress

30. Is the best description of you easygoing and relaxed? _____ (+3)

31. Is the best description of you aggressive or easily angered? _____ (–3)

32. Do you have a demanding job with little say over how things get done? _____ (–2)

(continued)

How Many More Years—Continued

Education

33. Do you have four or more years of college? _____ (+3)
34. Do you have one to three years of college? _____ (+2)
35. Do you have a high school education only? _____ (+1)

Weight

36. Have you always been within 5 percent of your ideal weight? (See height and weight chart on page 223.) _____ (+2)
37. Are you currently within 5 percent of your ideal weight, but were once more than 30 percent over? _____ (+1)
38. Have you always been from 5 to 30 percent overweight? _____ (–1)
39. Has your weight fluctuated by more than ten pounds several times since high school? _____ (–2)
40. Have you always been more than 30 percent overweight? _____ (–4)

Alcohol

41. Do you drink moderately (no more than two beers, two glasses of wine or two shots of whiskey a day on average), but not to the point of drunkenness? _____ (+2)
42. Do you abstain totally from alcohol? _____ (+1)
43. Do you regularly drink until intoxicated? _____ (–6)

Medical exams

44. Do you have an annual physical exam? _____ (+1)
45. Do you have a proctological exam every other year after age 40? _____ (+2)

How to Score

Begin with 72 (the average life expectancy for men). Adjust for your current age (add one point if you've passed the age of 30, two if you've passed 40 and so forth). Total your score from the questions above. Then add it all up.

_____72_____ Average life expectancy

+ _____ Age adjustment

+ _____ Score from questions above

= _____ Total (estimated life expectancy)

Improving with Age

That's not to say that you can smoke like a chimney, drink like a fish, eat like a pig and just psych your sofa-slugging self into being the George Burns of your block. You have to practice a healthy lifestyle to avoid most of the conditions that cause us to look and feel old. But even so, why is it that some guys follow the rules and still get old while others age slower than Dick Clark?

It may be a matter of self-perception. "People who live long and healthy lives have a purpose in life; they have a reason to get out of bed each morning," says Walter Bortz, M.D., clinical associate professor of medicine at Stanford University in Stanford, California, and author of *We Live Too Short and Die Too Long.* "My friend George Sheehan (the late *Runner's World* columnist) used to say 'Make yourself indispensable.' My granddad used to say 'Make yourself necessary.' People who live long and productive lives don't feel old because they make themselves necessary."

And so should you.

A good first step is to realize that getting older, while having its drawbacks, also has certain advantages—beyond looking "distinguished" as you gray. So before checking out the sticker prices of red convertibles, keep a few things in mind about middle age and beyond.

Emotionally, you're at your most stable—or you should be. Maybe you can't bench-press as much as some pimply faced teen at the gym, but does your wife or sweetheart care? Maybe your hair is thinning or you need bifocals, but will your kids love you any less because of it? With all due respect to your fraternity brothers, your current support group is probably more loving and understanding than what you got in those bulla-bulla days, and hey, at least you don't have to arm-wrestle for the last beer. Plus, with each passing year comes the added maturity to see things more rationally and with the experience lacking in someone 10 or 20 years younger.

Financially, you're at the prime of your career and earning potential. No longer green and still not ready to be sent to greener pastures, your worth on the job skyrockets, and promotions come more readily than they did a decade ago. After all, you're taken more seriously now. And as a result, you're able to buy those finer things in life: a nice car, a nice house or apartment, even bookshelves that don't involve concrete blocks.

And intellectually, you've never been more capable. In fact, practical problem-solving ability peaks during your forties, according to research at the University of Wisconsin. (Yes, it's even greater than in your teens, twenties or thirties.) So even though brain cells are dying, experience and common sense—the stuff that comes only with age—more than make up the difference. This seems to hold true well past the middle years.

Case in point: Researchers at the University of Southern California and the University of Missouri timed a group of typists ranging from college age to well into their sixties. They expected a blowout by the younger folks, since their fingers are more nimble and their reaction times are faster. But everyone typed an average of 60 words per minute. The older typists, it seemed, achieved their speed with cunning: They read ahead in the text and typed smarter, saving a millisecond here and a nanosecond there.

See the Glass Half-Full

There are other studies, all of which prove the same point. Maybe you've lost something in certain aspects, but you've gained so much more in others. And once you realize this and can see your future through optimistic eyes, you'll minimize your chances of feeling old. Not only will optimism help you be a little happier with the inevitable, it also may actually help you live longer.

Another case in point: According to a study at Brown University in Providence, Rhode Island, blaming your aches and pains on age itself, rather than on the actual cause—like playing basketball for too long or the fact that you caught a virus—may make you die sooner. Researchers surveyed nearly 1,400 people over age 70 who were experiencing health problems. Those who blamed their ailing health on "old age" had a 78 percent greater risk of dying in the near future than those who cited a specific, non-aging reason. "Once you say a problem is due to old age . . . you've given up, in a way," explains William Rakowski, Ph.D., assistant professor of medical science at the Center for Gerontology and Health Care Research at Brown University.

Of course, optimists are made, not born. "The right attitude needs to be cultivated," says Dr. Douglas. "It's done so in realizing that the world doesn't come to an end if your team doesn't win the pennant or if the Republicans or Democrats don't get into the White House. It's going out and running the best race you can run."

And that's something to keep in mind as you are about to run the most challenging laps of your life.

"There are obvious things you can do to look and feel younger and live longer: Don't smoke. Exercise regularly. Eat a good diet and use alcohol in moderation. But most people know about that," adds Huber Warner, Ph.D., deputy associate director of the Biology of Aging Program at the National Institute on Aging in Bethesda, Maryland. "To me, one secret to aging well is the ability to come to grips with a decline in physical function that is real but still being able to use what you have to maintain function as well as possible. Maybe you'll never be a champion pole vaulter, but realize that even though you may be older, you can still do a lot of things—and still do them well."

Part II
Stop the Age Robbers

AGE SPOTS

Who Says You Can't Reverse Time?

Sometimes they're called age spots, sometimes liver spots. But these harmless brown marks on the face and the backs of the hands, among other places, have nothing to do with your liver and are only indirectly related to age. But they can make you feel older, because they commonly appear on older skin.

Doctors call them solar lentigos, and they crop up on skin that has been exposed to the sun for years. Because it often takes decades for them to form, in a sense they're related to age. But if your skin is always covered, you could live to be 100 years old without developing a single spot, says Karen Burke, M.D., Ph.D., a dermatologist in private practice in New York City.

Age spots are your skin's defensive response to too much sun. Your skin tries to protect itself by producing more melanin, the same pigment of which freckles are made.

But freckles and age spots are quite different. "Freckles appear when you're young, they're worse in the summer, and they tend to fade with age," says Nicholas Lowe, M.D., clinical professor of dermatology at the University of California, Los Angeles, UCLA School of Medicine.

"Age spots are generally larger, less regular in shape and darker than freckles," he says. "They also tend to hang around forever."

While sun is always the big culprit, certain other things can react with the sun to encourage the formation of age spots.

Top spotters include musk and bergamot oil, common ingredients in men's colognes and aftershaves and in some lotions. Certain oral medicines will do the same thing. These include tetracycline and some other antibiotics, some diuretics (water pills) and antipsychotic drugs such as chlorpromazine.

Skin contact with parsley, limes, parsnips and other foods that contain chemicals called psoralens may also lay the groundwork for age spots. Psoralens can cause the skin to be more sensitive to the sun, so the skin burns more easily, and when the little blisters from the burns heal, age spots may appear in their places.

First, Prevent New Ones

You can put the little spot factories in your skin out of business right now, doctors say. But it will take vigilance to keep them from gearing up again.

Screen yourself. The number one way to keep more age spots from forming is to use sunscreen. "Start using an SPF 15 or higher sunscreen on a daily basis," says John E. Wolf, Jr., M.D., professor and chairman of the dermatology department at Baylor College of Medicine in Houston. What's SPF? It stands for sun protection factor. SPF 15, for example, means you can stay out in

---

Is It Skin Cancer?

Age spots are harmless, and if you choose to ignore one, nothing will happen to you. Ignore a melanoma, however, and it can kill you.

Melanoma is a nasty form of cancer that appears as a discoloration on the skin. How can you tell a melanoma from an age spot?

Use this alphabetical checklist to help spot these potential killers, suggests Thomas Griffin, M.D., a dermatologist at Graduate Hospital of Philadelphia and clinical assistant professor of dermatology at the University of Pennsylvania School of Medicine, also in Philadelphia.

- *A* is for asymmetry. Be concerned if a brown spot or mole develops an irregular shape. Age spots are usually round.
- *B* is for border. Look for a jagged one; age spots are usually even.
- *C* is for color changes. It could mean trouble if a dark area arises within a mole or brown spot or if an area within a mole or brown spot begins to lighten. Age spots are usually one color.
- *D* is for diameter. A brown spot or mole that gets larger than a pencil eraser could be a melanoma.

If any of these characteristics is present, or if you're at all uncertain whether something is an age spot or a melanoma, get yourself to a doctor quickly, Dr. Griffin says. Though melanoma is dangerous, it's also curable if caught early.

the sun 15 times longer before burning than you could without the sunscreen.

Apply it to the backs of your hands and your face first thing in the morning, Dr. Wolf says. Keep a tube handy for reapplying after you wash your hands. If you see any new spots beginning, switch to a higher SPF.

Don't be too sensitive. If your skin produces age spots readily, you'll want to avoid musk and bergamot oil in your colognes, aftershaves and lotions. Do you have to give up your Night of the Musk Ox cologne? Not necessarily, but you would be better off applying it to unexposed skin rather than to your face and neck, suggests Dr. Burke. If you're on a sun-reactive medication, such as tetracycline, don't worry. Your new sunscreen ritual should keep you safe from new age spots.

Wash up. If you've handled any foods that contain psoralens, such as limes or parsley, wash your skin thoroughly and reapply sunscreen before going outdoors again, says Dr. Burke.

Out, Out, Damn Spots

What if you already have an age spot or two? In brief, you can bleach them, peel them, freeze them or zap 'em. If your age spots are mild, there are a few home treatments you can try. The rest will require a visit to your dermatologist.

Fade 'em. You've heard the ads for Porcelana since you were a kid. It's an old product, but it may work. Porcelana and other creams, including Esotérica and Palmer's Skin Success fade creams, contain hydroquinone, which interferes with your skin's production of melanin. Dr. Burke says these products work slowly, however. Prescription-strength hydroquinone preparations might work faster.

Ask for an Rx. More stubborn age spots respond well to prescription creams containing hydroquinone, Dr. Burke says. Ask your dermatologist about a prescription for Melanex or Eldoquin. Another prescription age spot eraser is tretinoin (Retin-A), which comes in cream or gel form. Better known for its acne- and wrinkle-removing abilities, Retin-A gradually returns skin to its normal state, and as it does so, age spots fade away. It can be used in conjunction with hydroquinone at your doctor's discretion, Dr. Burke says.

Bleach them away. A hair bleaching product that's at least 30 percent hydrogen peroxide can help fade away smaller age spots. The products with the highest percentages of peroxide are those for blonde shades, such as Nice 'n Easy 97 and 98 and Ultress 24, 25 and 26. You can buy these products at any pharmacy. Dr. Burke suggests dabbing on the peroxide with a cotton swab. You may have to use it daily for several weeks.

Peel them. Your doctor can treat age spots quickly by applying acid directly to the spots, says Dr. Wolf. Trichloroacetic acid, frequently used in chemical peels, might be appropriate treatment if you have just a few spots that aren't too dark. Drawbacks? Acid peels are mildly painful, and they sometimes work too well, leaving white spots where the brown spots were.

Freeze them. Your doctor may also suggest freezing the spots with liquid nitrogen. As with the chemical peel, liquid nitrogen can create white spots, Dr. Wolf says. Liquid nitrogen also stings—but no more than, say, a punch in the arm from your kid brother.

Zap 'em. With a laser, that is. The state-of-the-art treatment for age spots is the laser, says Dr. Lowe. "These lasers can be set to destroy only the pigment cells. The great thing about this treatment is that in the hands of an expert, you don't run the risk of having white spots where the dark spots had been." Does the laser treatment hurt? Only about as much as the snap of a rubber band, says Dr. Lowe. Keep in mind that laser treatment is the most expensive weapon against age spots.

Remember that with all these treatments, it is essential to keep using sunscreen. Otherwise, new age spots are sure to form.

ALLERGIES

Escape from Snivelization

Springtime at last, with its flowers, grasses and weeds.

And all that pollen floating through the air, stuffing up your nose, making you sneeze uncontrollably and turning your leisurely stroll through the park into a mad sprint for a box of tissues. In ten minutes, you go from lively to grumpy, ready to crawl back indoors, close the windows and hibernate next to a packet of sinus tablets.

Seasonal allergies like this affect an estimated 45 to 50 million Americans, or one in every five, according to the National Institutes of Health. But pollen isn't your only allergy enemy. Dozens and dozens of things can trigger allergic reactions, from dust mites, mold and pet dander to shrimp and peanuts. Even a pair of latex gloves or a condom can cause trouble.

And allergies aren't always something to just sneeze at, either. In cases of asthma and severe food allergies, they can prove deadly.

"Fortunately, there's a lot you can do to improve things," says Harold S. Nelson, M.D., senior staff physician at the National Jewish Center for Immunology and Respiratory Medicine in Denver. "Although they seem terrible when you have them, allergies really don't have to dominate your life."

A Case of Mistaken Identity

When it comes to fighting disease, your immune system is usually pretty darned sharp. It can quickly identify harmful foreign substances such as germs and viruses and whip them with lethal efficiency.

But sometimes your body gets a little confused. For reasons nobody quite understands, your immune system can misidentify harmless substances such as mold, pollen and food by-products and attack them. Mast cells, part of your immune system, attach to these substances, which are known as allergens. The

21

mast cells then release powerful chemicals called allergic mediators, including histamine, to combat the allergens.

The result, Dr. Nelson says, is a classic case of allergy symptoms: a stuffed-up nose, sneezing and watery eyes. If you have contact (skin) allergies, you can end up with a rash or hives. A food allergy can cause stomach cramps, nausea and vomiting. And 5 to 12 hours later, when other parts of the immune system join the battle, a second wave of similar symptoms can strike.

Heredity is behind many allergies. You can inherit the ability to produce an antibody called immunoglobulin E, or IgE, says allergist David Tinkelman, M.D., clinical professor of pediatrics in the Department of Allergy and Immunology at the Medical College of Georgia in Augusta. If you don't inherit IgE, he says, you are less likely to develop allergies.

Food allergies are rarer than you may think. Only 0.1 to 5 percent of the population suffers from them, Dr. Nelson says—and most people outgrow them by age three. Still, some adults are highly allergic to nuts, seafood, milk, eggs or other foods. And in some cases, the reactions worsen over time.

It's not likely that you're going to develop new allergies after age 30, Dr. Nelson says, unless you are exposed to some new allergen such as a pet or a pollen. The good news is that allergies tend to subside at about age 55, says Edward O'Connell, M.D., professor of pediatrics, allergy and immunology at Mayo Medical School in Rochester, Minnesota. That's because your immune system begins to decline, making it less likely to attack an invading mold spore or another allergen.

More Than a Little Trouble

Allergies are usually just an annoyance. You can take an over-the-counter or prescription medication, and the symptoms will probably subside, Dr. Nelson says. But some allergies can be much more serious.

In the case of bee stings and other unfortunate insect encounters, about 1 percent of the population can develop a dangerous allergic reaction called anaphylaxis, according to Susan Rudd Wynn, M.D., an allergist with Fort Worth Allergy and Asthma Associates in Fort Worth, Texas.

If you have this reaction shortly after a bee sting, you may notice symptoms such as itchy palms, tightness in your chest, hoarseness or even a feeling of impending doom. "If so, get yourself to an emergency room fast," Dr. Wynn says. "Anaphylaxis is not something to mess around with." In fact, she says, as many as 50 people a year die of the reaction, many because their throats swell shut and they suffocate. In rare cases, food allergies can cause anaphylaxis as well, Dr. Wynn says.

There's no test to predict anaphylaxis. But doctors can give adrenaline self-injection kits to people known to have severe allergic reactions. "That can buy you some valuable time, so you can get to the hospital for further treatment," Dr. Wynn says.

There's also some evidence that men with allergies may be at higher risk of developing certain cancers, including prostate cancer. A six-year study of more than 34,000 Seventh-Day Adventists in California showed that men with one allergy are 1.4 times more likely to develop prostate cancer, 2.2 times more likely to develop cancer in the lymph glands and 4.4 times more likely to develop tumors. Researchers don't understand the possible link between allergies and cancer. In fact, Dr. Nelson says other studies have shown that the chances of developing some types of cancer actually seem to decrease in people with allergies. "That whole area is really up for grabs," he says.

Sniffle Stoppers

The best advice for whipping allergies? Avoid whatever makes you sneeze or break out. An allergist can perform simple blood or skin tests to pinpoint your allergies. "Once you know what causes you problems, you can try to stay away from it," Dr. Wynn says.

Here are some tips on keeping your allergies at bay.

Choose your weapon. Two types of over-the-counter medication attack allergy symptoms. Antihistamines relieve sneezing, itching and a runny nose. And decongestants help unclog a stuffed-up nose. Some medicines combine both; read the label to find out what you need.

"The big drawback of antihistamines is that they can make you drowsy," says Edward Philpot, M.D., assistant clinical professor of medicine in the Department of Rheumatology, Allergy and Immunology at the University of California, Davis, School of Medicine. "If all you have is a stuffy nose, just

Thinking of You—Achoo!

She's the woman of your dreams. Except that every time you dream of her, your nose stuffs up and you sneeze for 20 minutes. What's going on here?

"The sneezing could result from your being turned on to her," says Martin Valentine, M.D., an allergy expert and professor of medicine at the Johns Hopkins Asthma and Allergy Center in Baltimore. He explains that the thought of someone special could cause blood vessels in your nose to widen, which in turn might make you congested and induce sneezing. Consider, too, that strong emotions can also worsen the symptoms of asthma sufferers.

take a decongestant." Or if you need an antihistamine, try one of the newer prescription antihistamines such as terfenadine (Seldane), which don't make you drowsy.

If you're unhappy with the effectiveness of one antihistamine, try different brands until you find one that works.

Go on the attack. If you know the pollen count is high, or if you're going to visit Aunt Jane and her blasted cat, take your medication before symptoms arrive. "It's much more effective that way," Dr. Philpot says. "It gives the antihistamine a jump on your allergies." Make sure you take the medicine at least 30 minutes to an hour before you're exposed to allergens.

Avoid alcohol. Alcohol can worsen symptoms such as congestion, Dr. Wynn says, and mixing alcohol with antihistamines can cause serious health problems. Read the label on your allergy medication before drinking anything.

Be doggone careful. Dander from dogs and cats is a major household allergen. If you're allergic to dander, the simplest way to ease the problem is to send Fido or Fifi packing. But that's hard to do emotionally—and it may be unnecessary. Dr. Nelson says taking these steps might correct the problem and still let Rover stay over.

- Keep pets out of your bedroom.
- Confine them to parts of the house that don't have carpeting.
- Bathe pets weekly to wash the dander away.

Bust the dust. The biggest enemy in your house is also the smallest. The dust mite is a microscopic organism, but under magnification, it looks like the Beast That Ate Coney Island. Breathing these little buggers can cause all sorts of allergy symptoms. To help reduce the problem, the experts suggest these steps.

- Cover your pillowcases and mattress in plastic covers. Wash sheets, mattress pads and blankets every week in water that is at least 130°F.
- Clean house regularly. Vacuum at least once a week, and keep clutter to a minimum—it just collects dust.
- Choose hardwood or vinyl floors over carpet whenever possible. A study at the University of Virginia in Charlottesville found that carpeting attracts and keeps allergens at 100 times the rate of bare polished floors. Use washable area rugs instead, especially in the bathroom.

Starve your food allergy. Unfortunately, the only way you're going to avoid a food allergy is to avoid the food that's causing it. If you're not exactly sure which food causes problems, Dr. Nelson says a doctor can perform tests to check your sensitivity. You can also keep a food diary, noting what you eat each day and keeping track of when you have an allergic reaction. That should help you narrow down the source of the allergy.

Lay off the latex. A study of more than 1,000 U.S. Army dentists found that between 9 and 14 percent of people may be allergic to the latex found in

Can You Be Allergic to Cold?

You walk down the driveway on a cold winter morning to fetch the newspaper. Two minutes later, you break out in hives. Why?

It's rare but possible to be allergic to sudden drops in temperature, says Martin Valentine, M.D., an allergy expert and professor of medicine at the Johns Hopkins Asthma and Allergy Center in Baltimore. A 30°F drop—such as when you leave your warm house to fetch the paper—can cause hives and swelling that can last for up to two hours. Drastic changes, such as jumping into a frigid swimming pool, can cause shock in some people.

If you think you're allergic to cold, try placing a sandwich bag full of ice on your arm for 30 seconds to two minutes. An itchy welt will form if you're allergic. Your doctor can prescribe the proper antihistamine medication to help you deal with the problem, Dr. Valentine says.

gloves. Other studies found similar allergies to rubber products ranging from boots to condoms.

The bottom line? If one brand of glove, condom or whatever gives you a rash, try another. Since manufacturers use different additives in their products, Dr. Nelson says it may help to sample brands until you find one that doesn't bother you.

Sleep in. Pollen counts usually peak in the early morning, between the hours of 5:00 A.M. and 8:00 A.M. If you can stay inside until mid-morning, Dr. Philpot says you'll be better off. And no matter how nice it feels outside, don't sleep with the windows open on high-pollen days. "You'll guarantee yourself a miserable wake-up call," he says.

Halt the humidity Keep your house or apartment dry to cut back on allergens. That means running the air conditioner, which dries the air as it cools it, or using a dehumidifier. A humidifier or vaporizer is a bad idea. "Dust mites just love the extra moisture from a humidifier," Dr. Wynn says. "And so does mold. If you have allergies, just forget the humidifier altogether."

Uproot your problem. The American Lung Association says the following plants can cause big-time allergies: oak and walnut trees, juniper, cypress, privet shrubs and all types of Bermuda grass. If you're looking for sneezeless replacements for your yard, try these: mulberry, fir, pear and silk trees; hibiscus, yucca and pyracantha shrubs; and dichondra, Irish moss and bunchgrass lawns.

You can obtain a complete list by writing to the American Lung Association of California, 424 Pendleton Way, Oakland, CA 94621. Enclose a self-addressed, stamped envelope.

Give it a shot. If your allergies resist every trick, you may need allergy shots, Dr. Philpot says. Doctors can inject you with small quantities of what you're allergic to, helping your body build immunity to the allergen. This is usually a last resort, since you may need from six months to a year of weekly shots plus another shot each month for up to five years.

"It takes a commitment," Dr. Philpot says. "But it's the only thing that helps some allergy sufferers." Dr. Philpot recommends that you steer clear of corticosteroid injections, which he says can suppress your immune system and linger in your body. "They're like using a bazooka to rid your house of termites," he says. "You'll get rid of the termites, but you'll damage the house pretty badly, too."

ANGER

You Can Learn to Be Cool

As men, we do a lot of things right. But traditionally, being angry hasn't been one of them.

Not that we have any trouble getting angry. Heck, we're experts at that. "We know from various studies that men are more likely to get angry over trivial things, such as having someone get in front of them in line or being stuck in traffic," says Sandra Thomas, R.N., Ph.D., an anger researcher and director of the Center for Nursing Research at the University of Tennessee, Knoxville. "For most women, these aren't triggers of anger; they just cause some momentary annoyance."

It's how we get angry that causes us problems. "A man who is angry for one reason or another will go home and kick the dog," says Sidney B. Simon, Ed.D., a counselor and professor emeritus of psychological education at the University of Massachusetts at Amherst and an author who specializes in anger and forgiveness.

Wrong Targets

Unfortunately, the hurt doesn't end with Fido. Men have long had a reputation for venting their anger—often at the wrong targets. Some @#$%*& jerks cut us off on the highway, and we go home and take it out on the kids. Our #@&^%$* bosses pass us up for promotions, and we treat our wives as though they're responsible.

Being that we're now sensitive, 1990s kind of guys, this sort of behavior makes us feel embarrassed, hurt, ashamed and a host of other not-so-great emotions. Problem is, since this sensitivity stuff is all new to us (after all, we were raised to not express our emotions as easily as women), we sometimes channel all these feelings into only one emotion—anger—rather than experiencing and addressing them directly, says Roland D. Maiuro, Ph.D., director of the Harborview Anger Management and Domestic Violence Program in Seattle. Women, on the other hand, tend to experience a fuller range of emotions.

"In our society, we're programmed to be macho, Rocky Balboa–like protectors and providers," adds Dr. Simon. "We fear that if we show any weakness, we will somehow lose our manhood. Men resist appearing to be wimps in any form." So we dig in our heels and try to rationalize why the dog deserved a wing tip on its backside, why the kids needed to be yelled at or why our better halves don't support us as they should. This, of course, leads to more arguments and anger. And more trouble.

A Is for Aging

"When you get angry, there are various physiological changes in the body, because anger triggers the fight-or-flight response," says Christopher Peterson, Ph.D., author of *Health and Optimism* and professor of psychology at the University of Michigan in Ann Arbor. "The adrenaline gets hyped up, your heart beats faster, your respiration becomes more rapid and shallow, and your digestion stops." This is why we usually feel like smashing a wall or someone's face.

Of course, we usually hurt ourselves more than we hurt anyone else. Getting angry frequently has clearly been established as a contributing factor to higher rates of heart disease, high blood pressure and other life-threatening illnesses, especially if you have a Type A personality and get angry easily. It also affects our mental capabilities. "All emotions have some influence on the way we think, but strong emotions can actually slow your ability to rationalize, solve problems and make decisions," says Mara Julius, Sc.D., a psychosocial epidemi-

Tame Your Temper at the Table

The wrong diet can make you feel grumpy as well as look lumpy, according to researchers at the State University of New York at Stony Brook and Oregon Health Sciences University in Portland.

After studying 156 women and 149 men for five years, they noted that people who consumed the typical high-fat American diet were more easily angered than those who changed to healthier diets. Those who switched to low-fat eating showed less anger and were less likely to get depressed.

Researchers believe that reducing the amount of fat in the diet and in the bloodstream plays a role: The less fat there is, the better the overall mood.

ologist at the University of Michigan School of Public Health who for more than 20 years has studied how coping with anger affects the health of men and women. "When you're feeling anger, rage or hostility, it overwhelms you. In some people, it slows down the thinking process; in others, it stops the thinking process completely."

Adds Dr. Peterson, "Anger also causes us to lose our sense of humor and to alienate people. It takes its toll on our energy, creativity and all those other things that might keep us feeling young."

Extinguishing the Ire

But since we're all going to get angry at some point, we might as well do it right. Here's how, according to Dr. Julius: Get angry when you're provoked, but don't stay that way. Cool off and identify the source of your anger. Remove the source by identifying the underlying problem.

If anger is handled correctly, says Dr. Julius, we can lessen or avoid the health problems brought on by it—from elevated blood pressure, obesity and depression to heart problems and cancer. "You become ill during chronic prolongation of anger," she says. "In other words, it's not so much getting angry that hurts. The damage is done when you stay angry. If you get angry and deal with it quickly and effectively, the damage is minimal, if anything."

So here's how to blow your top without blowing it.

Choose your targets. "It's important that you express your anger, but there are constraints against expression in a lot of situations," says Dr. Thomas. "For instance, it's usually disadvantageous to express your feelings in the workplace to your supervisor or even to your co-workers. Even if you're doing everything right, speaking in a totally rational and low-key manner, the other person is likely to get defensive and later engage in vindictive behavior."

You have to be careful with whom you share your feelings, or they might come back to haunt you. Dr. Thomas's advice: "Pick a close friend, confidant or someone else you can trust—and not necessarily the subject of your anger— to tell how you feel."

Mind your I's and you's It's always better to express your feelings rather than to tell others how they should have behaved, says Dr. Maiuro. One way is to concentrate on giving "I" messages. For instance, it's better to say "I was angry that you didn't drop off the car" than "You said you'd drop off the car, and you didn't." "You" messages sound accusatory and put people on the defensive, setting up rather than solving arguments.

Get busy to chill out. Since we're quick to fly off the handle when we're angry, it's advised that we use this sudden burst of energy positively. "One thing that's really effective is to do something physical," says Dr. Thomas. Reason: Exercise channels the adrenaline from your fight-or-flight response more positively than does idle stewing, allowing you to think more clearly about how to deal with your anger.

Take a zen-minute break. The workplace is one of our most frequent sources of anger, but it's not always practical to leave the office to go running. "In situations where you can't exercise, find a quiet spot and meditate, breathe deeply or practice some other type of relaxation technique," says Dr. Thomas.

Don't sweat the small stuff. A lot of our anger is over things we can't do anything about. "Take traffic, for instance," says Dr. Julius. "Everybody gets angry at traffic, so I won't say 'Don't get angry when you're stuck in traffic.' But you don't have to be consumed by that anger if you do what you can but realize that it's all you can do."

For instance, do what you can to avoid traffic by rescheduling your commuting time or taking a bus or train. "But realize that you alone cannot stop traffic, so being angry about it is a waste of your energy. Instead, channel your feelings into using this wasted time more effectively—by listening to music or audio books in your car, planning out your schedule or some other activity," suggests Dr. Julius.

And count your blessings. "It's also important to realize the trade-offs— to count your blessings, so to speak," adds Dr. Julius. "When you're stuck in traffic, think of all the positive things: the fact that you own a car and that along with city traffic come some advantages—museums, good restaurants, parks." It takes some time to do this, but it helps put things in perspective. When you're angry at your kids or wife, thinking about how lucky you are to have them eases your anger.

Write it out. Worried about saying something stupid? Then say nothing— out loud, at least. Nobody says you have to talk to express yourself. "Respond in writing," says Jerry L. Deffenbacher, Ph.D., professor of psychology at Colorado State University in Fort Collins. "That gives you a chance to collect yourself and to get your act together to respond more rationally. And you'll feel in control by halting the immediate confrontation."

Surround yourself with happy people. Monkey see, monkey do. "If you want to not be angry, try to associate with non-angry people," advises Dr. Peterson. "These ways of feeling and acting are contagious. The trick, of course, is to surround yourself not with some annoyingly positive Pollyanna people but with rational people who see solutions to problems."

Be a joiner. Some anger stems from loneliness, so adding to your social calendar can help. "Sometimes you have to force yourself to get involved. You may not like everyone, and they might not like you, but being active breaks up depression, and depression can leave many people angry," says Dr. Peterson. "Besides, joining clubs and other groups helps you see the accomplishments in your life, which can defuse feelings of anger, loneliness and depression."

Have a good cry. It's a great emotional release and a lot healthier than venting at the wrong person. "When children get angry, both boys and girls cry. Unfortunately, society starts giving boys the message that they shouldn't cry or they'll be sissies," says Dr. Thomas. "So boys learn to not do it, and as a result, they suffer as men."

ARRHYTHMIAS

When the Heart Goes a Little Crazy

During a particularly stressful time at work, did you feel a pounding in your chest so loud that you wondered if it could be heard throughout the entire office? Or during an intense game of touch football, did you notice your heartbeat accelerating into a sprint?

Welcome to the world of arrhythmias, disturbances of your heartbeat's normal rhythm. Your heart is a real workaholic, beating about 100,000 times a day. With a rigorous schedule like that, no wonder it occasionally blips, bumps and jumps a bit out of kilter. Most often it will set itself back on course before you even have time to get anxious about what has just happened.

But occasionally, those little quirks of the heart are more than just harmless oddities. Certain forms of arrhythmia can sap your energy, leaving you feeling timeworn and worn out. On occasion, big disturbances in the heart's rhythm can threaten the heart—and your life.

Serious arrhythmias are more likely to happen with increasing age. "In general, when arrhythmias begin later in life, they should be investigated much more carefully and treated more seriously," says Marianne J. Legato, M.D., associate professor of clinical medicine at Columbia University College of Physicians and Surgeons in New York City.

A Look inside the Chest

True, no matter what your age, the vast majority of ticker tremors aren't a sign of impending doom. Most commonly, they involve an extra *lub-dub* or two that you may not even be aware of, unless you feel a fluttering in your chest.

"At some time in our lives, everyone has extra beats," says Gerald Pohost, M.D., director of the Division of Cardiovascular Disease at the University of Alabama School of Medicine in Birmingham. "And certainly, the vast majority of these extra beats are harmless."

But if you have coronary artery disease—in particular, the buildup of plaque, which consists of fatty and other deposits that can play a role in a heart attack—the heart may not be getting sufficient blood and oxygen. This can cause arrhythmias that may pose a serious and or even a life-threatening problem. And since coronary artery disease tends to become more common as people age, potentially serious rhythm disorders are more prevalent as time marches on.

If you have had a heart attack, your doctor may have already cautioned you that the injured heart muscle is more likely to cause anarchy in the heart's routine electrical impulses, producing dangerous abnormal beats called ventricular arrhythmias. When this happens, the heart can accelerate from a jog to a sprint, beating at a frantic pace of perhaps 150 to 300 times per minute instead of the normal 60 to 100. At its worst, this condition can deteriorate into such serious quivers and quakes that the heart will no longer pump blood adequately—and sudden death may be the result. Sure, it sounds alarming. But don't panic. Remember, most irregular heartbeats are not a cause for concern—and if you take control of your health, you can reduce your chances of developing serious arrhythmias.

Righting Your Rhythm

Since many worrisome heartbeats are closely intertwined with coronary disease, probably your best defense against those unwanted shivers and shudders of the heart is to prevent heart problems in the first place. Even if you've experienced palpitations, you might be able to keep them to a minimum through lifestyle changes. Here are some ways to do that, either by preventing arrhythmias altogether or by cutting down on their frequency.

Snuff out smoking. Cigarettes are an important contributor to heart disease. They can also provoke certain types of irregular heartbeat. If you nix the nicotine in your life, your heart will have an easier time maintaining a steady beat, says Richard Helfant, M.D., vice chairman of medicine and director of the Cardiology Training Program at the University of California, Irvine, Medical Center.

Learn some stress busters. Many experts believe that stress plays a role in the development of coronary artery disease as well as contributes to arrhythmias. To silence stress, try a lot of exercise, warm baths, massages and creative hobbies, says Fredric J. Pashkow, M.D., medical director of the Cardiac Health Improvement and Rehabilitation Program at the Cleveland Clinic Foundation in Cleveland.

Don't soak yourself in coffee. One British study of 7,300 people found that nine or more cups of coffee may provoke some people's hearts to skip beats. Some smaller studies suggest that lesser amounts of coffee may have similar effects, particularly in those people unaccustomed to drinking lots of caffeine. If you're prone to irregular heartbeats, do not overdo the caffeine.

Imbibe with caution. Binges of heavy drinking can increase your chances of arrhythmias even if you don't have heart disease. In one U.S. study, six or more drinks a day increased the risk of very rapid heartbeat associated with an irregularity called supraventricular tachyarrhythmia. Some doctors call this syndrome holiday heart because it often happens in people who consume more alcohol than they're used to during the holidays.

Professional Beat Keepers

It might happen quite unexpectedly. During a routine physical exam, your doctor may order an electrocardiogram—a test that measures the smoothness of your heartbeat—and discover a serious rhythm disorder that he thinks needs medication to control. He may also diagnose arrhythmias if you complain of palpitations and light-headedness. There are several options when more than lifestyle changes are required to control an irregular heartbeat.

Drugs are one. "Medications are able to control many arrhythmias and their symptoms. Some of the newer drugs are quite effective," says Dr. Pohost. Although these medications can help prevent sudden death by stabilizing the electrical activity of the heart, they must be chosen carefully by your doctor, since they may cause side effects of their own, such as aggravated arrhythmias, gastrointestinal upsets and low blood pressure. In many cases, people end up taking these drugs for the rest of their lives.

Your doctor might also recommend an implantable cardiac defibrillator. This relatively new battery-driven device is surgically placed right into your chest or abdomen, where it will monitor your heartbeat. If the beat becomes dangerously fast or chaotic, it will zap the heart with a shock that might feel like a slap or a thump in the chest. This is meant to startle your heart back to normal activity.

How successful are these devices? One study found that among 650 patients (average age 60 years), the implantable defibrillators kept 60 percent of them alive for at least ten years. The researchers estimated that virtually all of them would have died without this high-tech hardware.

When your heartbeat just won't shape up, doctors have another hi-tech option, called catheter ablation, at their disposal. This treatment is reserved for particular types of rhythm disorder that may be resistant to other therapies. It is particularly useful for conditions in which the abnormal heartbeat originates in the heart's upper chambers. It involves threading a thin tube through one of your veins and into the heart.

Once this catheter is properly positioned, a mild radio-frequency current is activated to kill tiny areas of the heart tissue that are causing the arrhythmias. By destroying cells in a section of tissue no bigger than ⅕ inch in diameter, this procedure eliminates the wacky impulses that cause certain types of high-risk arrhythmias.

ARTHRITIS

Ensuring a Pain-Free Tomorrow

An estimated 31 million Americans have been diagnosed with arthritis. And those are just the people who are smart enough to see their doctors about that blasted pain in their joints, tendons and muscles.

Six million more of us suffer quietly, paying the price for a long-ago football injury, years of carrying around an extra 20 pounds or just bad luck.

That's because despite its reputation for being as much a part of growing old as gray hair, arthritis is an equal opportunity deployer—of pain. "Many people aren't surprised to hear that arthritis is the single leading cause of disability in people over age 45," says Paul Caldron, D.O., a clinical rheumatologist and researcher at the Arthritis Center in Phoenix. "But they are surprised to learn it's the single leading cause of disability among all ages."

A Burden to Body and Mind

At best, arthritis can slow down your movements and cause some pain; at worst, it can cause agony and even debilitate to the point where sufferers need hospitalization or around-the-clock care, says Jeffrey R. Lisse, M.D., director of the Division of Rheumatology and associate professor of medicine at the University of Texas Medical Branch at Galveston. Because of the pain, arthritis can also make you lose sleep and hamper your sex life. It can even lead to weakness in your cardiovascular system, because people with arthritis often become sedentary when exercise is too painful.

But arthritis ages more than just the body. "Depression is almost universal among arthritis patients," says Dr. Lisse. "But a lot of people with arthritis also get what's known as learned helplessness. That occurs when someone starts out healthy and able to do things for himself, but over time, as the pain gets worse, he is less able to take care of himself. Someone else must assume these functions, so the person with arthritis winds up more and more helpless. In fact, some of the youngest patients in nursing homes are people suffering from severe arthritis, who are there because of the inability to care for themselves."

Adds Arthur Grayzel, M.D., vice president of medical affairs for the Arthritis Foundation, "I think that society almost expects people to have arthritis when they're old, so when an elderly man limps or uses a cane, it might not surprise anyone. But when you're young and your body image is very different, the effects can be devastating. The fact is, a lot of people who have arthritis—athletes, movies stars and others in the public eye—won't admit it because it seems to have a negative image. Having arthritis makes you seem old before your time."

Different Types, Same Symptoms

Most people know arthritis causes painful, stiff and sometimes swollen joints. But arthritis can also affect muscles and tendons, which may not swell but still hurt. And while technically there are more than 100 different forms of arthritis, the most common are osteoarthritis and rheumatoid arthritis.

You may already be familiar with osteoarthritis, the most common type, which affects about 16 million Americans. This is often caused or aggravated by athletic injury. "That's not to say that if you play sports, you'll get arthritis. But those who have experienced repeated injury to a joint, no matter how minor, have an increased chance of getting osteoarthritis," says Dr. Caldron.

About four million American men have osteoarthritis, which results when cartilage in the joints deteriorates. Besides injury, this form of arthritis is caused by overweight or other stress on joints. It's typically localized to a certain area, such as the fingers, knees, feet, hips or back. Osteoarthritis usually strikes men in their forties and fifties.

The other major form of this disease is rheumatoid arthritis. It usually strikes in a man's twenties and thirties and causes more serious pain in more than one part of the body. "What's really sad is that many people have significant pain and loss of function, and there's nothing you can do to prevent it, since we don't know what causes it," says Dr. Grayzel. "It strikes women three times more often than men, but when you're talking about a disease that affects nearly 2½ million Americans, we're still talking about over 600,000 men." Unlike osteoarthritis, rheumatoid arthritis is caused by chronic inflammation in the joints. It is thought to be caused by an immunity disorder.

So Long, Suffering

You may not be able to prevent arthritis, but you can lessen its aging effects on you. So even if you have never been bothered with arthritis pain, you are just beginning to feel some morning stiffness or evening pain or you have a full-fledged case of arthritis, here's how to deal with it.

Lose weight. "Being overweight is a major risk factor, especially for arthritis of the knees and hips," says Dr. Grayzel. "Even when you're in your twenties or thirties, you should try to reduce your weight close to the normal range for your height. If you're 20 percent overweight or more, you're a prime candidate for osteoarthritis. But any weight loss helps. If you lose just ten pounds and keep it off for ten years, no matter your current weight, you can cut your risk of osteoarthritis in your knees by 50 percent."

Watch what you eat. Various studies show that food plays a crucial role in the severity of arthritis. Norwegian researchers discovered that patients with rheumatoid arthritis saw dramatic improvements in their conditions within one month of beginning vegetarian diets. Other scientists have found that omega-3 fatty acids, abundant in cold-water fish such as salmon, herring and sardines, also ease rheumatoid arthritis pain.

In addition, "a diet low in saturated fat and animal fat seems to be helpful," says Dr. Caldron. "Eating a lot of fresh fruits and vegetables and non–red meat sources of fat such as fish and chicken may cause the body to produce fewer pro-inflammatory substances. That's not to say a diet will cure arthritis, but it may modify the effects of arthritis.

"Some people react to certain foods, almost like an allergy," says Dr. Caldron. "It may result from wheat or citrus fruits, lentils or even alcohol. The problem is, there's no way to test for this. But if you notice a significant reaction and more pain consistently within 48 hours after eating a certain food, eliminate it from your diet."

Get physical. Regular exercise to build your muscles and flexibility can keep osteoarthritis at bay or lessen its effects. Exercise is also recommended for rheumatoid arthritis, although workouts should be under a doctor's supervision and emphasize range-of-motion exercises.

"Exercise improves strength and flexibility, so less stress is placed on the joints, and they can move easier and more efficiently," says John H. Klippel, M.D., clinical director of the National Institute of Arthritis and Musculoskeletal and Skin Diseases in Bethesda, Maryland. "Inactivity, on the other hand, actually encourages pain, stiffness and other symptoms."

Weight lifting is particularly useful because it builds muscle tone, which is especially important for arthritis sufferers. Emphasize building the abdominal muscles to reduce back pain and the thigh muscles for knee pain, advises Dr. Grayzel. Meanwhile, aerobic exercise such as running, bicycling and swimming is also helpful for improving flexibility.

Slow down when you have to. When a joint is swollen and inflamed, continuing to use it doesn't help. "Don't exercise through the pain," says Dr. Grayzel. "Otherwise, you'll just hurt more." So even if you're on a regular exercise program, skip a day (or two) when your joints or muscles begin to hurt.

Get in gear. "A frequent cause of osteoarthritis is injury, so you should take full advantage of the various protective equipment for athletics," says Dr. Caldron. "By wearing protective gear, you'll lessen the likelihood of injuring or reinjuring joints, tendons and muscles, which reduces the risk of osteoarthritis." Anything that cushions these areas, such as the elbow and knee pads used for football, hockey and basketball, will help.

Turn up the heat. For immediate relief, many people find that placing warm, moist heat directly on inflamed areas helps reduce pain, says Dr. Lisse. Hot water bottles, heating blankets and hot baths help. But use heat judiciously—no more than 10 to 15 minutes at a time. And be sure to take a break for at least one hour before reapplying. Over-the-counter analgesic balms such as Ben-Gay can also help ease pain when joints are hot, tender and swollen. But don't use them with heat, cautions Dr. Caldron. The two together may cause nasty reactions such as burning and blistering.

Or chill out to prevent pain. Ice, meanwhile, is sometimes recommended to prevent pain when joints are overworked or overused. Dr. Lisse suggests that you wrap some ice in a towel and gently apply it to your joints several times a day, 15 minutes on and 15 minutes off.

Also practice the other way to cool off—by finding ways to deal with the stresses in your life. When you're tensed up, you hurt more. But anything you can do to learn to relax—whether it's listening to music, meditating or taking up a hobby—can help, especially when pain is severe.

BACK PAIN

Taking On the Ache— And Winning

After a weekend of hauling boxes up to the attic, you wish you were a spineless amoeba. That way, you wouldn't have to endure the miserable, wrenching back pain that hobbles you so much your spine feels as old as the pyramids and as fragile as King Tut's mummy.

"A 30-year-old guy who has an aching back and limited mobility can feel like a 90-year-old," says Joseph Sasso, D.C., president of the Federation of Straight Chiropractors and Organizations.

At least 70 percent of men will have back pain at some point in their lives. Of those, 14 percent will have severe pain that lasts at least two weeks, and up to 7 percent will have chronic pain that can last for more than six months, according to Gunnar B. J. Andersson, M.D., Ph.D., professor and associate chairman of the Department of Orthopedic Surgery at Rush-Presbyterian–St. Luke's Medical Center in Chicago. Nearly 400,000 back injuries occur on the job each year, and that results in more lost productivity than any other medical condition. Back pain is the most frequent cause of restricted activity among people under age 45 and the second most common reason (after cold and flu) that people see doctors, according to the American Academy of Orthopaedic Surgeons. It is also the fifth leading cause of hospitalization and the third most common reason for surgery, Dr. Andersson says.

"Sleep, sex, sitting—I can't imagine any activity that isn't affected by the back. It's involved in almost everything we do. You can't get in and out of a car, run, jump or walk. Until you have back pain, you don't realize everything that a back does for you," says Alan Bensman, M.D., a physiatrist at Rehabilitative Health Services in Minneapolis.

Twist and Shout

Most men experience their first bouts of back pain between the ages of 30 and 45, says Dan Futch, D.C., chief of the chiropractic staff at Group Health Cooperative HMO in Madison, Wisconsin.

"Those ages are the window of opportunity for back pain," he says. "About the same time you start getting gray hairs, you'll probably start noticing twinges of pain in your back."

The thirties and forties are when arthritis and other types of natural degeneration in the small joints of the back begin to catch up with us, says Robert Waldrip, M.D., an orthopedic spine surgeon in private practice in Phoenix. Spinal stenosis, for example, a narrowing of the canal in the vertebrae that surround the spinal cord, puts pressure on nerves in the lower back and causes pain. In other cases, the problem is a herniated disk. Disks are small pads made of a tough, elastic outer covering (called the annulus) and a soft center. The disks act like shock absorbers between the vertebrae. Over time, a disk can herniate, meaning that the annulus has torn and the soft center has extended out to press against a nerve root, causing horrible pain. Poor posture also increases strain on the back and can aggravate arthritis and lead to disk problems.

But by far, the most common cause of back pain is muscle strain. As we get older, many of us get less and less exercise. Instead of being weekend warriors, we become Sunday spectators. As a result, the muscles in the abdomen and back that support the spine weaken and get out of shape, Dr. Bensman says. So things that you used to do with ease, such as lifting a bag of groceries out of your car, helping a friend move a hefty sofa or dancing the limbo, suddenly make you feel like you have a dozen knives sticking in your back.

Lifting something when your back is out of shape is like pulling a guy out of the stands at a professional football game and asking him to be starting quarterback. You're probably going to get hurt, because you're straining your back in ways that it's not prepared for.

Of course, even well-conditioned athletes such as Wayne Gretzky and Jose Canseco can get back pain, but in general, the better conditioned you are, the less likely your spine will cause havoc.

See your doctor if the pain is so intense you can't move, if it spreads to your legs or buttocks, if your legs or feet feel numb or tingly, if you lose control of your bladder or bowel movements or if you also have a fever or abdominal pain.

Keeping Your Spine Sublime

Often back pain is easily relieved without surgery or drugs, Dr. Waldrip says. In fact, 60 percent of people with acute back pain return to work within one week, and 90 percent are back on the job within six weeks. Here are some tips for preventing and treating back pain.

Do an early morning stretch. "I tell my patients to always start off their days by stretching while they're still in bed," Dr. Bensman says. "Remember that you've been lying prone for eight hours, and if you jump right up, you may be looking at a sore back." So before you get up, slowly stretch your arms over your head, then gently pull your knees up to your chest one at a time. When you're ready to sit up, roll to the side of the bed and use your arm to help prop yourself up. Put your hands on your buttocks and slowly lean back to extend your spine.

Walk away from it. Walking keeps your back healthy by conditioning your whole body. It strengthens the postural muscles of the buttocks, legs, back and abdomen. A brisk stroll may also help your body release endorphins, hormones that subdue pain. Swimming, bicycling and running are good, too. Try walking or another aerobic exercise for 20 minutes a day, three times a week, says Dr. Futch.

Take a break. Sitting puts more strain on your back than standing. If you must sit at your desk for an extended time or you're traveling by plane, train or car, change position often and give your back a break by standing up and walking around every hour or so, says Augustus A. White III, M.D., professor of orthopedic surgery at Harvard Medical School in Boston and author of *Your Aching Back*.

Leave your luggage lie. Instead of leaping out of the car or airplane and grabbing your bags, take a couple of minutes to stretch, Dr. Bensman suggests. Slowly bring your knees toward your chest and gently swing your arms around to loosen up stiff muscles. Avoid lifting with overstretched arms and try to keep the bags close to your body. Consider getting a collapsible luggage carrier with wheels.

Kneel, don't bend. Avoid bending over at the waist to pick up something. That creates tension in the back and increases your risk of injury, Dr. Futch says. Instead, use long-handled tools and kneel on a cushion or knee pad to garden, vacuum or do other "low-level" activities.

Let your legs do the work. If you're lifting something—no matter if it weighs 5 pounds or 50—bend your knees, keep your back straight and lift with your legs. "The legs are much stronger than the back and can lift a lot more weight without strain," Dr. Futch says.

Test the load. "How many of us have strained back muscles when we tried to pick up boxes that we thought were empty but were actually filled with encyclopedias?" asks Dr. Sasso. Always nudge a box with your foot or cautiously lift it an inch or so before really trying to heft it. If it's too heavy for you, don't be macho—ask for help.

Turn your back on heavy lifting. If you can't find someone to help you move a heavy object, try this maneuver as a last resort: If the object is setting at table height, turn your back to it to drag or lift it. You can also use this technique for raising windows. This position reduces the pressure that would be exerted on your spine by forcing you to use your legs for leverage.

Straighten up. Maintaining good posture is one of the best ways to prevent back pain, Dr. Futch says. To improve your posture, try this. Stand against a wall

Lifting 101: Back to Basics

We all think we know how to do it. After all, you've hoisted, hauled and hefted things for years. But even if lifting seems like a mundane part of life, doing it wrong can send a painful shock wave rippling through the sturdiest of spines. To prevent that, the American Academy of Orthopaedic Surgeons suggests that you follow these guidelines when lifting.

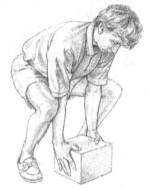

Stand as close as you can to the object you want to lift (left). Separate your feet shoulder-width apart to give yourself a solid base of support. Bend at the knees, tighten your stomach muscles and lift with your legs as you stand up. Don't bend at the waist, and don't try to lift an object that is too heavy or an awkward shape by yourself.

When you're holding an object, keep your knees slightly bent to maintain your balance (right). Point your toes in the direction you want to move. Avoid twisting your torso. Instead, pivot on your feet. Keep the object close to you when moving.

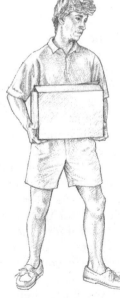

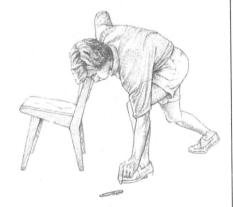

To lift a very light object such as a pencil off the floor, lean over, slightly bend one knee and extend the other leg behind you (above). Hold on to a nearby chair or table for support as you reach down for the pencil.

or sit in a dining room chair, making sure that your shoulders and buttocks touch the wall or your chair. Slip your arm into the space between your lower back and the wall or chair. If there is a point where your hand isn't touching both your back and the wall or chair, tilt your hips so that the extra space is eliminated. Hold that position for a count of 20 while looking in a mirror to see what your posture looks like. Try to maintain that posture for the rest of the day. Do that exercise once a day for three weeks to ensure that good posture will become a habit.

Check your mattress. Your mattress should provide proper support, be level and not sag. So if you feel like you're sleeping in the middle of a pita bread, it's probably time to get a new mattress, Dr. Sasso says.

"A bed loses a tremendous amount of firmness as it ages," Dr. Bensman says. "A mattress is like a pair of shoes. It may have fit your needs at one time, but that doesn't mean it's always going to fit."

Roll it up. A lumbar roll, a round foam rubber pad that can be purchased at most medical supply stores, can help you maintain the natural curve in the small of your spine and prevent lower back pain, says Hamilton Hall, M.D., director of the Canadian Back Institute in Toronto. Whenever you sit, stick the roll between your lower back and the chair.

Dress for success. Wearing tight pants can prevent you from using proper biomechanics such as bending your knees, especially when lifting, Dr. White says. Try wearing looser-fitting clothing for a month.

Forgo the tobacco. Smoking decreases blood flow to the back and can weaken disks, Dr. Bensman says. So if you smoke, quit.

Do the big chill. Apply ice to your aching back as soon as possible to reduce pain and swelling, Dr. Bensman says. Wrap an ice pack in a pillowcase or towel (never place the ice directly on your skin) and put it on the sore spot for ten minutes each hour until the ache subsides.

Then warm it up. Once ice relieves the swelling—usually within 48 hours—you can begin using heat. Heat increases blood flow to the wound, relaxes tissues and can improve your mobility, Dr. Bensman says. Apply a warm washcloth—it should be about skin temperature—to your back for 5 to 10 minutes every hour, or take a warm 15-minute shower or dip in a whirlpool.

Reach for over-the-counter relief. Taking one or two aspirin or ibuprofen tablets every four to six hours can relieve pain and reduce swelling, Dr. Bensman says. Don't exceed the manufacturer's recommended dosage.

Put up your feet. When minor back pain strikes, lie on the floor and put your legs up on a chair so that your thighs stay at a 90-degree angle to your hips and your calves rest at a 90-degree angle to your thighs. This position relaxes key back muscles and is one of the least stressful for your spine, Dr. White says.

Keep moving. Although lengthy bed rest was once recommended for back pain, doctors now believe that the more active you are, the sooner you'll recover. In fact, two weeks of bed rest weakens muscles and the spine, and that can actually slow your recovery and make you more likely to have a relapse, Dr. Hall says. So don't stay in bed for more than two days, and make sure you get up at least once an hour to walk or stretch.

Get manipulated. Chiropractors are gaining respectability in the medical community, Dr. Bensman says. An analysis of 25 studies of spinal manipulation—the heart and soul of chiropractic treatment—found that manipulation does provide at least some short-term relief for uncomplicated, acute back pain.

"Sure, chiropractors work," Dr. Bensman says. "They're becoming quite knowledgeable and offering some real benefits." In a typical case, a chiropractor may do a series of thrusts with the heels of his hands along the troubled area of your spine. Ask your doctor for a referral to a chiropractor in your area.

Get a second opinion. More than 400,000 surgeries, such as spinal fusion and disk removal or destruction, are done each year to relieve back pain, according to the American Academy of Orthopaedic Surgeons. Yet a Blue Cross and Blue Shield study found that almost 13 percent of spine operations are performed for inappropriate reasons. Get at least one other opinion if your doctor has suggested surgery, Dr. White says.

Eight Exercises to Minimize Back Pain

If you want a large return for a small investment, try these exercises recommended by the American Academy of Orthopaedic Surgeons. By strengthening and stretching your back, stomach, hip and thigh muscles, they will help keep your back feeling strong and flexible.

Check with your doctor before starting any exercise program.

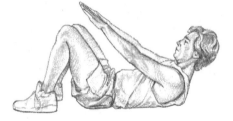

Lie on your back with your knees bent and your feet flat on the floor. Slowly raise your head and shoulders off the floor, and reach forward toward your knees with both hands (left). Hold for a count of ten. Lie back down, and repeat five times.

Lying on your stomach, tighten the muscles in one leg and raise it from the floor (right). Hold for a count of ten and return your leg to the floor. Repeat with the other leg. Do five repetitions with each leg.

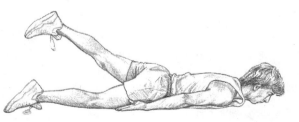

(continued)

Eight Exercises—Continued

Lie on your back with your arms at your sides. Lift one leg off the floor and hold it for a count of ten (right). Return it to the floor and lift the other leg. Repeat five times with each leg. If this is too difficult, keep one knee bent while raising the other leg.

Stand with your back against a wall and your feet shoulder-width apart. Slide down into a crouch, with your knees bent to about 90 degrees (left). Hold for a count of five and slide back up the wall. Repeat five times.

Holding on to the back of a chair, lift one leg backward (right). Keep your knee straight. Lower the leg slowly and repeat with the other leg. Do five repetitions with each leg.

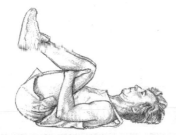

On the floor or on your bed, lie on your back with your knees bent and your feet flat. Raise both your knees toward your chest (above). Put both hands under your knees and gently pull your knees as close to your chest as possible. (If you feel pain when you do this, try pulling your knees apart.) Do not raise your head. Lower your legs without straightening them. Start with five repetitions several times a day.

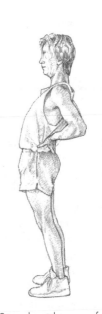

Stand with your feet slightly apart. Place your hands in the small of your back (above). Keeping your knees straight, bend backward at the waist as far as possible and hold the position for one or two seconds.

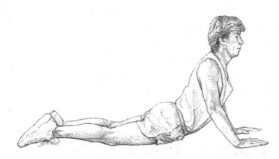

Lie on your stomach with your hands under your shoulders and your elbows bent. Push up with your arms (above). Raise the top half of your body as high as possible, allowing your hips and legs to remain flat on the floor or bed. Hold the position for one or two seconds. Repeat ten times several times a day.

BALDNESS

A Brush with Destiny

You teased Dad about his bald spot for years. He just sat there in his easy chair, reading the paper, taking it like a man, as you colored his scalp with crayons or tapped on it like a bongo drum.

But one day he reached his limit. Pop leaped from the La-Z-Boy, looked you square in the eye and said "Someday, son, this won't seem so funny."

He sure got that right.

You're not bald yet, but your hair is definitely starting to go. You wear baseball caps everywhere and switch hairstyles twice a month. Lately, you've been thinking about drugs that stimulate hair growth, transplants—even a toupee.

Sure, you'd like to laugh it off. But it's not that easy. You look a little older with every lost lock of hair. And looking old is making you feel old. How long will it be before some kid starts using your head for a tom-tom?

Fortunately, there are more options than ever for dealing with baldness.

"Things are definitely looking up for men losing hair," says Dominic A. Brandy, M.D., medical director of Dominic A. Brandy, M.D., and Associates, a permanent hair restoration practice in Pittsburgh. "The bottom line is that you don't have to surrender to baldness if you don't want to."

Bad Roots? Blame Your Family

The great majority of hair loss in men—perhaps 85 percent—has genetic roots. Forget the old saw about baldness coming only from your mother's side. Researchers now say you can inherit baldness from your father (revenge is his) as well.

This genetic form of baldness is called hereditary alopecia, or male pattern baldness. The telltale signs are a receding hairline, a growing bald spot on the crown or both.

No one is absolutely sure what causes hair to stop growing. Current wisdom holds that the male hormone testosterone, or perhaps a by-product of testosterone, may be the problem. Whatever the cause, individual hair strands thin gradually, and follicles eventually stop producing them altogether.

Men can start balding as early as age 18 or as late as their fifties or sixties. Only 12 percent of men are balding at 25—but the figure jumps to 37 percent at 35 and 45 percent at 45. Two-thirds of all men are bald or balding by 65.

Generally, guys who start balding earlier will lose more hair, and at a faster rate, than men whose balding is delayed.

You shouldn't always blame your genes for thinning hair, however. Marty Sawaya, M.D., Ph.D., assistant professor of dermatology at the University of Florida Health Science Center in Gainesville, says a number of nonhereditary factors can cause hair to thin as well. Potential culprits include:

- Drugs such as beta-blockers (often used for high blood pressure) and some vitamin A–derived medications such as the anti-acne drug isotretinoin (Accutane) and the antipsoriasis drug etretinate.
- Conditions such as arthritis and lupus.
- Major stress events, such as a divorce or the death of a loved one.
- Fad and crash diets that don't give you adequate protein.
- Anabolic steroids, such as those prescribed to men with hormone imbalances and sometimes used by Arnold Schwarzenegger wanna-be's.

Sometimes nonhereditary causes result in only temporary hair loss. Dr. Sawaya says a thorough medical exam, improved diet, better stress management and medical treatment can help regrowth in some cases.

Patching It Up

Undoing hereditary hair loss is a bit more tricky. Ken Hashimoto, M.D., professor of dermatology at Wayne State University School of Medicine in Detroit,

---

Are You Really Losing It?

Don't panic if you keep finding hair in the sink or on your brush. Non-balding men typically lose 50 to 100 hairs from their heads each day, according to Marty Sawaya, M.D., Ph.D., assistant professor of dermatology at the University of Florida Health Sciences Center in Gainesville. That many hairs a day isn't much, seeing as adults have more than 100,000 hairs on their heads.

If you're afraid you're losing hair, try this simple test. Grab a handful and give a firm but gentle pull. If more than a half-dozen hairs fall out, you may be in the early stages of male pattern baldness.

stresses that miracle hair treatments—massages, topical creams, megavitamins and the rest—do absolutely no good.

What will work? Consider these options.

Hair transplant. This practice has been around since the 1950s. The old method involved moving large plugs of hair (8 to 20 hairs at a time) from the back of a patient's head and embedding them in a balding area. This sometimes resulted in the "doll's hair" look, with uneven, unnatural hairlines.

New micrografting surgical techniques allow doctors to transplant as few as one hair at a time, creating a more feathered, natural look. "When it's done properly, nobody will ever know," Dr. Brandy says. "It's not cheap—but doctors can do things now that make your hair look absolutely natural." The procedure is basically painless, since doctors use local anesthesia. A complete transplant can take from one to three visits over several months and will typically cost $5,000 to $15,000.

Hair-lift. This procedure is used to fill in a large bald spot on the crown of a man's head. A surgeon cuts bald scalp from the top of the head, then stretches the

Minoxidil: Hair Loss Hero (sometimes)

In 1988, thin-haired American men joyfully welcomed minoxidil—hailed as the world's first true baldness buster.

Turns out that many of them were expecting a bit too much.

"Minoxidil is not a miracle baldness cure," says Harry L. Roth, M.D., clinical professor of dermatology at the University of California, San Francisco. "This drug works in a number of cases, but it's clearly not for everyone."

Minoxidil is most effective on men under 30 years of age who have been losing hair for less than five years. Dr. Roth says prime candidates have bald spots that are two inches across or smaller. Minoxidil does nothing to restore receding hairlines, though in some cases it may keep them from fading further.

Even among the best candidates, only one in three will experience optimal results (a doubling of hair density). Another 40 percent can expect increased density but will still be left with a partial bald spot.

"I tell my patients to expect their baldness to slow down," says Dominic A. Brandy, M.D., medical director of Dominic A. Brandy, M.D., and Associates, a permanent hair restoration practice in Pittsburgh. "But anything more than that is really a bonus."

Cost can also be a concern. Minoxidil runs about $600 for a year's supply—and you must use the product forever. If you stop the treat-

hair-covered scalp from the back and sides over the bald spot. The results, Dr. Brandy says, can be dramatic.

A stronger anesthesia is used for hair-lifts than for transplants. Dr. Brandy says it has the same effect as the gas a dentist uses on a patient having his wisdom teeth pulled. The procedure takes one or two treatments. Costs generally run from $3,500 to $5,000.

Scalp reduction. This is a scaled-down version of the hair-lift. If your bald spot is smaller, removing it could cost about $3,000.

Researchers are also trying an experimental procedure that involves cutting flaps of tissue from the back of a man's head, then sewing the whole piece onto his balding upper forehead.

Hair weave. This is a cosmetic treatment, not a surgical procedure. Technicians splice natural or synthetic extensions to existing hair to make it look more full. It may be cheaper in the short run—costs can start at as little as several hundred dollars—but it has to be tightened, or adjusted, every four to six weeks, as hair grows.

ments, you'll lose everything you had gained within six months.

Officials from the Upjohn Company, manufacturer of the minoxidil-based prescription treatment called Rogaine topical solution (minoxidil 2 percent), say they have tried from the beginning to steer away completely bald men. "Guys who are totally bald just aren't going to benefit from our product," says company spokesman Jeff Palmer.

Upjohn continues to refine Rogaine, which is the only government-approved drug for baldness. Meanwhile, other researchers are evaluating these alternative treatments. Some may not be available yet.

Aromatase. Balding men appear to be deficient in this enzyme—which, when present in high-enough levels, causes follicles to grow hair. Researchers are working to refine a method of restoring aromatase levels.

Tricomin solution. This new drug seems to work by stimulating the growth of new hair follicles and by preventing existing follicles from becoming dormant, according to Karen Hedine, vice president of business development for the drug's maker, ProCyte of Kirkland, Washington.

Diazoxide. Like Rogaine, this drug appears to work by dilating blood vessels in the scalp.

Electrical stimulation. Tests involving low-current doses of electricity to men's scalps have shown promise in Canadian tests. Researchers predict treatments could be available in the United States in a few years.

"Hair weaves can look pretty good, but I don't really recommend them," Dr. Brandy says. "You have to keep going back periodically for tightening, which can be expensive. I think results are better with the other procedures."

Toupee. "Rugs" are out of vogue with many younger guys. But if you're willing to spend some money (more than $1,000 in most cases), you can find a natural hair or synthetic hairpiece that doesn't look like it was just peeled off a weasel's back.

Bald Is Beautiful

If all these options seem a little drastic, you may want to think about trying life au naturel. Millions of men lose their hair, after all, and most adjust just fine.

In fact, some guys think baldness is a sign of maturity, wisdom—even virility. "Baldness is the trend of the 1990s," says John Capps III, founder of Bald-Headed Men of America, a self-help group that claims more than 20,000 members. "These days, what's in your head is much more important than what's on it."

Group members say they're out to fight society's notion that bald men are unattractive and past their primes. Capps, who founded the group in 1972, says an increasing percentage of members are guys under age 40. "They are seeing that hair is not the most important part of them," he says. "When people look at you and form an impression, they're looking at your smile, your handshake and the twinkle in your eye long before they're looking at your forehead."

If you like, group members will meet with you one-on-one, either by telephone or in person, to discuss how to deal with your thinning hair. Capps stresses that it's not a professional counseling service but says the informal chats seem to help some guys.

For more information on Bald-Headed Men of America, write to Capps at 102 Bald Drive (really), Morehead City (really), NC 28557.

Thickening the Plot

Finally, if you're not willing to drop thousands of dollars—but you're not quite ready to part with your youthful mane—try these hairstyling tips, courtesy of George Roberson, author of *Men's Hair*.

Keep it short. Clipping your hair to a length of ½ to 1 inch will make it look neat and natural.

Forget the comb-over. You won't fool anyone by growing a foot-long piece of hair on the side of your head and plastering it over your bald spot.

Try hair elsewhere. A neat beard and moustache can draw people's eyes south, from your forehead to your face.

Remember the critical conditioner. Some conditioners give hair the illusion of greater thickness. Some experts suggest trying a leave-in conditioner that may add a tiny amount of thickness to individual hairs.

Change your goop. Switch from an oily groomer (such as Brylcreem) to a non-oily one (such as Dep or Tenax).

BODY IMAGE

Liking the Man in the Mirror

As you stroll onto the beach, you take a quick wistful look at the young women in their string bikinis, splashing sunscreen on their sleek bodies. You suck in your stomach as best you can as you stake your claim to a spot nearby while your wife dashes off for a swim.

After a few moments, one of the young women says something to you, and to your surprise, you actually say something flirtatious in reply. You know it's just innocent fun, but you feel like a teen again, chatting with these women half your age. But then a pair of young guys who look like tanned Greek gods emerge from the surf and flop in the sand next to the girls.

"What's up?" one of the guys says.

"Nothing much. We were just teasing that old guy over there," the blonde says, smiling at you.

You laugh nervously, but inside you feel like dog meat. Okay, so you've put on a few pounds, and your hair is thinning and getting a little gray. But old guy? Later you tell your wife the whole story. She laughs and says you look fine just as you are. But you don't believe her, and after that day, no matter how many people tell you how good you look, you don't believe them. Even now when you look in the mirror, you can see changes looming and wonder how long before all vestiges of your youthfulness vanish completely.

"Body image has a total impact on how we feel about aging," says Mary Huntington Lehner, clinical director of the Rocky Mountain Treatment Center in Great Falls, Montana. "There's a direct connection between your self-esteem and your body image. The better your self-esteem, the better you'll feel about what is happening to your body as you journey through life."

But even if you have terrific self-esteem, battling gray hair, crow's-feet and extra pounds in a society that worships youth and vigor can be demoralizing, says Ann Kearney-Cooke, Ph.D., a Cincinnati psychologist in private practice who specializes in body image problems and eating disorders.

Model Behavior

From the tan, square-jawed male models in TV commercials to the tough, muscular heroes of action-adventure movies, men are bombarded with the message that if you're not young, tall, ruggedly handsome and a perfect physical specimen, you don't measure up, psychologists say.

"In the eyes of society, when you're 20, you're hot; when you're 40, you're not; and when you're 60, you're shot," says Stanley Teitelbaum, Ph.D., a clinical psychologist in private practice in New York City.

That not-so-subtle vision is reflected in clothing store mannequins, whose proportions have bypassed the longtime industry standard of 38 regular and which now stand 6 feet 2 inches tall with a 42-inch chest and easily fill a size 42 suit, according to Judith Rodin, Ph.D., author of *Bodytraps* and professor of psychiatry and medicine at Yale University School of Medicine in New Haven, Connecticut. These images set a standard that men feel compelled to meet, Dr. Kearney-Cooke says.

"Men are increasingly self-conscious about their bodies," Dr. Kearney-Cooke says. "It used to be that men were concerned about how their bodies functioned and women were concerned about how they looked. Now both men and women are concerned about their looks."

How Bad Is It?

A growing number of men believe looking young and attractive is important. At the same time, more and more guys are displeased with their appearance.

In a 1989 survey of 1,000 men ages 18 to 60, Dr. Kearney-Cooke and Ruth Striegel-Moore, Ph.D., associate professor of psychology at Wesleyan University in Middletown, Connecticut, found that 63 percent believed that being attractive was very important compared with only 29 percent of guys in a similar survey conducted in 1973. In addition, 49 percent of the men in the 1989 survey said they were very self-conscious about their appearance, and 91 percent wanted to change their bodies.

In 15 years, the number of men displeased with their overall appearance increased from about one in seven to one in three. So what exactly do men dislike about their bodies? Just about everything from head to toe. In a study at Old Dominion University in Norfolk, Virginia, about 40 percent of the 103 balding men who participated said hair loss made them look older and feel less attractive. About 60 percent spent time looking at their bald spots in the mirror and wondering what others would think.

"I treat a lot of men who have problems surrounding hair loss," Dr. Teitelbaum says. "They see themselves starting to bald, and they get frantic. They get frightened because losing hair represents losing something that they believe is prized and valued by our youth-oriented culture."

In addition, 33 percent of men are dissatisfied with their muscle tone, 28 percent dislike their chest sizes, and 20 percent are dissatisfied with their faces, according to Dr. Rodin.

But the thing most men would change is weight. About 50 percent are concerned about beer bellies, and 41 percent are dissatisfied with their overall weight, according to Dr. Rodin.

But not all are worried about fat. Some men want to gain weight. In fact, men who have poor body images are just as likely to be worried about being underweight as they are about being overweight, according to research conducted at the University of Michigan in Ann Arbor.

"When I was growing up, I can't recall any man being weight-conscious unless he was really obese," Dr. Teitelbaum says. "Now men talk about it as much as women do. Years ago, diets and concerns about weight were considered to be a woman's problem. Men didn't discuss it. Now they talk about it openly."

Making That Change

It's probably not surprising that middle-aged men are starting to keep plastic surgeons busy. Most guys who opt for plastic surgery get face-lifts, liposuctions, eye-lifts, nose reshapings and dermabrasions, according to the American Society of Plastic and Reconstructive Surgeons. Of the 394,911 cosmetic surgery procedures that the organization logged in 1992, 49,848—or 13 percent—were done on men.

Here's Looking at You

Of course, good looks don't guarantee that you will have a good body image or that you will age more gracefully than others. "Some men age better than others and make the necessary shifts into new phases of the life cycle. Some can't handle it at all," Dr. Teitelbaum says. "This task is hardest for middle-aged men who have relied heavily upon their looks to get by in the world. If your looks are your calling card—if they are what other people have applauded you for throughout your life—it can be devastating when you start to lose them."

While body image can be a problem throughout a man's life, worries about it usually level off as a man reaches his fifties. "As men get older, they're more concerned about having healthy bodies than looking good," Dr. Kearney-Cooke says.

The best reward for improving your body image at any age is that you'll feel more comfortable with yourself, and as a result, more people will want to be around you. "Then a good body image can definitely make you feel younger," says Debbie Then, Ph.D., a social psychologist in Stanford, California. "The more positive you are, the more outgoing you'll be. And that's important, because it's been shown that people who have more friends and acquaintances are healthier."

Here are some tips to help you feel better about your body.

Look from the inside out. "You aren't your body. You just happen to be in your body," says Susan Olson, Ph.D., director of psychological services at the Southwest Bariatric Nutrition Center in Tempe, Arizona. "Try not to look at yourself as just a physical being, because that's going to pass." Find other reasons for liking yourself, such as a solid career or a good sense of humor.

Find a hero. Find a picture in a magazine of a man who has features similar to yours, cut it out and put it on your mirror for inspiration, Dr. Olson suggests. The fact that he isn't perfect should make you feel better about yourself, she says.

Give yourself a hug. Dr. Olson suggests that every time you look in a mirror, say to yourself "I love you; I think you're absolutely handsome." "That affirmation may seem ridiculous, but it's important, because you're not going to believe those words coming from anyone else until you believe them from yourself," she says.

Look back. Find a favorite picture of yourself from each decade of your life. "Looking at those pictures will help you realize that you were a better-looking person than you may have thought you were at the time," says Ann Meissner, Ph.D., a psychologist in private practice in St. Paul, Minnesota. "It will also make you think twice about how accurate your judgments are about yourself now."

Look ahead. Conjure up an image of yourself 5, 10 or 20 years from now. How do you look? How does it feel? Keep doing it until you find an image of yourself that feels comfortable, says Rita Freedman, Ph.D., author of *Bodylove*.

Graduate to a new image. Forget about the good-looking, athletic guy who got all the girls when you were in high school. "You're not in high school anymore. Your sense of what is fun and who is attractive is different at 40 than it was in high school," says Leonard Felder, Ph.D., author of *A Fresh Start: How to Let Go of Emotional Baggage*. "So stop judging yourself based on your old high school standards."

Try some soul food. If you're working on changing your appearance, commit yourself to two other goals that aren't related to your body, Dr. Kearney-Cooke says. So if you're trying to flatten your abdominal muscles, for example, then also coach a Little League baseball team or take an automotive repair class. "It helps you see yourself as a whole person," she says.

Sweat it out. Regular exercise such as walking, bicycling, swimming or weight training can help you stay fit—and improve your body image—when you do it for at least 20 minutes a day, three times a week. "There's no question that people who exercise have better body images," says Mark Leary, Ph.D., professor of psychology at Wake Forest University in Winston-Salem, North Carolina. "Exercise helps people maintain their weight as they age, makes them feel better and also counteracts many of the effects of aging. You walk more erect and have better stamina."

Please yourself first. If you do decide to make changes in your body, do it for yourself; you'll enjoy it more. "As we get older, we cling to this idea that your physique has to look like it did when you were 22. In fact, your friends and family probably don't care if you have the body of a 22-year-old. They just want you to have a decent 40-year-old body," Dr. Leary says.

Ask the tough questions. If you're concerned that a woman you're interested in dating has a problem with balding, potbellies or whatever physical feature you're self-conscious about, ask her, Dr. Felder suggests. "If she is honest and says no, she doesn't have a problem with it, then you have to ask yourself why you are creating a problem in your mind if it doesn't exist in hers," he explains. "If she does have a problem with it, you can either let her go or find a compromise, such as losing some weight, that will work for both of you."

Dress for success. "Appearance does count at any age, but you don't have obsess about it. Just make the most of what you do have," Dr. Then says. "For health reasons, exercise, eat a balanced diet, maintain a weight that is right for your proportions and practice good grooming. Wear clothes that complement your looks, but realize that you don't have to look like the guys in fashion magazines to have a happy, successful life. Try to be the best possible version of yourself."

BURNOUT

Time to Climb out of Your Rut

Lately, you're as cranky and easily irritated as an arthritic lap dog. You have lost your youthful resilience and spend most of your time fighting a losing battle with ever-increasing bouts of fatigue. Not only can you tell what day of the week it is by what strain of flu you have, but your body has become a playground for all manner of backache, chest pain and headache.

What's going on? Did you go to bed one night and age 30 years in your sleep? Or are you experiencing a syndrome known as burnout? Undoubtedly, it's the latter. Burnout is a kind of stress/boredom/frustration cocktail that can leave you feeling tired, irritable, achy and old.

"Burnout can certainly make you feel old before your time," says C. David Jenkins, Ph.D., professor of preventive medicine and community health at the University of Texas Medical Branch at Galveston. "Burnout tends to drain people of the physiological and mental reserves that are, in youth, typically there to keep them going. Luckily, burnout does not necessarily age people or take years off their lives in a permanent fashion. It can be reversed."

But to understand how to beat or even prevent burnout, you need to know how most men set themselves up for burnout without even realizing it.

No Variety, No Spark

If you are dying for a good case of burnout, there are a number of ways you can accomplish it. But contrary to popular belief, one of them is not trying to do too many things. "Burnout does not occur by having too many pots boiling on your stove," says Faye Crosby, Ph.D., professor of psychology at Smith College in Northampton, Massachusetts, and author of *Juggling*. "Many times it occurs because you have only one pot boiling constantly and can never take it over to the sink to fill it up. Eventually, all the water boils away."

According to Dr. Crosby, variety is a basic human need and a good way of vaccinating yourself against burnout. But variety is not achieved merely by doing different activities. The activities have to answer different needs. "At work, our activities tend to be very agenda-oriented; things need to get done by a set time for a definite purpose," notes Dr. Crosby. "At home, our activities are much more socioemotional. They please us, they make us feel good, they answer emotional needs without having specific agendas."

The problems start when there's too much agenda and not enough emotional outlet. And it's a setup all too familiar for men. "For the most part, if you ask a man to tell you about himself, he'll tell you what he does for a living rather than about his family or hobbies," notes Herbert J. Freudenberger, Ph.D., author of *Burnout: The High Cost of High Achievement* and the originator of the term *burnout*. "And while things are slowly changing, men are still cast in the singular role of worker/provider. They typically do not take advantage of the nurturing role in the home that women enjoy and therefore have fewer places to renew themselves when constant focus on the job burns them out."

Perfectionism Can Hurt

Just to the right of the "one pot boiling for too long" road to burnout is Perfection Alley. "Many times the men who most frequently suffer from burnout are the perfectionists who cannot delegate," says Dr. Freudenberger. "They give themselves absolutely no latitude when it comes to making mistakes. But to be a perfectionist is to make unrealistic demands on yourself and to set impossible goals. You might be able to do it for awhile, but in the long run, burnout is almost a certainty."

It is no coincidence, then, that one of the highest burnout ratios is found among air traffic controllers, a profession of mostly males who work under conditions in which anything short of constant perfection could amount to loss of life. So great is the pressure they're under not to make mistakes that by the time they reach their mid-forties, many of these guys have had to leave their jobs, says Dr. Jenkins, who participated in a definitive study of air traffic controllers and burnout. "And in fact, it seems that the professions most prone to burnout are the ones where constant vigilance is demanded and where the cost of mistakes is horrendous," he says.

But not everyone works in an environment demanding such enforced perfection. Some people do it to themselves, wrongly convincing themselves that every little mistake they make could mean disaster.

Overwork, Underappreciation

Another good way to burn out is to do everything yourself: Never delegate, never let anything out of your sight. A somewhat apocryphal story attributed to Lee Iacocca relates the time when one of his senior vice presidents at Chrysler was bragging about the fact that he hadn't had a vacation in two years. But instead of praising the executive for his sense of duty, Iacocca fired him, saying that "anyone who can't take a vacation in two years has something seriously wrong with him."

Dr. Crosby agrees. "As a matter of fact, if you can't get away from your home and office for at least five days each year without worrying that everything is going to fall apart, you have a serious problem."

Burnout can also result from a lack of positive reinforcement and social support. "One of the big complaints we heard from our air traffic controllers was that since they were expected to turn in flawless performances as a matter of course, they rarely received compliments for outstanding work during periods of heavy traffic," notes Dr. Jenkins. "But in situations similar to this, when support groups were developed to provide feedback and praise, burnout, as measured by job turnover and employee satisfaction, seemed to decrease."

Signs of Trouble

How do you know if you have burnout? One way to tell is to take the test below. Another is to listen to whether your friends say you've changed. "But

Are You Burning Out?

Feeling like an ornery old workhorse lately? It could be burnout.

The following self-test, developed by Herbert J. Freudenberger, Ph.D., and included in his book *Burnout: The High Cost of High Achievement*, may give you the answer. When taking this test, consider changes in your behavior over the past six months. Give yourself about 30 seconds before answering each question and then rate your response from 1 to 5. One means little or no change; 5 means a great deal of change.

1. Do you tire more easily? Feel fatigued rather than energetic?
2. Are people annoying you by telling you "You don't look so good lately"?
3. Are you working harder and harder and accomplishing less and less?
4. Are you increasingly cynical and disenchanted?
5. Are you often invaded by a sadness you can't explain?
6. Are you forgetting deadlines, appointments, personal possessions?
7. Are you increasingly irritable? More short-tempered? More disappointed in the people around you?
8. Are you seeing close friends and family members less frequently?

you probably won't," says Dr. Freudenberger. "A major coping mechanism that I've noticed in burnout patients is denial—denial that this is happening, denial that this is something they need help to overcome." In other words, the person who knows the least about burnout is the one suffering from it.

But if you won't listen to your friends, at least listen to your body. "One of the first signs we noticed in the air traffic controllers who were burning out was a sense of fatigue," says Dr. Jenkins. "And I'm talking about a pervasive mental and physical fatigue that a good night's sleep will not get rid of."

Chest pains are another mile marker on the road to burnout. "I received a call from the hospital about a man who had checked in the day before with chest pain, severe pain on his left side, terrible headaches and shortness of breath," recalls Dr. Freudenberger. "He thought he was having a coronary. But a series of tests turned up nothing. Upon exploring what was going on in his life, both at work and at home, we quickly realized the problem to be a stress response to burnout."

Gastrointestinal problems, backache, headache, sleep disturbances and a higher incidence of minor illnesses such as colds are some of the body's other responses to burnout. So are skin disorders, adds Dr. Freudenberger. "I see this quite a bit in accountants, who, during periods of the year when they are

9. Are you too busy to do even routine things such as making phone calls, reading reports or sending out Christmas cards?
10. Are you suffering from physical complaints—aches, pains, headaches, lingering colds?
11. Do you feel disoriented when the activity of the day comes to a halt?
12. Is joy elusive?
13. Are you unable to laugh at a joke about yourself?
14. Does sex seem like more trouble than it's worth?
15. Do you have very little to say to people?

Scoring

Add up your answers.

0 to 25. You're doing fine.

26 to 35. There are things you should be watching.

36 to 50. You are a candidate.

51 to 65. You're burning out.

Over 65. You are in a dangerous place, threatening to your physical and mental well-being.

putting in up to 20 hours a day, come to me with acne, eczema and hives."

On the mental front, a lack of resilience, characterized by a feeling of being whipped, can be a harbinger of burnout. "Our air traffic controllers called it bounce-back," says Dr. Jenkins. "They couldn't bounce back from a taxing period of heavy controlling and face the next period of activity with any sense of ease, comfort and casualness. They were drained."

Depression and increased irritability are also possibilities for those who are burning out. "But more interesting is the development of a superperson personality," notes Dr. Freudenberger. "The person feels he can handle everything, needs no help and may actually become arrogant about it."

The Solution

Whether burnout has made you move, think and feel like a cranky Methuselah on a bad day or you just want to make sure you never end up aging 30 years in as many weeks, the following tips will help you "de-burnout" your life.

Listen to your friends. "The first step to curing burnout is to admit the problem exists," says Dr. Freudenberger. "But that's harder than it sounds, because of the denial mechanism people often use to cope with burnout. So listen to your friends and family members. Pay attention when they say you've changed. You may not notice it yourself, but burnout can be very apparent to those close to you as well as to co-workers who can see the transformation."

Diversify. "Just as a bank must diversify its holdings so that it doesn't have to depend on one source for its profits, people have to diversify their emotional portfolios," says Dr. Crosby. "This means looking at your activities and making sure that you participate in some that are goal-oriented and some where the aim is to feel good and have fun. I actually encourage people to list them in two columns. If you have 2 items in one column and 40 in the other, things are out of whack, and you need to do some account balancing."

Stop being perfect. The trick is to give yourself a little leeway when you can. "Take stock of your situation and see what mistakes you can and can't make," says Dr. Crosby. "Not every miscalculation you make is going to plummet the world into Armageddon. In other words, don't sweat the small stuff." And that goes for all activities, work-related and otherwise.

Know your needs. "If you know that you need positive feedback to replenish yourself, then don't just ignore that fact," counsels Dr. Freudenberger. "Actively solicit feedback from family and friends and in the workplace." Tell them that you would occasionally like to hear "Good job!" when you've done something well. Or find a support group that you can share your feelings, achievements and gripes with. It doesn't have to be anything formal. A few people going through the same things as you will do just fine.

Volunteer. "Volunteering is a very important anti-burnout device," says Dr.

Crosby. "Whether you're at work or at home, worrying over a set of marketing reports or putting up aluminum siding, you have to drop what you're doing, mentally change gears and go interact with a whole new set of people in a whole new environment."

"It doesn't matter if you work in a soup kitchen twice a week, collect clothes or deliver meals. You receive gratification that you are doing something for someone else," adds Dr. Freudenberger. "You may also receive some very important perspective on your life by seeing those less fortunate than you."

Take five. Dr. Crosby prescribes a five-day vacation alone at least once a year. That means leaving the wife, the kids, the dog, the goldfish—everything—behind. They'll get on just fine without you for five days. "As a matter of fact," adds Dr. Crosby, "if you feel that the world will fall apart if you leave for five days, you have a good indicator that you are taking things far too seriously and are probably heading for burnout."

Take 15. "You also have to set aside some relaxation time during the course of the day," says Dr. Freudenberger. "And I mean every day, both at work and at home. When people tell me they can't do that, I make them actually take apart their days piece by piece, and they suddenly find all sorts of little opportunities for 15-minute breaks. And that's all it really takes."

Take off the red cape. Stop trying to be Superman. "The trick is to allow yourself the occasional mistake—to recognize pressure release points where mistakes will not mean the end of the world," Dr. Crosby says. In other words, handing in that report a day late won't push the company into bankruptcy.

BURSITIS AND TENDINITIS

Waylay the Scourge of Weekend Warriors

You decide to show the frisky kid down the block a thing or two about shooting hoops—for four hours. You till your garden all afternoon. You run up 17 flights of stairs when the office elevator is on the blink.

What do these iron-man actions have in common? They're all terrific ways to get a raging case of bursitis or tendinitis. These painful conditions overlap so often that doctors frequently diagnose them as bursitis/tendinitis, because it can be hard to tell where one leaves off and the other begins.

And they can happen most often to men in their forties, particularly to those haven't made a point of maintaining flexibility. Without regular stretching, muscles and tendons get tighter and rub together more, increasing the risk of inflammation.

Once you have bursitis or tendinitis, you find yourself moving in slow motion, because a sudden move can feel as though you've just been jabbed with a red-hot poker. It can hit you in any joint you take for granted.

Here's why it hurts.

The No-Use Syndrome

Your bursae are tiny fluid-filled sacs that cushion the spaces where muscle passes over bone and where two muscles rub together. In your kneecaps and elbows, they form cushions between skin and bone. They can get inflamed when you injure or overwork an out-of-condition joint or even when you're fighting fit, if you suddenly accelerate your workout beyond what you're used to, says Pekka Mooar, M.D., director of the Delaware Valley Sports Medicine Center in Philadelphia.

If you have tendinitis, it is not really your tendon but a ring of tissue around the tendon where it attaches to a bone or muscle that hurts. The pain is caused by overuse of the tendon, which produces inflammation.

"We all get more aches and pains with age; there's no controversy about that," says Phillip E. Higgs, M.D., a reconstructive surgeon at Washington University School of Medicine in St. Louis. But if you stay limber over the years, a burst of effort is much less likely to bring on bursitis and tendinitis, he says.

It is too little exercise, not aging itself, that increases your risk of these painful ailments. That's what Dr. Higgs and his colleagues concluded after counting cases of bursitis and tendinitis in a study of 157 poultry workers and 118 data processors. Although the workers ranged in age from 20 to 71, the younger workers who didn't exercise much had nearly the same number of inflammations as older workers who got little exercise.

Bursitis and tendinitis vary a great deal from person to person, Dr. Higgs says. For example, one day of all-out sports may cause symptoms in one person, while another has no trouble until after years on an assembly line.

The Consequences of Abuse

Shoulders, elbows, hips, knees and ankles are especially vulnerable to bursitis and tendinitis. For men, shoulders are the usual problem area, because we tend to do more throwing or to have jobs that require a lot of overhead lifting. Women tend to get pain in the hips, because women's hips are set wider than ours, which puts more stress on their joints.

Any activity that requires repetitive motion or pressure, from working on an assembly line to carpentry to letting Rover haul hard on a leash, increases your risk.

Bursitis and tendinitis are also caused by overdoing a favorite sport. Tennis can do in elbows and wrists; swimming or shooting hoops can irritate the shoulder bursae; running can aggravate ankles and Achilles tendons, particularly if you run on hard surfaces in the wrong shoes. And skiing can cause hips and knees to flare up.

Bursitis is often missed as a cause of lower back pain, experts say. And it often accompanies the disorder called fibromyalgia, which causes muscle pain and stiffness throughout the body.

Fortunately, bursitis and tendinitis are very treatable. And you can head them off at the pass.

Shock-Absorbing Your Joints

The most important thing is to get into condition gradually and to ease into vigorous exercise gently, says Stephen M. Campbell, M.D., a rheumatologist at Oregon Health Sciences University in Portland.

Start with a stretch. "In preparation for vigorous activity, you need to do

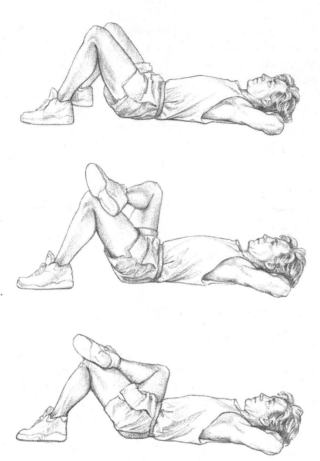

Lie flat on your back with your knees bent and your feet flat on the floor (top). Clasp your hands behind your head. Cross your right leg over your left leg, placing your right foot on the outside of your left leg just below the left knee (middle). Do a gentle pelvic tilt (that is, press the curve of your back toward the floor). Keeping your shoulders and upper back stationary, use your right foot to steadily pull your left knee toward the floor on your right side (bottom). You should feel a stretch in your left lower back or outer thigh as you try to touch your left knee to the floor. Hold for six seconds. Return to the starting position. Relax. Repeat the exercise using your left foot on the outside of your right leg (just below the right knee) to pull your right knee toward the floor on your left side. Repeat three to five times, twice daily.

more stretches of the muscles you'll be using," says Dr. Mooar. "Hold a slow, sustained stretch for ten seconds, and don't bounce. Repeat the stretch three to five times before exercising." And don't do high-speed stretches, or you risk tearing muscle fibers or ligaments, he says. If you're unsure which stretching exercise is best for you, check with a trainer. The one shown above can get you started.

Ease into new activities. If you take up a new sport, work at gradually increasing the strength and flexibility of the muscles you'll be using, says Dr. Mooar. If you choose tennis, for example, take it one set at a time at first. "Don't pick up a racket and play lots of sets at once, because your shoulder is going to feel like it's falling off," he says.

Precondition your joints. If your job or hobby calls for repetitive motion, ask a trainer to recommend strengthening and endurance exercises targeted for that motion, Dr. Mooar says. "If you do this," he says, "you can stop bursitis and tendinitis from happening over and over." Many people develop chronic inflammation from reinjuring their joints, he says.

Use office technology. Typing and filing can trigger problems in your wrists and back. Use a keyboard wrist rest for typing, says Dr. Campbell. And check that your chair is well adjusted so that your back is supported and your arms and wrists are level with each other.

Go easy on your knees. There is little but a tiny bursa between your

Wise Up Your Workouts

Let bursitis or tendinitis spoil your participation in your favorite sport? No way! You can sidestep them both with gradual conditioning. Or if bursitis or tendinitis has already hit, learn how to stage a careful comeback. Here's some advice for various activities.

Weight lifting. Learn proper form carefully and at your own pace from a trainer; don't push yourself to the limit. Always warm up and stretch before you lift and cool down after, says Robert L. Swezey, M.D., medical director of the Arthritis and Back Pain Center in Santa Monica, California.

Tennis. To avoid serving up wrist pain or tennis elbow, choose a large-handled racquet, decrease the string tension and wear an elastic band around your forearm to support the muscles, says Stephen M. Campbell, M.D., a rheumatologist at Oregon Health Sciences University in Portland. If your shoulder is the problem, modify your serve to avoid vigorously swinging your arm over your head.

Running. Condition yourself gradually before running longer distances, says Dr. Campbell. Don't run too vigorously if you're just starting, avoid hard surfaces and wear shoes with soft soles and high-quality insoles and arch supports.

Swimming. Although swimming is very gentle on most joints, the shoulder can get too much of a workout, Dr. Campbell says. To prevent or heal shoulder bursitis or tendinitis, avoid the freestyle, or crawl, and butterfly strokes, he says. Use the breaststroke or sidestroke or a kickboard instead.

Returning to training. After a bout of bursitis or tendinitis, it's crucial to wait until all the pain has gone for restarting vigorous workouts, says Dr. Campbell. Once you get your doctor's okay to start again, exercise at a lower frequency and intensity, and recondition your injured joint over weeks or months, he says.

kneecap and the skin over it, says Dr. Mooar. So if you're doing cleaning or gardening on your knees, kneel on a piece of foam rubber or wear knee pads to cushion them. Many garden centers, sporting goods stores and hardware stores carry foam rubber or knee pads.

Bouncing Back

If you already have bursitis or tendinitis, the first thing to ask yourself is, what have you done differently? "You're overdoing whatever it is," says Dr. Campbell. "First, stop it." Then:

Put it on ice. "Apply a paper cup full of ice to the painful area," says Robert L. Swezey, M.D., medical director of the Arthritis and Back Pain Center in Santa Monica, California. Rub the icy bottom or side of the cup into the sore spot for two to five minutes, three or four times a day, to control the inflammation, he says.

Switch off with heat. After the ice, apply a microwavable heat pack or electric heating pad to soothe the pain, says Dr. Campbell. Microwavable packs are available at most pharmacies, he says.

Bundle up for bed. Wear a flannel shirt or a wool sweater at night to keep a painful shoulder extra warm. If you sleep shirtless in a cool room, your morning stiffness and soreness will be greater.

Use the right pain reliever. Choose an aspirin or ibuprofen pain reliever for the pain, says Dr. Campbell. Aspirin and ibuprofen block the production of chemicals called prostaglandins, which contribute to swelling and pain in inflamed tissue. Acetaminophen won't control inflammation because it does not block prostaglandins.

Swing your shoulder. Sometimes bursitis or tendinitis in the shoulder progresses to a painful condition called adhesive capsulitis, or frozen shoulder. When this happens, the shoulder's range of motion is severely restricted, and the joint is nearly immobile. To avoid frozen shoulder, you need to start moving your shoulder as soon as the acute pain has passed, says Dr. Campbell. Lie facedown on a cushioned surface such as a bed, and hang the affected arm over the side. Gently swing your arm like a pendulum, gradually increasing the range until you can swing it in a full circle. Do this for 15 to 30 minutes, three to five times a week, to restore your range of motion, he says.

Check out chiropractic care. If your pain won't quit, a technique called friction massage may clear up the problem, says Warren I. Hammer, D.C., a chiropractor in private practice in Norwalk, Connecticut. When inflammation is chronic, fibrous adhesions don't allow the bursae to glide smoothly. Friction massage can break down those adhesions, says Dr. Hammer, relieving the cause of bursitis pain. "Also, an inflamed tendon becomes thicker and shorter, which creates further inflammation in the bursa it's rubbing over," Dr. Hammer says. "The deep pressure of massage across the bursa and tendon can lengthen the tendon fibers again." Use ice to calm the inflammation before chiropractic treatment, he says.

Thawing the Freeze

If bursitis or tendinitis lingers too long, you can wind up with a painful, "frozen" joint or restricted motion. Here's how your doctor can help.

Get prescription relief. If you have no history of stomach problems, your doctor can recommend prescription-strength non-steroidal anti-inflammatory drugs (NSAIDs) for pain, says Dr. Campbell. Like aspirin and ibuprofen, NSAIDs work by blocking the production of prostaglandins. But they can also irritate the stomach lining like aspirin does, so they are usually not prescribed for long periods.

Be cautious about injections. Nearly the last resort for pain, steroids are "shortcuts, not cures," says Dr. Mooar. Most doctors recommend injecting a painful joint, tendon or bursa no more than twice a year. Frequent injections can weaken or rupture a tendon.

"Most people are overinjected with cortisone-like drugs," says Dr. Swezey. "Most doctors use 10 to 20 milligrams for bursal injections, but I've found that 2½ milligrams works quite well."

Keep surgery as a last resort. For extremely severe bursitis, your doctor may use a needle to draw fluid off a painful joint or recommend that an orthopedic surgeon remove an inflamed bursa entirely, says Dr. Mooar. But before consenting to surgery, you should seek a second opinion.

CAFFEINE

You Command the Supply

If you're like most guys, mornings are a two-part affair: B.C. (before caffeine) and A.D. (awake from the dead). A slug of coffee or strong tea can clear your head, jump-start your body and help you deal with the knuckle-heads lying in wait at work.

Just be careful not to overdo it. Health experts warn that caffeine overload may turn you into a fatigued, trembling insomniac zombie with raging heart-burn and diarrhea—not exactly the ideal picture of youth and vitality.

"Take it easy with caffeine," says Mary Sullivan, R.D., a registered di-etitian and nutrition support specialist at the University of Chicago Hospitals. "It can really help you sharpen your mind and body when taken in small amounts. But it may also cause some harm if you have an excessive amount in your diet."

Grounds for Concern

Caffeine stimulates the central nervous system, triggering the release of adrenaline into your bloodstream and raising blood sugar levels. That can make you more alert and focused and help you ease into the day.

At normal levels—the average American man consumes about 200 milli-grams of caffeine per day, the amount found in about two five-ounce cups of coffee—that's about the end of the story. But push caffeine intake further, and you may be pushing your luck.

If you're counting sheep at night and flopping facedown at your desk during the day, caffeine may be the culprit. "Too much caffeine is one of the first things I check for when someone complains of fatigue or insomnia," says

Richard Podell, M.D., clinical professor of family medicine at the University of Medicine and Dentistry of New Jersey Robert Wood Johnson Medical School in Piscataway.

Caffeine can interrupt your sleep patterns at night, robbing you of your deepest, most restful sleep. Dr. Podell says that can create a nasty cycle: poor sleep at night, luring you to take more caffeine during the day, leading to even worse sleep and making you crave caffeine even more the next day. "You have to get off somewhere," Dr. Podell says, "or your sleep and energy levels may just get worse."

For years, the scientific world has bombarded the public with other claims about the ill effects of caffeine, ranging from increased cholesterol levels to pancreatic cancer. Research has been inconclusive at best and contradictory at worst. In part, that's because caffeine studies almost always use coffee. And coffee may contain other substances that cause problems.

"We need more conclusive studies to see just what is a coffee problem and what is a caffeine problem," says Manfred Kroger, Ph.D., professor of food science at the Pennsylvania State University in University Park. "Right now, the issue is too confused to make a specific statement—other than that you should take both caffeine and coffee in moderation."

So how much caffeine is too much? "Two cups of coffee a day is probably not going to cause any problems," Dr. Kroger says.

Again, that means about 200 milligrams of caffeine a day—the equivalent of four cans of cola, three cups of tea or three pounds of milk chocolate (skipping coffee is not a valid medical excuse to eat three pounds of chocolate, in case you were wondering).

"Just use your head," Sullivan says. "If you're having trouble sleeping or feeling jittery, it's probably a good idea to cut back, whatever your intake level."

Controlling the Kick

Life without caffeine? Sure. And while we're at it, let's just drop baseball and dating from life as well.

Look, nobody's saying you can't enjoy a mug of coffee or a can of cola. But if caffeine is bothering you, or if you're worried about caffeine's possible long-term consequences, try some of these tips.

Nix the nightcap. Beware caffeine's long-lasting jolt. Studies show that caffeine stays in your system longer than most other stimulants. Half the caffeine you drink in a cup of coffee may still be coursing through your veins five hours later. So if you're having problems sleeping, Sullivan says you should avoid caffeine starting in the late afternoon.

Cut where you can. There's nothing wimpy about drinking decaffeinated coffee. In fact, switching to "unleaded" may be the single fastest way to cut your caffeine intake. Still, Dr. Kroger warns that decaf may contain harmful elements of regular coffee that have yet to be investigated fully. "Switching to decaf is not an invitation to continue drinking ten cups a day," Dr. Kroger says.

Other alternatives? Try the new half-decaf, half-regular coffees on the market. Or switch to coffee made from arabica beans. These beans can contain about one-third less caffeine than the cheaper robusta beans, which are often used in instant coffees.

Sullivan also suggests avoiding other caffeine sources whenever possible. Soft drinks contain only one-third to one-half as much caffeine as coffee—but drinking a caffeine-free brand can still cut your caffeine intake by as much as 60 milligrams, Sullivan says.

Be careful with dark chocolate, too. You'd need to eat more than a pound of

Caffeine Count

How many milligrams of caffeine are in that drink or chocolate bar? Here are the numbers.

Food/Beverage	Caffeine (mg.)
COFFEE (PER 5-OZ. CUP)	
Drip	115
Percolated	80
Instant	68–98
Decaffeinated	4
TEAS (PER 5-OZ. CUP)	
Tetley	64
Lipton	52
Tender Leaf	33
Constant Comment	29
SOFT DRINKS (PER 12-OZ. CAN)	
Tab	57
Mountain Dew	54
Coca-Cola	46
Diet Coke	46
Pepsi	38
Diet Pepsi	36
CHOCOLATES (PER 1 OZ.)	
Ghirardelli dark chocolate	24
Hershey's milk chocolate	4

A Hidden Kick

Some over-the-counter drugs contain surprising amounts of caffeine. The following table shows the caffeine content of one tablet of each nonprescription medication.

Drug	Caffeine (mg.)
Maximum Strength No Doz	200
Vivarin	200
No Doz	100
Aspirin Free Excedrin	65
Excedrin Extra Strength	65
Anacin (regular strength)	32
Maximum Strength Anacin	32

Hershey's milk chocolate to get the same amount of caffeine found in a cup of percolated coffee—but just three ounces of Ghirardelli dark chocolate contains nearly a cup of coffee's worth of caffeine by itself.

Read the label. Anyone who has ever pulled an all-nighter knows that pep pills such as No Doz and Vivarin are absolutely stuffed with caffeine. That's the whole point. But you may be surprised to find that some analgesics (such as Anacin and Excedrin) contain as much caffeine as a typical can of cola. If you're caffeine-sensitive, check the small print on your box of aspirin.

Break your routine. Maybe you're not hooked on caffeine. Maybe you're hooked on a routine. "If you find yourself picking up a mug of coffee every time you sit down to a task, you probably just have a bad habit," Sullivan says. "Ask yourself if you really want that cup or whether you can do without it."

You could also try putting something else in your mug (water, perhaps, since most of us don't drink enough anyway).

Back off slowly. If you think too much caffeine makes you crazy, just try going cold turkey. You could end up with a whole new set of problems—headache, anxiety and feelings of depression. Dr. Podell suggests reducing caffeine intake gradually, over a few days or a week. That could ease withdrawal symptoms, which may occur even in moderate caffeine users.

CANCER

Putting Up a Good Fight

When a guy is told he has cancer, a lot of questions zip through his mind: "Am I going to die?" "What am I going to tell people?" "How are we going to pay the bills?" "Will I lose my hair?" "Will I be sick to my stomach?"

Cancer is a particularly powerful ager. It's a fearsome predator that can cause debilitating pain and suck youth and vigor out of any one of us.

The disease can actually accelerate the aging process by causing chemical changes in the body that lead to painful joints, dulled appetite, weight loss, weakness, fatigue and loss of stamina, says Ernest Rosenbaum, M.D., an oncologist at the University of California, San Francisco/Mount Zion.

"Cancer drains you. If you have cancer, you can feel aged and older very quickly," says Charles B. Simone, M.D., an oncologist in Princeton, New Jersey, and author of *Cancer and Nutrition*.

One Name, Many Diseases

Cancer is life-threatening because its abnormal cells grow uncontrollably, can spread throughout the body and can damage surrounding normal cells, says John Laszlo, M.D., national vice president for research at the American Cancer Society. It is actually not one disease but an array of more than 100 kinds of malignancy that attack different organs of the body in a variety of ways. So lung cancer, for example, may spread to other tissues in a slightly different way than colon cancer.

"There's this perception that cancer is a single entity and that we're going to find some magic pill that will totally prevent the disease or will be the ultimate cure for all forms of cancer. Unfortunately, cancer is more complicated than that," says Ronald Ross, M.D., director of cancer cause and prevention research at the University of Southern California Kenneth Norris, Jr., Comprehensive Cancer Center in Los Angeles.

Researchers suspect that 5 to 10 percent of cancers may be inherited, meaning that the disease is passed on from one generation to another through an abnormal gene. But in the vast majority of cases, cancer develops through a complex series of steps that often includes prolonged exposure to carcinogens, which are cancer-causing substances such as tobacco and asbestos, Dr. Laszlo says. These carcinogens usually affect cells in specific organs. Asbestos, for example, increases a person's risk of lung cancer, while excessive sun exposure is linked to increased risk of skin cancer.

Some researchers believe that carcinogens cause the formation of free radicals, unstable oxygen molecules that can damage the string of DNA molecules that tell cells how to reproduce. Once the DNA is damaged in critical places, a cancer cell may form.

"The free radicals that cause aging are the same things that cause cancer," Dr. Simone says. "How do we prevent that? We need to decrease our exposure to the things that cause free radicals, including fatty foods, tobacco and alcohol."

Each year, about 632,000 new cases of cancer are diagnosed among American men, according to the American Cancer Society. The most common types of cancer in males are found in the prostate, colon and rectum, lungs and bladder. In men younger than age 35, cancers of the skin and testicles as well as lymphomas such as Hodgkin's disease are the three most prevalent.

Cancer kills about 283,000 men annually and is the second leading cause of death for Americans of all ages. By the year 2000, cancer is expected to affect

Seven Signs You Shouldn't Ignore

Here are seven common warning signs of cancer. If you develop any of them, contact your doctor immediately.

1. A lump or thickening in the breast (yes, even in men)
2. A change in a wart or a mole
3. A sore that doesn't heal
4. A change in bowel or bladder habits
5. A persistent cough or hoarseness
6. Constant indigestion or trouble swallowing
7. Unusual bleeding or discharge

two in every five Americans and will surpass heart disease as the nation's leading killer, Dr. Simone says.

But having cancer isn't an automatic death sentence. In fact, more than half of all Americans diagnosed with cancer survive it, according to the American Cancer Society. If detected early, some types of cancer, such as those of the skin and prostate, have five-year survival rates topping 90 percent. If a patient appears free of cancer symptoms for five years, doctors may consider him "cured," although some cancers may relapse after ten or more years.

"We've made slow, steady progress against cancer in the past 50 years. Step-by-step, we're winning this war," says Harmon Eyre, M.D., the American Cancer Society's deputy executive vice president for research and medical affairs.

Most cancers occur in men older than age 50, and 66 percent of cancer deaths occur after 65. In fact, of the 200,000 cases of prostate cancer—the most common cancer among men—diagnosed each year, less than 200 are among men younger than 45.

"For the most part, the young don't have to fear cancer. It's something that lurks in the distant future, sometimes up to 30 or 40 years away," says Carl Mansfield, M.D., professor and chairman of the Department of Radiation Oncology and Nuclear Medicine at Thomas Jefferson University Hospital in Philadelphia.

What You Can Do

However, some cancers can take more than 30 years to develop. So what you do now can have a tremendous impact on your ability to have a long, healthy and cancer-free life, Dr. Lazlo says. In fact, oncologists estimate that perhaps 50 percent of cancers could be prevented if men made just a few simple adjustments in their lifestyles. Here's where to start.

Become an ex-smoker. Lung cancer was a rare disease before cigarette smoking became popular. Now it is the leading cause of cancer-related deaths and is expected to kill nearly 94,000 American men annually, says Dennis Ahnen, M.D., associate director for cancer prevention and control at the University of Colorado Cancer Center in Denver. Smokers are ten times more likely to develop lung cancer, and up to 30 percent of all cancer deaths are caused by smoking, says Dr. Rosenbaum, author of *You Can Prevent Cancer*. The American Cancer Society estimates that 90 percent of lung cancers, 75 percent of cancers of the mouth, larynx and esophagus and about 50 percent of bladder and pancreatic cancers could be prevented if guys would quit using tobacco. The most important thing that a man can do to prevent cancer is to not smoke, Dr. Ross says.

Watch out for passive smoke, too. Up to 8,000 lung cancer deaths a year among nonsmokers can be attributed to secondhand smoke, Dr. Simone says. In a preliminary study of five nonsmoking men who were exposed to heavy cigarette smoke for three hours on each of two days, which were six months apart, researchers at the American Health Foundation in Valhalla, New York, found high levels of lung carcinogens in the men's urine 24 hours later. In addition, researchers at the University of California, Berkeley/University of California, San Francisco Preventive Medicine Residency Program found that restaurant workers are exposed to twice as much passive smoke as people who live in households where at least one person smokes. Bartenders are exposed to 4½ times as much passive smoke. Compared with the general population, these food service workers were found to be 50 percent more likely to develop lung cancer, a difference attributable, at least in part, to passive smoking in the workplace. Avoid smoky bars and always ask to be seated in nonsmoking sections of restaurants, Dr. Simone suggests. If people in your household smoke, ask them to quit or establish an area where they can smoke without endangering you.

Go light on the booze. Heavy alcohol consumption increases your risk for cancers of the liver, mouth, esophagus and larynx. Researchers speculate that alcohol doesn't cause cancer directly but paves the way for tumors by generating free radicals. Most experts recommend that you limit yourself daily to no more than one 12-ounce beer, one 5-ounce glass of wine or a cocktail made with 1½ ounces (or one shot) of liquor.

Fill up on fiber. Men who eat lots of fibrous fruits, vegetables and whole grains, such as broccoli, brussels sprouts, cabbage, apples, bananas, mangoes and whole-wheat cereals and breads, have fewer colon and rectal cancers than men who don't eat these foods, Dr. Simone says. Fiber helps speed stool through your body and reduce exposure of your digestive tract to carcinogens.

The National Cancer Institute recommends that men eat at least 20 to 30 grams of fiber a day. If you start your day with a cereal that has at least 7 grams of fiber per serving, add another 3 grams of fiber by topping your cereal with one medium sliced banana and two tablespoons of raisins. Then you're halfway to the minimum daily recommendation of 20 grams, says Gladys Block, Ph.D., professor of public health nutrition at the University of California, Berkeley. Then all you need to do is make sure you have three more servings of fruits, vegetables and/or grains through the rest of the day. Beans, for example, are particularly high in fiber.

Think like a vegetarian. Eat at least five servings of fruits and vegetables a day, Dr. Rosenbaum says. These foods contain antioxidant vitamins and minerals such as beta-carotene, selenium and vitamins A and E that combat the formation of free radicals.

For example, in a study comparing 351 men who had bladder cancer with 855 men who didn't have the disease, researchers at the State University of New York at Buffalo found that men who ate the most fruits and vegetables had a 60 percent lower risk of developing this type of cancer, which strikes 38,000 men annually. The researchers speculate that beta-carotene and other carotenes are the most likely disease fighters.

Take a supplement. Supplements containing vitamins C and E and other

This Exam Could Save Your Life

We hate to bring it up, but have you felt your testicles lately? If you haven't, you could be missing a chance to detect one of the more treatable and curable cancers.

Although testicular cancer accounts for only 1 percent of cancers in all men, it is one of the most common cancers to occur in guys in their twenties and thirties. If it is detected early, however, it is nearly 100 percent curable, says Ernest Rosenbaum, M.D., an oncologist at the University of California, San Francisco/Mount Zion.

Because the most common symptom is a small, painless lump in the testicle, it's important to do a monthly testicle exam.

"Men may feel uncomfortable doing testicular exams the first couple of times, but that feeling should pass," Dr. Rosenbaum says.

Here are some tips for doing a self-exam, recommended by the National Cancer Institute.

- Try to do the exam after you've taken a warm bath or shower. The heat will relax the scrotum, the sac of skin surrounding the testicles, and make it easier for you to find anything unusual.
- Gently examine each testicle with both hands. Place your index and middle fingers underneath and your thumbs on top of a testicle.
- Roll the testicle between your fingers. It should feel smooth and firm. One testicle may be larger than the other; this is normal. Feel for any abnormal lumps; most are about the size of a pea.

If you do feel a lump, see your doctor. You may have just an infection. If it is cancer, your doctor may recommend removing the testicle. Testicular cancer seldom occurs in both testicles, and only one is needed for sexual function.

antioxidant vitamins and minerals can help neutralize certain carcinogens such as the nitrites found in bacon, sausage, hot dogs and cured meats, according to Kedar N. Prasad, Ph.D., director of the Center for Vitamins and Cancer Research at the University of Colorado Health Sciences Center in Denver and author of *Vitamins in Cancer Prevention and Treatment*. Supplements can also strengthen your body's immune system so that it can destroy newly formed cancer cells before they multiply, Dr. Prasad says. He suggests taking 15 milligrams of beta-carotene once a day, 2,500 IU of vitamin A twice a day, 500 milligrams of vitamin C twice a day, 200 milligrams (or 134 IU) of vitamin E twice a day and 50 micrograms of selenium twice a day.

Trim the fat. A high-fat diet, like many American men eat, is believed to trigger cancer. Researchers aren't certain why fat promotes tumors, but several factors could play a role, Dr. Mansfield says. Some suspect that fatty foods spark the production of bile acids that interact with bacteria in the colon to form carcinogens. It could also be that fat cells are more susceptible to carcinogens than other cells. Whatever the cause, many experts suggest slashing your dietary fat consumption to no more than 25 percent of calories. To do that, eat more fruits, vegetables and whole-grain foods, trim all visible fat from meats and eat no more than one three-ounce serving of red meat, fish or poultry a day.

Throw the deep fryer away. Frying simply adds more fat to food, and fat promotes cancer. Broil, steam, bake or boil your food instead, Dr. Mansfield says. Brown or sauté in nonstick pans, or use vegetable spray or chicken broth.

Go easy on the barbecue. The smoke and heat of charbroiling creates several cancer-causing substances, including nitrosamine, one of the most potent carcinogens known, Dr. Mansfield says. If you like to barbecue, do it carefully and sparingly, Dr. Prasad suggests. Place the grill as far above the coals as possible, and wrap aluminum foil around the grill to prevent fat from dripping onto the flame and causing excessive smoke and charring.

Trim your waistline. If you're overweight, you could be producing excessive amounts of estrogen. Although estrogen is a female reproductive hormone, men produce it, too, and it is believed to alter cell structure and has been linked to an increased risk of cancer, Dr. Mansfield says. Keep your weight within the range suggested by your family physician.

Pump it up. In a long-term study, researchers at Harvard University in Cambridge, Massachusetts, tracked cancer rates among 17,148 college graduates. After 23 years, the researchers concluded that the men who expended at least 1,000 calories a week (walking up one flight of stairs daily expends about 28 calories per week) were up to 50 percent less likely than sedentary men to develop colon cancer. Regular aerobic exercise such as swimming, walking or running for 20 minutes a day, at least three times a week, can speed up your digestion and reduce the amount of time that carcinogens have to do their nasty work in the colon and rectum, Dr. Simone says.

Stay in the shadows. Skin cancer, one of the most common cancers (it affects more than 700,000 Americans), is caused primarily by sunburn. To prevent skin cancer, avoid prolonged sun exposure, wear hats, long-sleeved shirts and pants and apply sunblock to exposed skin when you're outdoors, says Dr. Rosenbaum. The sunblock you choose should have a sun protection factor (SPF) of at least 15.

Compile your family tree. Although less than 10 percent of cancers have genetic roots, finding out if cancer runs in your family can help your doctor evaluate your risk and recommend ways to prevent the disease or detect it early, Dr. Rosenbaum says. Include as many relatives on both sides of your family as you can. If someone had cancer, jot down the age at which they were diagnosed and the organ in which it originated.

You Have It—Now What?

Nobody wants to hear his doctor tell him that he has cancer, but if you are diagnosed with it, don't panic, oncologists say.

"For many cancers, cure is clearly possible," says Dr. Erye. "The majority of individuals in this country who have cancer can expect to live normal life spans."

Treatments include surgery, radiation, chemotherapy and immunotherapy, which consists of injections of proteins and antibodies that assist or stimulate the immune system to fight the cancer. Which treatments are right for you will depend on the type of cancer, its size, how fast it is growing and whether it has spread beyond the original site.

Although many cancer treatments, particularly chemotherapy, have traditionally been arduous, new techniques are easing the process, Dr. Ahnen says. "I think we're much better at treating the side effects, particularly the nausea and vomiting associated with chemotherapy," Dr. Ahnen says. "We now have potent medicines that can prevent these symptoms."

But whatever type of cancer you have, the psychological strain can be enormous.

"It feels unfair," says Karen Syrjala, Ph.D., a psychologist at the Fred Hutchinson Cancer Research Center in Seattle. "They think 'At 30 or 40, how can this be happening to me?' It's not really what you planned to be doing with your life at that point, so it feels like an intrusion. It feels wrong. The whole family can feel that way."

Even the closest of friends and family may start distancing themselves from a guy who has cancer because of their own dread of cancer or fears that he will die, Dr. Mansfield says. As a result, the man with cancer often ends up socially isolated.

Here are some strategies for coping with the ups and downs of cancer treatment.

Become a know-it-all. Find out everything you can about your cancer and treatment. Ask your doctors and nurses question after question. "The first thing to do is gather information, so you understand what is happening to you and what your options are," Dr. Syrjala says. "Any time you know that you have options, you're going to feel more in control of the situation."

Don't blame yourself. "That's something that men sometimes do," Dr. Syrjala says. "You didn't cause your cancer. Yes, there are things you can do to reduce your chances of getting cancer, but nothing will absolutely prevent it."

Have a daily chuckle. A sense of humor is extremely important because it can help you cope with the worst aspects of cancer and its treatment, Dr. Syrjala says. Make time to watch funny movies or have a good laugh with a friend.

Don't be a passive patient. Treatment shouldn't be something that your doctor does to you; it should be something in which you have an active role. Think about what you can do for yourself that might help you recover, says Dr. Syrjala, and discuss it with your doctor.

Be honest with your doctor. Your oncologist won't know if a treatment is bothering you unless you speak up. If you don't have a good relationship with your physician, consider seeing someone else, Dr. Syrjala says.

Talk about it. "It's helpful to talk about your fears and sadness, because if you talk about them, you might find out there's something you can do about them," Dr. Syrjala says. "If you don't talk about your fears, you tend to not do anything about them. Sometimes talking takes away the power of your fears." Counseling may help.

Get some support. Find a support group for people with your type of cancer. "People in support groups live longer," Dr. Syrjala says. "We don't know why, but clearly, there is something about sharing your experiences with people who are in similar circumstances that can help you live a longer, more fulfilling life." Your doctor or local affiliate of the American Cancer Society should be able to help you find such a group.

Keep eating. Up to 40 percent of men who have cancer actually die of malnutrition, Dr. Simone says. That's because cancer cells release a hormone called cachectin that suppresses the appetite. That loss of appetite is compounded by some types of cancer treatment that can cause nausea and vomiting, such as chemotherapy. "The foundation of healing is good nutrition. I tell my patients that even if a meal seems unappetizing, try to eat some of it. Just chew and swallow, because you need that food," Dr. Mansfield says. He suggests eating small meals such as half a sandwich and a glass of orange juice several times a day and nibbling on healthy snacks such as carrots, apples and other fruits and vegetables.

CHOLESTEROL

A Highly Important Matter

Life used to be so simple: You'd pick up a few items at the grocery, throw a steak on the grill when you got home and enjoy your dinner with a can of beer and reruns of "Quantum Leap" to keep you company.

But today, it's hard to put a steak on the barbie with a clear conscience. *Cholesterol* has become the buzzword of our time, and it's difficult to go anywhere without being reminded of it. Packages on supermarket shelves proudly proclaim that their products have no cholesterol. An evening of television just isn't complete without a few 30-second commercials that make you cringe with guilt if you're munching on high-fat snack foods. And your own doctor probably preaches the gospel of getting your cholesterol to unfathomable depths.

So what's it all about? Ask any doctor worth his stethoscope, and he'll confirm what you probably already know: Cholesterol is a major contributor to heart disease, one of America's most dreaded aging-related health problems. Yes, some men continue to live in a state of denial about their health, but the ramifications of ignoring cholesterol are pretty daunting—and they grow even more daunting as you approach middle age.

The Heart Connection

In the late 1940s, the people of Framingham, Massachusetts, agreed to become guinea pigs for some of the nation's top researchers, who proceeded to poke and probe the bodies and nearly every morsel of food consumed by these willing test subjects. The researchers' mission: to find out what factors contribute to heart disease.

One factor they've paid a lot of attention to is cholesterol. They found that as blood cholesterol levels increase, so does the risk of heart disease. And in which group in Framingham was that connection the strongest? Sorry to say, it was men between ages 40 and 59.

Consider these facts: One in six men between 45 and 64 years old has some type of heart disease or has had a stroke. Each year, nearly one million men have heart attacks, which claim more male lives than any other single cause. A staggering 95 million American adults have blood cholesterol levels considered either borderline high or high.

Just reading these statistics is probably enough to give you chest pains. Hopefully, it's also enough to get you to take cholesterol more seriously. The good news is that you can slash your chances of having a heart attack if you find out your cholesterol reading and, if need be, hammer it into submission rather than letting it hammer you.

Just what is cholesterol anyway? Despite the bad rap that cholesterol has received (and deserves), it's much more than a devious monster doing only life-threatening dirty work. In fact, cholesterol is a waxy substance produced naturally by the liver. It is present in every cell in the body and is essential to human life. But it's also consumed in the diet, coming exclusively from animal products. When it joins forces with the saturated fat you eat, together they can deliver a double jolt of trouble.

As cholesterol and fat navigate through your bloodstream, they inevitably run aground against the walls of your arteries, dropping anchor and narrowing your arteries and impeding the flow of blood to your heart. At its worst, this ominous process, called atherosclerosis, can lead to agonizing angina (chest pain) and a heart attack.

It Takes All Kinds

You're probably aware that most talks about cholesterol eventually introduce a parade of abbreviations, such as *LDL* and *HDL*. When you get your cholesterol checked, your doctor should measure not only the total cholesterol level in your bloodstream but also your HDL (high-density lipoprotein) level. If these tests show signs of potential trouble, your doctor should decide to check your LDL (low-density lipoprotein) level, too, since evaluating all these numbers can be important in determining your risk.

Let's look more closely at these cholesterol factions. Cholesterol maneuvers through your bloodstream by catching rides on cooperative molecules called lipoproteins. While the cholesterol transported on LDLs is responsible for the bombing raids on your artery linings, the HDLs do just the opposite, actually kidnapping cholesterol and banishing it from the body. Like a Hail Mary pass that connects in the final seconds of the fourth quarter, HDLs can come to your rescue. For that reason, the more of them you have, the better.

Unfortunately, too many of America's bloodstreams have too many LDLs and too few HDLs, a combination that gives unhealthy total cholesterol numbers. In the United States, the average total cholesterol is about 206, which is higher than the desirable level of less than 200 (we're talking milligrams of cholesterol per deciliter of blood).

Make a Big Difference

As you move through adulthood, your cholesterol level will tend to rise, unless you take some action to stop that trend in its tracks. By making some painless lifestyle adjustments, your cholesterol count can win big.

And how large is the payoff? Studies in men show that for every 1 percent cut in your cholesterol level, you can deflate your chances of a heart attack by 2 percent. With dietary changes alone, you can whittle away an average of 10 percent of your cholesterol reading, which would improve your chances of dodging heart disease by 20 percent.

Even if your cholesterol count is already at a stratospheric level, that's no reason to be discouraged. In fact, the higher your cholesterol count, the greater impact a heart-healthy diet can have, says Margo Denke, M.D., assistant professor of medicine at the University of Texas Southwestern Medical Center at Dallas's Center for Human Nutrition and a member of the nutrition committee of the American Heart Association. For example, someone with a cholesterol reading of 280 may be able to steamroll 25 percent off the top by eating right. Not bad! If you want to keep your ticker pumping right, that's a bottom line you can't afford to ignore.

Here are some cholesterol busters that can help keep a normal cholesterol level where it is or deliver a knockout punch to a bloated cholesterol count.

Watch the fat. "Decreasing saturated fat is the most effective anticholesterol strategy you can use," says Karen Miller-Kovach, R.D., chief nutritionist at Weight Watchers International in Jericho, New York. That is, eat less of the kind of fat you find in red meat, butter, cheese, whole milk and ice cream. Saturated fat raises LDL and total cholesterol levels. Conversely, eating monounsaturated fat—the good fat—helps decrease cholesterol.

"When you switch from a diet high in saturated fat to one high in monounsaturated fat, and your weight stays about the same, your LDL cholesterol will fall while the HDL cholesterol remains stable," says Robert Rosenson, M.D., director of the Preventive Cardiology Center at Rush-Presbyterian–St. Luke's Medical Center in Chicago. "That's why olive oil is so popular, since it's high in monounsaturates." Better yet, find a way to get more fatty fish, such as salmon and tuna, into your diet. They are brimming with monounsaturates.

Eat less cholesterol. As important as reducing saturated fat can be, don't forget about dietary cholesterol. The cholesterol in your blood that isn't produced by your own body comes from your diet. Here's how to keep it under control.

Try to eliminate organ meats (such as liver) from your diet. Limit the amount of lean meat, poultry and fish to three ounces per day. And when it comes to eggs, limit your consumption of yolks to no more than two a week. Avoid commercial cakes, cookies and pies; instead, make your own using egg whites or egg substitute.

Finally, when you're going through the buffet line, reach with gusto for vegetables, fruits and grains, which contain absolutely no dietary cholesterol. But show some willpower in holding out against high-fat salad dressings, sauces and butter.

Feed on fiber. As foods high in fat and cholesterol make a quick exodus from your diet, fill the void with foods high in soluble fiber, including dried beans, citrus fruits, peas, apples and lentils. Adding soluble fiber to your diet could help reduce your blood cholesterol by another 5 to 10 percent.

Feel your oats. Oat bran has been on a roll for years. But how much is

Playing the Cholesterol Numbers Game

Once you've passed your 20th birthday, doctors recommend that you celebrate with a cholesterol test. As the years go by, you should get one at least every five years.

One of the readings that this test will produce is your total blood cholesterol level. Here's a look at what that number means (all numbers refer to milligrams per deciliter of blood).

Less than 200—desirable
200 to 239—borderline high
240 and above—high

Even if your total cholesterol count earns a blue ribbon, you still need to have it measured regularly, along with a check of your HDL (high-density lipoprotein) cholesterol, the good kind. Sometimes a high HDL level will help compensate for a total cholesterol number in the "borderline high" range (although you're still well advised to get your total cholesterol as low as possible). If your HDL reading is less than 35, it falls into the "low" category, and you need to work at raising it. (Your best options are losing weight, exercising more, quitting smoking and cutting back on how much sugar you eat.)

And what about LDL (low-density lipoprotein) cholesterol, the bad kind? If your other tests reveal potential trouble, your doctor should use the data from your cholesterol test to calculate your LDL level, too. Below 130 is considered desirable.

Finally, to help interpret what all these numbers mean, your doctor may determine your cholesterol ratio, which is the ratio between your total cholesterol and your HDL number. If this ratio is 3.5 to 1 or lower, you are doing just fine.

hype, and how much holds water? Researchers at the University of Minnesota in Minneapolis reviewed all the studies examining the power of oats and reached an artery-cleansing conclusion: Add 1⅓ cups of oat bran cereal (or three packets of instant oatmeal) to your daily diet, and watch your cholesterol level dip by 2 to 3 percent. If your cholesterol level is already high, you'll reap even more benefits, with oat bran skimming 6 to 7 percent off the top.

Shape up. You don't need to compete in a triathlon for the good of your cholesterol. About 20 minutes of exercise, three times a week, should be your goal. "We've learned that even moderate aerobic exercise (brisk walking, jogging, swimming) raises HDLs, although this often takes six months to a year to occur," says Dr. Rosenson.

Control your girth. If the spare tire around your midsection seems to be overinflating, there are more than cosmetic reasons to chip away at that unattractive gut. In ever-widening research on ever-widening waistlines, Dr. Denke has found that excess body weight can boost total cholesterol in men while suppressing HDL cholesterol. As your love handles shrink, however, you'll get a handle on your cholesterol again, and your HDLs will tend to rise, too.

Bag the cigarettes. There are a lot of good reasons to quit smoking, and here's one more: Smoking can lower your HDL reading, something no health-conscious person can afford to do.

But even if you're a chain-smoker, there's some encouraging news—if you're willing to toss out your cigarettes for good. By stopping smoking, says Dr. Rosenson, you can reverse the decline in your HDL level in about 60 days. It doesn't take years to eliminate smoking's dirty work.

Toast to moderation. It's almost too good to be true: A drink or two of any alcoholic beverage each day can raise the HDL component of your cholesterol count. Even so, don't go to extremes toasting this newfound knowledge quite yet, since there's too much of a downside to drinking excessively. And besides, alcoholic drinks are brimming with calories, so they can defeat your efforts at losing weight.

Another option? Drink grape juice—the purple kind. Grape skin contains a cholesterol-lowering ingredient, according to Leroy Creasy, Ph.D., professor of pomology at Cornell University College of Agriculture and Life Sciences in Ithaca, New York.

How Magical Is Medicine?

For some people, even heroic efforts at lowering high cholesterol run aground. They may need help from anticholesterol medications, which can cut cholesterol readings by an average of 20 percent. Before you take these medications, however, most experts advise you to try a more conservative approach (diet, exercise, weight loss) for about six months. If that doesn't work, drugs may be the answer, particularly if your LDL cholesterol is still high, you have other risk factors for heart disease (such as family history or high blood pressure) or you already have heart disease.

Nicotinic acid and bile acid binders may be your doctor's first medication choices.

Nicotinic acid (such as Niacor) is one form of niacin, the vitamin that can be purchased without a prescription. But since you need to take nicotinic acid in high doses for it to make a difference in your cholesterol reading, doctors consider it a drug. So should you. High doses can cause serious side effects. Make sure that you take only the prescription form of the drug, and relay any problems to your doctor.

"Flushing and stomach upset can occur with niacin," cautions Richard Helfant, M.D., vice chairman of medicine and director of the Cardiology Training Program at the University of California, Irvine, Medical Center. He suggests avoiding niacin completely if you have diabetes, ulcers, liver disease or major heart rhythm problems.

Other medications have potential side effects, too, so your doctor should monitor you closely when you're taking them. Some of these prescription drugs, including the bile acid binders cholestyramine (such as Questran) and colestipol hydrochloride (Colestid), are available in powder form. Most others, including lovastatin (Mevacor) and gemfibrozil (Lopid), come as pills. Some of these drugs—nicotinic acid and bile acid binders—have been around long enough for research to show that they not only can bring your LDL cholesterol level to its knees but also can decrease your chances of developing heart disease.

Incidentally, even if your doctor prescribes medication, don't think that you're off the hook, Dr. Denke cautions. "Drugs aren't a substitute for healthier eating, losing weight, exercising and other lifestyle strategies that need to be part of getting your cholesterol under control."

Dental Problems

Keep Your Teeth Forever

They've carried you through the steaks, pretzels and caramels of life. In your young and stupid days, they may even have pried open a bottle or two. Surely, your teeth now deserve some care. That's particularly true if you don't want people soon calling you Pops.

Few things age a man faster than neglected teeth. When you were young, a little neglect might have led to an occasional filling. But as you age, neglected decay can set you up for a host of dental problems, such as periodontal disease. And if not arrested promptly, long-term neglect can eventually cause you to lose teeth entirely.

As you age, your teeth may start to show telltale signs of years of indulgence. Coffee, tobacco, red wine and food dyes can all work their way deep into microscopic cracks in the tooth enamel, resulting in brown or yellowish stains.

But what if you've always shown your dental hygienist scrupulously clean teeth? Sorry, but even if you're dedicated about dental care, age still changes your teeth. Years of chewing wears down tooth surfaces and actually shortens your teeth. Gums recede with age and wear. And even careful brushing has its downside if you've used the wrong technique for decades. Hard scrubbing wears down the translucent enamel coating of your teeth so that the yellowish material underneath, called dentin, begins to show through. Many otherwise natty men as young as age 40 are dismayed by their dingy teeth.

Know Your Enemy

When you were an adolescent, cavities were your main dental concern (and fear). But these days, your dentist will tell you that the greatest enemy to your mouth is not cavities but gum disease.

There's a little moat around each tooth that forms a tiny crevice between tooth and gum. When bacteria get in and linger, they cause inflammation, which eventually deepens the crevices into pockets. As the inflammation simmers, bone, gum and connective tissue may get eaten away, leaving you with less foundation to hold your teeth in place. All that simmering can also cause bad breath, soreness and bleeding.

The other enemy is cavities (yes, they still count). Cavities start when a sticky film called plaque builds up on your teeth, trapping bacteria and breeding decay. Even though you may not have gotten many new cavities in your first years of adulthood, hang on to that toothbrush. Many men heading into middle age start to get cavities along with gum disease. That's because as gums recede with age, the root (which has no protective enamel) is exposed to decay.

Your Daily Plan for a Perfect Mouth

One option you always have as you get older is to get wiser. If you update your cleaning methods and keep an educated eye on what goes in your mouth, you can flash that killer grin forever.

Swab the deck. Brushing is your number one defense against dental problems. "At a very minimum, be sure to brush after breakfast and before you go to bed at night," says Hazel Harper, D.D.S., associate professor of community dentistry at Howard University in Washington, D.C., and vice president of the National Dental Association. Of course, it's best to brush after every meal.

Brushing, done correctly, removes the bacteria and plaque responsible for so many dental woes. But you should forget the "berserk chain saw" approach. Correct brushing, says Dr. Harper, means holding the brush with the handle in your palm and your thumb extended to act as a brace. This palm-thumb grasp tilts the brush at an angle, so bristles reach the gums and just underneath the gums as well as the tooth surfaces. Gently vibrate the brush in a small back-and-forth motion, covering only three teeth at a time. Then with a flick of the wrist, roll the brush against the sides of your teeth to sweep debris and bacteria away from the gum line. Finish up by brushing your tongue—your best antidote to bad breath, Dr. Harper says.

Use the right brush. Get rid of that hard-tufted, frayed thing in the toothbrush holder, says Dr. Harper. You need to use a soft-bristle toothbrush, and you should replace it every three months—sooner if the bristles start to fray, she says.

Pick your paste. Any toothpaste with the American Dental Association's seal of approval will do the job with a minimal amount of abrasion. If you tend to build up tartar, try a tartar control toothpaste. Tartar, or hardened plaque, feels like a rough coating on your teeth, says Richard Price, D.D.S., clinical instructor of dentistry at Boston University's Henry Goldman School of Dentistry. "These pastes reduce the amount of tartar you get, and the tartar that does build up will be softened and easier to remove," he says.

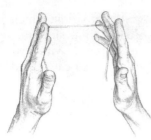 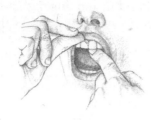 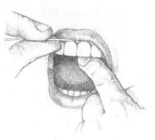

Break off about 18 inches of floss and wind most of it around one middle finger. Wind the rest around the middle finger of your other hand.

Using your thumbs and forefingers, slide about an inch of taut floss between your teeth. Gently curve the floss in a C shape around the tooth at the gum line.

Gently slide the floss up and down between the tooth and gum, making sure you go beneath the gum line. Repeat on the rest of your teeth with clean sections of floss.

Don't skip flossing. Floss daily to be sure of complete cleaning and healthy gums, says Dr. Price. Toothbrush bristles simply can't get into the crannies around teeth. It makes no difference what type of floss you use—waxed, unwaxed or flavored; just pick one that feels most comfortable to you, he says.

If big or stiff fingers or a dexterity problem makes the process unwieldy, try flossing one-handed. Wrap floss around the thumb and index finger of one hand, like you're forming a little slingshot, Dr. Price says. Or ask your dentist about flossing devices.

Know what's sticky. The foods that cling to your teeth are the foods that decay them, experts say. But it's hard to be sure which edibles in the following pairs are stickier: caramels or crackers? Hot-fudge sundaes or bread? Dried figs or puffed-oat cereal? Believe it or not, crackers, bread and cereal are the most likely to cling for long periods. Your best defense is to brush after every single snack, sugary or not. But if you can't get to a toothbrush soon, it's best to avoid the stickier foods.

Say cheese for dessert. It's an old custom in some cultures to serve cheese for dessert, and it might help cut cavities when you can't brush your teeth right after a meal. A few studies indicate that certain cheeses, particularly hard, aged ones such as Cheddar and Monterey Jack, may reduce cavity-causing bacteria. Just a small slice will do the job—and not add much fat or cholesterol to your diet.

Swish, swish. Regardless of what you've just eaten, if you can't brush right away, the next best thing is to find a sink and swish a mouthful of water around your teeth, says Andrew M. Lewis, D.D.S., a dentist in private practice in Beverly Hills. Swishing will remove most debris and also dilute the acids formed by food particles.

Facts about Fillings

"Whoaaaa, hold on there," you say to the dentist as he bears down on you with a mean-looking drill. "Whaddya mean I have cavities? I'm too old for that."

Sorry, buddy, but you're never too old for cavities.

Lots of men, middle-aged and beyond, get cavities, says Richard Price, D.D.S., clinical instructor of dentistry at Boston University's Henry Goldman School of Dentistry. One reason is that old fillings wear out. Although some may hang in there for decades, the average life span of silver fillings is about nine years. Beyond that, they tend to chip, crack and wear out.

"They're just replacement parts," says Dr. Price. "Any time you get a tooth drilled and filled, it will need to be drilled and filled for the rest of your life. It's like your warranty wearing out."

Sometimes adult men, even champion brushers and flossers, may acquire new cavities as well. The most common spot for these black holes is at the base of the teeth, where gums receding with age have exposed the sensitive roots to decay, says Dr. Price.

If you do need a filling—either a replacement or a new one—get ready to choose from a number of alternative materials.

Silver is by far the most common of the lot, because it's durable and affordable. The silver is mixed with mercury, which makes it easy to mold. The question has arisen from time to time whether this mercury, a poisonous metal, could leach into the body. Some men have even had perfectly good fillings removed because of the mercury scare.

That's a shame.

Yes, some mercury is released from silver fillings when you chew, but only minuscule amounts. Even less is absorbed by your body. "Nothing to worry about," says Joel M. Boriskin, D.D.S., chief of the Division of Dentistry at Alameda County Medical Center in Oakland, California. A number of studies measured the release of mercury from silver fillings and came to the same conclusion: There's no reason to be concerned unless your mouth is big enough (and rotten enough) to hold 1,000 fillings.

But just because silver is safe, that doesn't mean it's always the best. Gold, though expensive, is super strong and especially good for monster-size cavities. Fillings made from porcelain, quartz or acrylic, though not as durable as the metals, may be preferable for more visible fillings. They can be colored to match your own teeth.

Knockout Knowledge

Bam! If a tooth gets knocked out, all you need to know are two don'ts and two do's, says Andrew M. Lewis, D.D.S., a dentist in private practice in Beverly Hills. First, find the tooth. Then:

- Don't try to rinse or clean the tooth in any way.
- Don't try to put the tooth back in your mouth.
- Do put the tooth in cold milk if there's any handy.
- Do get yourself (and your milk-chilled tooth) to an emergency room or dentist's office pronto.

Follow these steps, and with luck, your tooth can be reimplanted successfully, Dr. Lewis says.

Heavy-Duty Home Care

If your dentist has noticed new cavities or early signs of gum disease, you needn't sit back in your rocker and let your teeth erode. There's a lot you can do to turn the tide at any age. Try these home treatments, with your dentist's guidance.

Sleep with some fluoride. "If you're prone to cavities, use an over-the-counter fluoride rinse every night," says Dr. Lewis. "You want to rinse and spit it out so that it's the last thing in your mouth just before you go to sleep." Fluoride actually remineralizes teeth, making them stronger and less prone to cavities and root sensitivity.

Plug in your toothbrush. Try an electric toothbrush if you have trouble brushing thoroughly by hand or you have gum problems, says Dr. Harper. The gentle vibration of the brush head massages gums as it cleans the teeth, she says. And research from the University of Alabama School of Dentistry in Birmingham has proven that electric toothbrushes are particularly effective against gingivitis.

Before you scout one out, check with your dentist. Many professionals recommend the newer breed of electric toothbrush, with bristles that rotate rather than vibrate. There are several brands for sale, including Interplak and the Braun Oral-B Plaque Remover.

Try an irrigator. An oral irrigator such as the Water Pik can help clean debris from between teeth and under gums, but use it cautiously, Dr. Harper says. "Sometimes irrigators aren't adjusted right, and the flow of water is strong enough to damage gum tissue," she says. Slow the flow if your gums feel sore or irritated after using your irrigator.

Help from the Pros

No amount of sink-side ambition can substitute for regular dental checkups, Dr. Harper says. To keep your teeth looking younger, see a dental hygienist twice a year for cleaning and your dentist at least once a year for an exam.

Your first stop is at the hygienist's chair for a professional cleaning to remove plaque and tartar, says Dr. Lewis. Once your teeth are clean as a whistle,

Facing the Fear

If you'd rather face an audit than go to the dentist, you are not alone. Wild fears about dentistry abound, even in men of otherwise great courage, says Mark Slovin, D.D.S., director of the Dental Phobia Clinic at the State University of New York at Stony Brook. Most of these fears are unfounded, he adds. Modern dentistry, while not always entirely painless, is no reason for panic. If you do panic, here's how to calm yourself.

Open up before you open wide. If you're afraid of the drill, own up. "A good dentist is able to understand the feelings and thoughts of a patient," says Arthur A. Weiner, D.M.D., associate clinical professor at Tufts University School of Dental Medicine in Boston. Don't hesitate to shop around for a dentist you're comfortable with.

Ask for a demo. Ask your dentist to explain unfamiliar procedures step-by-step and to demonstrate how he'll use the instruments. Ask what kind of sensations to expect while the work is being done.

Set up your signals. Ask your dentist to alert you to any upcoming pinching or pressure, so you can relax in the meantime, Dr. Weiner says. And agree on hand signals that will tell him when you want to sit up for a minute, pause or rinse.

Use relaxation techniques. Try deep breathing, concentrating on a pleasant image such as a day at the beach or listening to your favorite tunes on a headset to soothe your stay in the chair, says Dr. Slovin.

Ask for more pain relief. If you need extra anesthesia, go ahead and ask. Sedatives aren't a permanent solution, but they can get you through a procedure you need.

Seek professional help. If your fear is overwhelming, call your state dental society for help in finding a dental phobia clinic close to you. Or ask your dentist to recommend a psychological counselor who is familiar with dental phobias.

your dentist will examine your mouth. If cavities are cropping up more than they used to, he may apply a fluoride solution and prescribe a fluoride rinse or gel for you to use at home. But first, he'll fill any cavities.

And quicker than you might expect. With new, faster drills, your dentist can usually fill a cavity in about 15 minutes, a procedure that would have taken an hour 20 years ago, Dr. Harper says. What about pain? If reruns of the dental torture scene in *Marathon Man* are running through your head, don't worry—you won't need to outrun anything that awful. Modern dental procedures are light-years ahead of your worst dental memory.

On rare occasions, you may need a root canal to remove the pulp or nerve of a rotted tooth and fill the hole. Despite its painful reputation, a root canal done right can be no more uncomfortable than any other dental procedure, says Dr. Lewis.

For advancing gum disease, your dentist will refer you to a periodontist, or gum disease specialist. Treatment may involve oral antibiotics, antibacterial ointments squeezed into the gum pockets or, in severe cases, surgical removal of part of the infected gum or diseased bone.

And if stains or crooked teeth are your greatest dental problem, a cosmetic dentist can bring back that hungry-tiger gleam. Bleaching can whiten stains, and a variety of restorations can straighten a gapped or crooked grin. (For details, see Cosmetic Dentistry on page 404.)

DEPRESSION

The Sneaky Stealer of Spirit

All of us get the blues at one time or another. They could be triggered by anything from the death of your dog to knowing your softball team has a losing streak longer than Charlie Brown's. These gloomy feelings usually fade within short order, and you bounce back to your cheerful self. No big deal.

But if you're in a funk day after day—particularly if you can't put a handle on why—that's a big deal. Depression can sap your energy, crumple your posture, add wrinkles to your face and do a lot of other things that we associate with aging.

"Unquestionably, depression can make you look and feel older," says Harry Prosen, M.D., chairman of the Department of Psychiatry and Mental Health Sciences at the Medical College of Wisconsin in Milwaukee. "Some chronically depressed people can look very old and have stooped shoulders, furrowed lines around the eyes and all the other things that make a person looked aged. I've seen some depressed people who look like they're in their sixties when they're actually 35 or 40."

Yet relieving the strain of depression may be all you need to make yourself look years younger. "It's amazing how quickly the signs of aging can lift once the depression lifts," Dr. Prosen says.

A Heavy Toll

Depression can have an adverse effect on almost every part of the body. Let's start at that important spot below the belt. "It's well known that depression can suppress your libido, diminish sexual performance or cause impotence," Dr. Prosen says. "When you're depressed, the entire physiology of the body slows down. Swallowing, digestion, everything slows down or diminishes, and that includes sexual desire and arousal."

If that isn't enough to get your attention, consider that depression can make your immune system less vigilant, says Michael Irwin, M.D., associate professor of psychiatry at the University of California, San Diego, School of Medicine. In a study of depressed men in their early forties, Dr. Irwin found their natural killer cell activity had fallen to levels that you might normally find in men in their seventies. Reduced killer cell activity makes you more susceptible to infections, says Dr. Irwin.

Depression can also magnify the risk of developing atherosclerosis, a buildup of fatty plaque deposits on artery walls that contributes to coronary heart disease, says George Kaplan, Ph.D., an epidemiologist and chief of the Human Population Laboratory of the California Department of Health Services in Berkeley. In a study of Finnish men ages 42 to 60, Dr. Kaplan found that depressed men who had high levels of LDL (low-density lipoprotein) cholesterol—the bad kind—in their blood had twice as much plaque in their arteries as men who were not depressed.

Rheumatoid arthritis is yet another disease that can be aggravated or even triggered by depression, says Sanford Roth, M.D., a rheumatologist and medical director of the Arthritis Center in Phoenix. "It's not unusual for a person who suffers a devastating loss of a parent or spouse to develop a disease like rheuma-

Is It All in the Family?

You're not the only one who gets depressed. Grandpa, Pop, Uncle Leroy and your sister Vicki all regularly tumble into a funk that they can't seem to shake. What's going on here?

Men with family histories of depression are two to three times more likely to suffer recurrent bouts of depression than men who don't have family histories of depression, says Janice Peterson, M.D., a clinical psychiatrist at the University of Colorado Health Sciences Center in Denver. "There is well-documented evidence that like cancer, diabetes and high blood pressure, major depression has a genetic component," says Alan Mellow, M.D., Ph.D., assistant professor of psychiatry at the University of Michigan Medical School in Ann Arbor.

Okay, so you can't choose your parents. But knowing that your family has a history of depression should help you understand why you may feel on the downside more often than other people, Dr. Mellow says. So if you do feel despondent, especially if you have a family history of major depression, you should seek treatment, since you may be prone to more serious bouts of depression than other people.

toid arthritis," Dr. Roth says. "Because rheumatoid arthritis may have genetic roots, these people probably had the potential to develop the disease all along. It just took a depression to open it up."

Who Says We're Depressed?

Unfortunately, most men face a giant obstacle that prevents them from effectively fighting off this insidious agent. They think it isn't manly to admit they're depressed.

"Most guys have been taught that it's a sign of weakness to ask for help or to talk about their feelings, so they'll just try to tough it out when they're feeling depressed," says Dennis Gersten, M.D., a psychiatrist in private practice in San Diego.

And exactly how do guys tough it out? "Some men get angry and take out their frustrations on their families and others," says Bryan Cohen, psychotherapist and founding director of ManTalk, a counseling and resource center for men in Philadelphia. "But most men don't lash out. They feel a lot of shame and powerlessness about being depressed and take it out on themselves more than on other people. These men are prone to self-destructive behaviors such as alcohol and drug abuse."

Climbing out of the Hole

Obviously, guys who deal with depression by soaking their brains in beer aren't doing themselves any favors. There are much better, and much more effective, means for dealing with depression.

"It's been said that where there is depression, there is hope," says Dan Blazer, M.D., Ph.D., professor of psychiatry at Duke University Medical Center in Durham, North Carolina. "Depression is something that can be cured. You definitely don't have to just live with it."

Here are a few suggestions that can help lift you out of your black hole. If these don't help, it's a sign that you have a major depression. If that's the case, you should seek professional help.

Keep a goal in sight. "People who have dreams and visions of accomplishment are less likely to be depressed than those who don't have goals," Dr. Gersten says. Write down a list of goals that you want to achieve. Divide the list into sections that include things you want to do this week, this month, within a year and within five years. Put the list in a prominent place, such as on your refrigerator, and check off the goals as you achieve them. Try to update your list at least once a month.

Be a busy buckaroo. If you can keep yourself busy doing things such as yard work, racquetball or other activities, it will prevent you from dwelling on whatever is making you feel unhappy, says Linda George, Ph.D., professor of medical sociology at Duke University Medical Center.

When to Get Help

During his lifetime, a man has a 3 to 6 percent chance of having a major depression. Here's a list of symptoms, according to the American Psychiatric Association, that may help you determine the severity of a depression. If you have five or more of these symptoms in a two-week span, or if you have felt depressed for more than two weeks, you should seek the help of your doctor or a qualified therapist.

- You feel sad most of the day and have lost interest in pleasurable activities, including sex.
- You feel tired or lack energy to do day-to-day chores.
- You feel restless and can't sit still.
- You either have insomnia or oversleep.
- You have difficulty concentrating or making decisions.
- You have fluctuations in your appetite or weight.
- You feel hopeless, worthless and guilty.
- You think about death and suicide.

Exercise your funny bone. Humor is your best ally, Dr. Prosen says. Clip cartoons and funny articles out of newspapers and magazines and put them in a file you can flip through when you feel low.

Let the tears flow. Forget that old notion that big boys don't cry. Crying may be just the emotional release you need to snap out of your glum mood, says Kimberly Yonkers, M.D., assistant professor of psychiatry at the University of Texas Southwestern Medical Center at Dallas.

Lean on your pals. Friends and relatives have helped you survive hangovers, joked with you at weekend barbecues and shared the thrill of countless softball games. Now they can help you through this bleak time if you let them. "That doesn't mean you're asking them to solve your problems for you," Dr. George says. "It just means you're asking them to listen, let you get things off your chest and be supportive."

Put your negative thoughts on paper. Writing down your feelings when you're depressed can help you recognize faulty thought patterns and help you find ways to replace those thoughts with more uplifting ones, says Janice Peterson, M.D., a clinical psychiatrist at the University of Colorado Health Sciences Center in Denver. So for every negative thought you write down, such as "I'm the worst person in the world," also write down a positive one, such as "I have imperfections, but I also have a lot going for me." After a while, the positive thoughts might replace the negative ones in your mind.

Sweat it out. "Exercise is a fabulous way to relieve depression," Dr. Gersten says. "Aerobic exercise such as walking, running, swimming or bicycling chemically affects your brain in ways that can often reverse the effects of even a major depression." You don't have to run a marathon or bench-press 300 pounds to get a positive effect, either. Just 20 minutes a day of aerobic exercise, three times a week, may be all you need to fend off the blues.

Be a good actor. No, you don't have to bounce around like Bozo the Clown, but one great way to short-circuit depression is to act like a happy person for an hour, Dr Yonkers says. Then try it for another hour and so on. By the end of the day, you might be surprised to find you're not faking it anymore.

Get a load of carbos. Try eating at least one meal a day that is very high in complex carbohydrates, with little protein. Complex carbohydrates, such as those available in pasta and potatoes, may boost serotonin levels in your brain, says Judith Wurtman, Ph.D., a research scientist at the Massachusetts Institute of Technology in Cambridge and author of *Managing Your Mind with Mood and Food*. Serotonin is a brain chemical that keeps your moods stable.

Go easy on the booze. Although it may be tempting to drown your sorrows in a pitcher of beer, try not to overindulge, because alcohol is actually a depressant drug that can drag you further into the dumps. "Excessive drinking will also disrupt your sleep and may drive your friends and family away from you just when you need their support the most," Dr. Yonkers says.

See the light. Seasonal affective disorder can cause the symptoms of depression—all because of too little sunlight in the fall and winter, says Dan Oren, M.D., a senior clinical investigator with the National Institute of Mental Health in Rockville, Maryland. Try taking early morning walks, or ask your doctor if light therapy would help you.

Look in your medicine cabinet. Almost every drug has side effects, and one of those side effects can be depression. Ask your doctor if changing or adjusting your medications would help, Dr. Yonkers advises.

DIABETES

Arresting a Potential Killer

At this moment, more than three million men have no idea that they're about to become victims of a disease that can claim their sight, their manhood, their very lives—a disease that takes more than 160,000 lives a year, about half that number men. Yet many men shrug off any concerns about diabetes because its symptoms can go unnoticed. Besides, some guys still think it results from eating too much candy.

But it has nothing to do with extra helpings of sweets. Diabetes is the diagnosis when the body doesn't produce enough or properly use insulin, a hormone secreted by the pancreas that's needed to convert food into energy. The "sugar link" stems from the fact that much of what we eat for energy is broken down into a sugar called glucose, the fuel that's fed into every single cell to keep us alive. And people with diabetes must limit their sugar intakes because sweets can make blood sugar rise dramatically.

In healthy people, glucose is automatically absorbed by cells. The body uses exactly what it needs and stores the rest. But without insulin to unlock a cell's receptors so that glucose can enter, excess amounts of this sugar accumulate in the bloodstream, where it can cause a host of problems that age men before their time.

Nearly seven million guys have diabetes—and half of them are unaware of it. Most guys get diabetes, which is the fourth leading cause of death by disease in the United States, between the ages of 45 and 66. Yet even then, they face health risks normally associated with men much older: Men with diabetes face five times the risk of stroke and two to four times the risk of heart disease compared with men who don't have the disease. One in ten diabetes sufferers develops kidney disease, and between 15,000 and 39,000 a year lose their sight because of the disease.

"Any time you change the chemistry of the blood, you're going to change virtually every system affected by the blood," says Steve Manley, Ph.D., a psychologist in Denton, Texas, and staff psychologist at the Male Health Center in Dallas. "And that would be all of them."

Including your sexual organs. Diabetes can debilitate both the neurological system and the vascular system, and you need good nerves and blood flow to function sexually. The result: "Many men become impotent because of diabetes," says Dr. Manley. "I see men in their twenties who are sexually dysfunctional because of diabetes, since the disease can strike at any age. The effect is crisis."

The Brain Drain

For many guys, the aging isn't just in their bodies. "When your blood sugar is out of control, it has an effect on your cognitive function," says Patricia Stenger, R.N., a diabetes counselor and senior vice president for the American Diabetes Association. "You may have slower response time, and you feel sluggish and fatigued."

Adds Dr. Manley: "In effect, diabetes kicks you into a grief reaction, because you have lost something. Some people feel helpless and hopeless that their bodies somehow revolted against them. Some feel that they are no longer in control of their own destinies. They may lose belief, at least temporarily, that they are going to be okay at some point in the future. The disease begins to interact with their basic personalities."

Even eating presents its challenge. Diabetes sufferers must adhere to strict diets, in both what and when they eat. "Maybe they can have an infrequent piece of cake, on a child's birthday or an anniversary, but that's it," says Audrey Lally, R.D., a certified diabetes educator and nutrition specialist at the Mayo Clinic in Scottsdale, Arizona. "But for the most part, I discourage my patients with diabetes from ever using anything that contains large amounts of pure sugar."

And this regimen goes beyond the kitchen. No longer can guys with diabetes casually stroll barefoot on a summer's day. Because of nerve damage that could result in a loss of sensation in their legs and feet, they may be unaware of foot injuries. According to the American Diabetes Association, over 54,000 people with diabetes lose their feet or legs to amputation each year because of the disease.

Subtle Trouble

There are two types of diabetes. With Type I diabetes, which accounts for only 10 percent of cases, the body completely fails to produce insulin, so daily injections of this hormone are needed. Type I, often referred to as juvenile diabetes, is usually diagnosed during puberty, and the symptoms, which can mimic the flu, are sudden and very noticeable: extreme hunger and thirst, sudden weight loss and extreme fatigue and irritability.

In the more common Type II (or adult-onset) diabetes, the pancreas produces insulin, but not enough. There may be some symptoms—slow-healing cuts or bruises, recurring skin, gum or bladder infections or slight tingling or numbness in the hands or feet—but many guys don't really notice these subtle changes or simply shrug them off.

"Diabetes is a subtle disease that just creeps up on people—and the results can be devastating," says Xavier Pi-Sunyer, M.D., professor of medicine at Columbia University in New York City and past president of the American Diabetes Association. That's why it's important to get a blood screening for elevated glucose levels, especially if you have a family history of the disease, are overweight, are over age 40 or have any symptoms. "People may be unaware that they have the disease because they feel fine," adds Stenger.

Beating the Odds

"The best way to avoid diabetes is to watch your weight," says Lally. "That means eating a healthy diet that focuses on fruits and vegetables. Being overweight is the major risk factor for adult-onset diabetes. This is important for everyone but is essential if you have a family history of diabetes."

Even if you're among the 650,000 people diagnosed this year—that's one every 60 seconds—a healthy lifestyle may be all that's needed to get the upper hand on diabetes. Although some people with Type II diabetes require oral drugs or injections to stabilize their blood sugar, most can control the disease simply by adopting healthier lifestyles. By committing yourself to certain lifestyle changes, you may be able to reduce your need for medication—and possibly get off and stay off diabetes drugs for the rest of your life, says James Barnard, Ph.D., professor of physiological science at the University of California, Los Angeles. Here's how.

Eat right. That means low-fat and high-fiber, with at least five servings of fruits and vegetables a day, says Lally. For each extra 40 grams of fat eaten per day—the amount found in one fast-food burger and a large order of fries—your risk of developing diabetes rises threefold, and if you already have diabetes, you face a greater chance of complications, according to a study in the *American Journal of Epidemiology*. The problem: Dietary fat readily converts to body fat, and body fat induces cells to resist insulin, explains Frank Q. Nuttall, M.D., Ph.D., chief of the Endocrine, Metabolic and Nutrition Section of the Minneapolis Veterans Administration Medical Center.

Meanwhile, try to consume at least 25 grams of fiber daily from complex-carbohydrate foods, which help put the brakes on glucose entering your bloodstream and also keep cholesterol low—important for guys with diabetes, who face higher risk of heart disease. That's between two and three times what most men eat. The best sources of complex carbohydrates are potatoes, whole-grain breads, rice, pastas, legumes, oats and barley.

Time it right. "If you have diabetes, you need to eat every four or five hours," says Lally. Small meals are best, since large meals make it tougher for your body to meet the increased demand for insulin. The key is to evenly distribute your food throughout the day, so no single meal overwhelms the pancreas.

Avoid sugar and salt. It's a given that you should avoid sugar; even in tiny amounts, it can send your blood sugar sky-high. Of course, low sugar and low salt are good dietary rules for everyone to follow, but those with diabetes must be especially careful. Instead, satisfy your sweet tooth with artificial sweeteners such as aspartame (NutraSweet). But also be on the lookout for low-sodium or reduced-sodium products. Salty foods can raise blood pressure, a danger for people with diabetes.

Get your heart pumping. Regular aerobic exercise not only helps you control your weight but also makes cells more receptive to insulin. "You need to get your heart going and keep it going for at least 20 minutes," says Stenger. "You don't need to do anything fancy; a brisk walk is fine."

Meanwhile, researchers at Harvard University in Cambridge, Massachusetts, found that exercise is an excellent way to help prevent Type II diabetes. In their Physicians' Health Study of 22,000 doctors, researchers noted that guys who exercised at least five times a week lowered their risk of developing diabetes by more than 40 percent.

However, people with diabetes need to exercise with care. "The main concern for exercise and diabetes is the risk of hypoglycemia, or low blood sugar," says Greg Dwyer, Ph.D., professor of physical education at Ball State University in Muncie, Indiana. To avoid this, he suggests, stick to a routine requiring the same amount of exercise at the same time daily.

Pump some iron, too. Weight lifting also plays a role in improving glucose tolerance, the body's ability to metabolize sugar properly, according to a study by researchers at the University of Maryland College Park and Johns Hopkins University in Baltimore. However, check with your doctor before starting a weight-lifting program. Resistance training may cause surges in blood pressure.

Take vitamins E and C. These two antioxidants tend to be in short supply among people with diabetes—and Italian researchers have found that vitamin E helps improve the action of insulin. Good food sources include wheat germ, corn oil and nuts, but you should take a supplement containing 400 IU each day.

Meanwhile, because people with diabetes are prone to vascular disease, they may need to increase their intakes of vitamin C, suggests Ishwarial Jialal, M.D., assistant professor of internal medicine and clinical nutrition at the University of Texas Southwestern Medical Center at Dallas. The Recommended Dietary Allowance is 60 milligrams a day, but Dr. Jialal suggests a minimum of 120 milligrams of vitamin C daily, the amount you'd find in a guava or a glass of orange juice.

Pretend you have a headache. Aspirin can reduce the risk of heart attack and stroke among those with diabetes by as much as 20 percent, according to research conducted by the National Institutes of Health in Bethesda, Maryland, on 3,711 people with both types of the disease. "People with diabetes are much more likely to have cardiovascular disease, so the aspirin recommendation is even more relevant for them," says Frederick Ferris, M.D., chief of the Clinical Trials Branch at the National Institutes of Health. Most researchers recommend a daily dosage of one-half of an adult aspirin or one children's aspirin, but check with your doctor first: Aspirin therapy isn't suggested for people taking blood thinners or suffering from ulcers.

Share your feelings. Learning that you have diabetes can be quite a blow, and many guys, believe it or not, actually find comfort in sharing their experiences with others going through the same thing.

Meeting regularly with a support group can help you cope with the disease, mentally and physically; it's also a good way to beat depression. Call your local chapter of the American Diabetes Association for a list of support groups in your area.

Put a lid on stress. Even if you're not worried about depression, studies by researchers at Duke University in Durham, North Carolina, show that when you're under stress, certain hormones are activated that pump stored glucose into your bloodstream. Conversely, stress management and taking time to relax improve glucose control. While group therapy is one way to relax, others include meditation and yoga.

DIETING

There's a Better Way

One of your strong points is determination, right? So when you decide to drop a few years by dropping a few pounds, you go at it with teeth clenched.

What kind of rejuvenating diet did you say you were starting? The Nothing but Grapefruit Diet? The Magical Mystery Food Diet? The Drink Water until You Explode Diet?

How about none of them?

Diets don't work. Sure, you might lose some weight at first. But eventually, when you're so hungry that you could gnaw the hide off a bear, you'll go off the diet with a vengeance. And you'll usually regain more weight than you lost, says John Foreyt, Ph.D., director of the Nutrition Research Clinic at Baylor College of Medicine in Houston.

And if you want to slow the aging process, you should know that the net gain of body fat resulting from this cycle of lose and gain does just the opposite, putting a tremendous strain on your body. You see it in your skin as wrinkles and sagging, says George Blackburn, M.D., Ph.D., associate professor of surgery at Harvard Medical School and chief of the Nutrition/Metabolism Laboratory at New England Deaconess Hospital, both in Boston. But what you don't see is the aging on the inside—organs and systems that get old before their time.

Eating Your Heart Out

A lifetime of dieting may take a toll on your heart. Research done by Kelly Brownell, Ph.D., a psychologist and obesity researcher at Yale University in New Haven, Connecticut, found that repeated dieting can set you up for heart disease. Dr. Brownell's studies showed that people with big weight fluctuations have a 75 percent greater risk of dying from heart disease than people whose weights stay relatively steady. "A lot of weight fluctuation is required to put you in this category—not five pounds now and then," says Dr. Brownell.

Yo-yo dieting may also cause high blood pressure and redistribute fat to areas of the body where it does more damage, such as from the butt to the gut. (People with lots of abdominal fat, for instance, are more likely to develop heart disease, say experts.)

Weight a Minute

Remember, diets don't work. What works is slow, gradual weight loss based on lifestyle changes such as low-fat eating and exercise. Here's what to avoid.

Diet Pills—Are They Magic Bullets?

If you've had it with dieting, maybe you'd rather just pop a pill and wait for the weight to vanish. Sorry, it's not that simple.

"Some antidepressants can help people who have serious weight problems that include binge eating caused by behavioral or psychiatric disorders," says David Schlundt, Ph.D., a clinical psychologist and assistant professor of psychology at Vanderbilt University in Nashville. "But be sure to combine them with some form of psychotherapy."

What about over-the-counter diet pills? Most experts don't recommend them. Their active ingredient, phenylpropanolamine hydrochloride (PPA), is an adrenaline-like stimulant. "For people who aren't that healthy in the first place—who have high blood pressure, heart disease, asthma or diabetes—PPA can cause real problems," says Dr. Schlundt. Even low doses can raise blood pressure and increase heart rate. And large doses can cause anxiety, sleeplessness, even convulsions. PPA also has the potential for abuse, Dr. Schlundt points out. It gives you a "high" similar to that of speed or amphetamines that can become addictive.

For the seriously overweight, there may be a promising "fat blocker" pill on the horizon, says John Foreyt, Ph.D., director of the Nutrition Research Clinic at Baylor College of Medicine in Houston. It's called orlistat (Xenical), and it's being tested in the United States and Europe. "Orlistat is not for someone who needs to lose five or ten pounds but for moderate to severe obesity," he says. The drug works by blocking fat absorption.

"But no pill is a magic bullet," Dr. Foreyt says. "Even with orlistat, you still have to follow a low-fat diet and a sensible exercise program."

Go slowly. "Don't fall prey to weight loss schemes that promise speed," says Dr. Blackburn. The biggest virtue for successful weight loss is patience, because the only way to lose weight is slowly. "One-half to one pound per week is best," he says.

Never say never. Deprivation doesn't work, but lifestyle changes can, says Janet Polivy, Ph.D., a psychologist at the University of Toronto Faculty of Medicine. A good eating plan—one that is geared toward health, not toward weight loss—doesn't forbid occasional indulgences in high-fat favorites, she says. "If you're told to never eat fried foods, you'll feel terrible when you have some—which is inevitable—and you'll give up good eating because you'll feel like a failure."

Forget about fad food diets. "This concept is hogwash," Dr. Blackburn says. "There are no magical foods that cancel other calories consumed, such as grapefruit."

Don't trust testimonials. "Testimonials are a major approach of bogus weight loss schemes," says Terrence Kuske, M.D., a nutritionist and professor of medicine at the Medical College of Georgia in Augusta. A typical testimonial might look like this: "I lost my entire beer belly in only three weeks with Diet Dynamite! Bob C., Las Vegas." Chances are good that Bob C. doesn't exist—or, if he does, that he's related to the guy who runs this diet scheme. Legitimate weight loss programs are backed up by scientific studies, not by a testimonial from someone named Bob or Tod.

DIGESTIVE PROBLEMS

Easing Those Gut Reactions

As a schoolboy, you could swallow earthworms without blinking—or Pepto-Bismol. In college, there wasn't a five-alarm chili or barbecue on campus that you couldn't extinguish. Even as a bachelor, your digestive tract didn't so much as wince when you dined on leftovers that looked more like something from a petri dish.

But these days, your once cast-iron stomach is showing some signs of rust. Gas. Heartburn. Bloating. Cramps. Diarrhea. Constipation. And what can be even more embarrassing than these conditions is what brings them on: innocents such as an ordinary glass of milk, a burger without the fixings, the wrong kind of vegetable, even—get this—a slice of wimpy plain cheese pizza.

"Just as it takes longer to recover from a cold or an injury as you grow older, the same happens to your digestive system. Things just kind of slow down, and the repair mechanisms aren't quite the same as they used to be," says William B. Ruderman, M.D., chairperson of the Department of Gastroenterology at the Cleveland Clinic Florida in Fort Lauderdale. "You can't tolerate certain foods or the effects of alcohol as well as you used to. It certainly makes you feel your own mortality."

These problems have another impact as well. All those belches, rumbles and other internal actions wear more than just your digestive tract. "You may be hesitant to take a bus or go outdoors in case you have to go to the bathroom. You may not go to certain restaurants because you can't eat certain foods," says Devendra Mehta, M.D., a gastroenterologist and assistant professor of pediatrics at Hahnemann University Hospital in Philadelphia. "This can be very distressing at any age. But when you are young and have these problems, it disrupts your life."

Just because your innards may be out of kilter, however, it doesn't mean they have to stay that way. Whatever the problem, here's how to fix it.

Constipation: Unplug Your System

If you haven't been bothered by constipation, give yourself a few years. "Constipation gets a lot more common as you age," says Jorge Herrera, M.D., associate professor of medicine at the University of South Alabama College of Medicine in Mobile. "For one thing, as they get older, most people tend to eat less and become less active." And many medicines that people tend to take as they age for conditions such as heart disease and diabetes also cause constipation, says Dr. Herrera.

At any age, however, constipation can make you feel older. Whether you have to strain to move your bowels or simply don't feel the urge, constipation occupies your mind with thoughts of what you can't do, and because of that, your body may not feel like doing much of anything. Most guys over age 30 can expect at least an occasional bout with constipation—and more as they get older. But here's how to keep problems to a minimum, no matter what your age.

Bulk up your diet. "If you're eating the typical Western diet with a lot of processed foods, that will lead to constipation," says Dr. Mehta. "But a diet with lots of roughage and fiber that centers on plenty of fresh fruits and vegetables is the most important thing you can do to treat or avoid constipation, especially as you get older."

Experts say you need at least five servings a day in order to get the recommended minimum of 25 grams of fiber—about twice what's actually consumed by the typical American. Besides fresh produce, good sources of dietary fiber include whole-grain breads and cereals, pastas, brown rice, beans and bran.

Move your body. Any type of exercise speeds up gastrointestinal transit time, the amount of time it takes food to get from your mouth through the stomach and intestines. But researchers at the University of Maryland College Park found that men who undergo strength-training programs can improve their bowel transit times by about 56 percent compared with their pre-pumping days. Experts believe the contractions of abdominal muscles done in weight lifting help "squeeze" the waste through the intestines more quickly. Researchers also believe that any type of exercise has an effect on motilin, a gastrointestinal hormone that's related to faster transit time. Exercise also improves blood flow to the intestines, which improves bowel movements.

Get heavy into H_2O. "One reason why constipation is more common as you age is that generally, the older people get, the less they drink," says Dr. Mehta. "And the less you drink, the harder and less frequent stools become." Even if you don't have a problem with constipation, you'll help keep yourself regular by drinking at least six glasses of water or other nonalcoholic beverages each day.

Meanwhile, try to limit your intake of coffee, tea and alcohol. While caffeinated beverages actually speed bowel transit time (alcohol has no effect), these beverages are diuretics that can leave you dehydrated, and you need fluids in your system to aid bowel movements. And those with frequent constipation should avoid milk, cheese and other dairy products, which contain casein, an insoluble protein that tends to plug up the intestinal tract.

Heartburn: Put Out the Fire

You probably already know how heartburn makes you feel: like a frail, helpless old coot who has fallen victim because of a sandwich or blue plate special. Nothing can take the wind out of your sails—not to mention your appetite—faster than having to rest after each meal until the pain subsides or having to monitor your every bite in order to avoid the pain in the first place.

Heartburn occurs when stomach acids, in a process called reflux, splash up into the esophagus, says Sheila Rodriguez, Ph.D., gastrointestinal laboratory director for the Oklahoma Foundation for Digestive Research in Oklahoma City. Eating too fast or too much is one common cause, but pigging out isn't the only reason for this all-too-common after-dinner ailment. Heartburn can also be the primary symptom of other conditions, such as gastritis, an inflammation in the lining of the stomach.

"It's not that the natural aging process contributes to heartburn per se, but the condition does seem to be more of a problem as you get older," says Dr. Mehta. "One reason is that there's a clear association between heartburn and being overweight—and most men tend to gain weight as they get older. But another, less obvious factor is the same bacteria—*Helicobacter pylori*—that can cause ulcers." Also, after we're age 40, our esophageal muscles start to weaken, which can contribute to reflux. But here's how to take the fire out of heartburn.

Take smaller portions. Many guys with heartburn problems find that grazing helps extinguish that internal blaze. If you eat four or five smaller meals instead of three massive squares a day, your stomach churns out less acid, says Frank Hamilton, M.D., director of the Gastrointestinal Diseases Program at the National Institutes of Health in Bethesda, Maryland.

Down it with water. Drinking lots of water—especially with meals—helps wash stomach acids from the surface of the esophagus back into your stomach, says Ronald L. Hoffman, M.D., a physician in New York City and author of *Seven Weeks to a Settled Stomach*.

Know the offenders. Certain foods are more likely than others to bring on the symptoms of heartburn. According to Dr. Rodriguez, onions, chocolate and mints relax the lower esophageal sphincter, which allows stomach acids to wash up. Citrus fruits such as oranges and grapefruit, as well as tomato products, coffee and fried or fatty foods, can also cause trouble because they can irritate the esophageal lining, adds Dr. Hamilton.

Sleep on a slope. If heartburn troubles you often, place wooden or concrete blocks under the headboard of your bed so that you sleep on an incline, advises William Lipshultz, M.D., chief of gastroenterology at Pennsylvania Hospital in Philadelphia. If you raise the head of your bed by six inches, gravity makes it harder for stomach acid to flow.

If you must lie flat, lying on your left side might produce less heartburn, says Leo Katz, M.D., a gastroenterologist at Jefferson Medical College of Thomas Jefferson University in Philadelphia. In tests, he found that people who ate the same heartburn-producing meal usually got more heartburn when they lay on their right sides compared with their left sides. "We think it has something to do with the anatomy of the stomach and gravity," he says.

Lactose Intolerance: Douse Dairy Woes

Dare to eat dairy? Perhaps not. As much as 70 percent of the world's population has some symptoms of lactose intolerance, meaning these people experience ill effects from milk, ice cream and other dairy products. Symptoms include bloating, gas, stomach cramping and diarrhea, which can curtail your activities and hamper your lifestyle. Besides making you feel older, the symptoms often get worse as you grow older.

By about age eight, most of us start losing an enzyme called lactase, which helps us digest lactose, the sugar that makes milk taste sweet. Without the lactase, much of the lactose passes along your digestive system undigested, possibly sending your colon into spasms and churning up gas. "By age 20, lactose-intolerant people pretty much lose the ability to digest milk," says Dr. Herrera.

Lactose intolerance varies from person to person. Some guys may feel minor discomfort after a lot of dairy, while others may get major problems from just a sip or two of milk. So checking your individual tolerance, and staying within that range, is the best way for you to avoid trouble. While there are plenty of lactose-free products—you'll find them in your supermarket's dairy case—here's how you can have your (real) dairy and eat it, too.

Be a cocoa nut. Some research suggests that cocoa slows stomach emptying, which reduces the rate at which lactose reaches the colon, says Dennis A. Savaiano, Ph.D., professor of food science and nutrition and associate dean at the University of Minnesota College of Human Ecology in St. Paul. So by drinking chocolate milk or having chocolate ice cream, you may lessen, if not avoid, symptoms. But if you're making your own chocolate milk, use low-fat milk and powdered cocoa, which has no fat; chocolate syrup is loaded with fat.

Combine dining with dairy. Some people find they can go symptom-free if they have their dairy products with meals. That's because having food in your stomach slows the release of lactose into your intestines, says Douglas B. McGill, M.D., professor of medicine at Mayo Medical School/Mayo Clinic in Rochester, Minnesota. Still, it's not advisable to load up on several dairy products at one meal.

Choose the right yogurt. Yogurt may be one milk product you can eat without worry. But don't assume that all yogurt products are the same. "Some commercial brands add milk products, which can cause you problems," says Dr. Mehta. "The best thing is to make your own yogurt." You can find yogurt-making machines at cooking supply stores.

If you're buying yogurt, make sure you choose a brand whose label says it contains live active cultures. "As soon as the yogurt cultures pass into the intestine, they become active and start to break down the lactose," says Dr. McGill. Sorry, but frozen yogurt won't help, since there are too few bacteria to be helpful.

Diverticular Disease: Spare Your Colon

It's fine to act refined at the dinner table, but when you eat that way, don't count on your colon to keep its good manners. After decades of living off refined and processed foods and other low-fiber fare and trying to pass the hard, dry stools they create, the colon walls weaken and often develop tiny pouches called diverticula. While this condition, called diverticulosis, won't cause any symptoms for many people, some people may develop gas, cramping, severe indigestion or even constipation or diarrhea.

Since diverticulosis is the result of years of neglecting the needs of your colon, it usually strikes men over age 40—but it can make you feel decades older. Some men change their diets to avoid foods such as popcorn, seeds and nuts, since these can get caught in the pouches and cause pain. Other men, hampered by abdominal pain, reduce their physical activities or make other lifestyle changes.

About 5 percent of cases develop into the worst-case scenario, when diverticula rupture and cause serious infection or when they bleed, which can result in a significant hemorrhage. However, most guys with diverticulosis can control the problem themselves and stay as young as they should feel. Here's how.

Go for fiber. Eat more vegetables, more fresh fruits, more whole grains. If you don't eat much fiber now, you should work up to it gradually. "Eating too much fiber too soon can make symptoms worse," says Alex Aslan, M.D., a gastroenterologist in private practice in Fairfield, California. Start by adding a few small servings of fiber-rich foods—fruits, vegetables, pastas, brown rice, beans, bran or whole-grain cereals and breads—to your diet, and gradually include more each day for about six weeks until you consume at least 25 grams of fiber daily.

If you can't eat that much fiber, consider taking an over-the-counter fiber concentrate (such as Metamucil).

Don't smoke. Besides being the single worst thing for your overall health, smoking is terrible for those with diverticulosis, says Stephen B. Hanauer, M.D., professor of medicine in the Section of Gastroenterology at the University of Chicago Medical Center. Smoking may increase movement in your intestines, but the nicotine decreases blood supply, which causes or increases cramps.

Work it out. Any type of exercise helps by increasing activity in your intestines, which improves bowel function, says Dr. Aslan. Shoot for at least 20 minutes of continuous exercise no less than three times a week.

Irritable Bowel Syndrome: Grab Control

Here's a disease that some experts say might be as widespread as the common cold—and that causes even more misery. Doctors aren't sure what specifically causes irritable bowel syndrome (IBS) or even how to treat it. But IBS—sometimes called a spastic colon—is the diagnosis for people who are regularly annoyed with constipation, diarrhea, bloating, nausea or abdominal cramps, either singly or in some combination and usually with abdominal pain.

The good news (if there is any) is that you will probably outgrow your problem. "IBS is more of a problem in those in their twenties to fifties," says Dr. Mehta. "But at any age, it has some significant aging effects." Many patients find themselves planning their lives around these symptoms, he says. "You don't know whether you'll suddenly need to rush to the bathroom, so you plan your day-to-day activities with this in mind."

But having an irritable bowel doesn't have to put you in that mind-set. While you should see a doctor if you suspect that you have IBS, there are plenty of things you can do to lessen its symptoms.

Control your sweet tooth. Limiting the amount of sugar you eat is a key to putting the bite on IBS-triggered diarrhea. That's because sugars—especially fructose and the artificial sweetener sorbitol—aren't easily digested, which can cause the runs, says Dr. Hanauer. These sweeteners are in most sugar-free or low-calorie candy and gums as well as store-bought fruit juices. So if you like juice, make your own with a juicer.

Chill out. Being under stress makes IBS symptoms worse, and conversely, not being stressed out can help, adds Dr. Hanauer. He suggests that men under the gun manage their stress with the help of relaxation therapy techniques such as meditation, self-hypnosis, biofeedback and regular exercise. You can also keep a "stress diary" to help you determine the source of your difficulties.

Or warm up. Abdominal cramps may be relieved with a heating pad placed directly on the painful area, says Arvey I. Rogers, M.D., chief of gastroenterology at the Veterans Administration Medical Center in Miami. Just be sure to place it on the low setting to prevent burning your skin.

Cramps from an irritable gut may not respond to heat. See a doctor if your symptoms are persistent.

Watch what you drink. Coffee and other caffeinated drinks can aggravate IBS by speeding up motility, the pace at which stools move through the bowels—bad news if you're prone to diarrhea. Besides that, there's a chemical in coffee that can cause cramping, says Dr. Aslan. Meanwhile, milk may not be much better, because some people with IBS also have lactose intolerance.

Feast on fiber. A high-fiber diet tends to quiet that kvetching colon. Fiber increases stool production and reduces intestinal pressure, which can benefit those with either constipation or diarrhea (or both), says Dr. Hanauer. Those with IBS are advised to work up to eating 35 to 50 grams of fiber a day. Start by adding about three tablespoons of pure bran to your cereal each morning and eating at least four servings of fruits and vegetables each day. Grains and beans are great sources of fiber. Shoot for a cup of beans or other legumes a day. Other fiber-rich foods include whole-grain breads and cereals, pastas and brown rice. But add fiber to your diet gradually to help avoid its gassy side effects.

Ax fat. Fatty foods can make your stomach empty more slowly, causing nausea and bloating, says Dr. Aslan. So avoid cheeses, ice cream, rich desserts, fried foods and fatty meats such as hot dogs, sausage and bacon.

Inflammatory Bowel Disease:
Soothe the Intestines

Inflammatory bowel disease is a catch-all for two similar conditions: Crohn's disease, a chronic inflammation of the intestinal tract; and ulcerative colitis, in which the large intestine gets inflamed and riddled with ulcers. In each case, the main complaints consist of some combination of abdominal pain, rectal bleeding, cramps, weight loss, diarrhea and sometimes fever along with malabsorption, or the inability to take up and use nutrients from food. This, of course, can leave you feeling weak and fatigued, especially when you consider that a bout with inflammatory bowel disease (IBD) can last two or three weeks or longer.

So what causes IBD? Most research points to either a glitch in the immune system or an inherited genetic defect or weakness in the gut, since IBD tends to run in families. But IBD doesn't have to cost you your youthful vitality. With appropriate measures, you can still stay in the game. Here's how.

Eat light. "Avoid great blowout meals," advises Sidney Phillips, M.D., director of the Gastroenterology Research Unit at the Mayo Clinic. The more you eat, the harder your already inflamed intestines have to work.

Grab some shut-eye. Never pass up an opportunity to nap. While your symptoms are acting up, it's important to get as much sleep as possible to keep you from getting excessively tired, mentally or physically, says Dr. Phillips.

Know when to ease off. If your symptoms are mild, a high-fiber diet is important. Eating plenty of fruits, vegetables and whole-grain breads and pastas can help control constipation and diarrhea by absorbing the extra water in your intestines, says Samuel Meyers, M.D., clinical professor of medicine at Mount Sinai School of Medicine of the City University of New York in New York City. But when symptoms get severe, hold off on fiber until things improve. Too much fiber during a bout with IBD can actually make things worse.

Soothe your symptoms with nonprescription medication. Many IBD symptoms can be kept in check with over-the-counter antacids and diarrhea medications, says Dr. Phillips. Of course, most guys with IBD also need prescription medications to see them through the worst days.

DOUBLE CHIN

Growing a Beard Isn't Your Only Option

Gravity—what a bummer. It's the only thing standing between you and a roster spot with the Boston Celtics. It's constantly trying to pull your chest into your waistline. And now it's grabbing hold of your chin, adding an unwanted extra layer to that youthful Dick Tracy jawline.

"There's no question. A double chin makes some men feel like they're aging," says Robert Kotler, M.D., a facial cosmetic surgeon and clinical instructor in surgery at the University of California, Los Angeles.

"Every time they look in the mirror, they see it. When they feel tight around the shirt collar, they get reminded of it. And it's telling them that maybe they're not as young as they used to be."

Jaw Droppers

Three factors contribute to double chins: body fat, anatomy and time. Men store fat on their necks just as easily as on their bellies, Dr. Kotler says. So if you pack on a few extra pounds, there's a good chance some of it will settle under your chin.

But overweight people aren't the only ones in danger. Even thin people get double chins, usually because of the shape of the jaw and throat. "The less sharp the angle between the jawline and neckline, the greater the risk of a fleshy neck," says Dr. Kotler. "But the lower your Adam's apple is in your neck, the more likely you are to get a sag in your chin."

Age also increases the odds. Men's skin starts to lose its elasticity after 40 to 50 years. So even if you are fit and firm and have a profile like Dudley Do-Right himself, you may still show a slight double chin because of looser skin, Dr. Kotler says.

From a health perspective, none of this really matters. There's nothing dangerous about a double chin unless you're seriously overweight, Dr. Kotler says. Even then, it's a symptom of obesity, not a problem by itself. "For most men, double chins are just an unfortunate part of the aging process," Dr. Kotler says. "It means buying a bigger shirt size or being a little more self-conscious about your looks. But in the overall scheme of things, there are more important things to worry about."

Keeping Your Chin Up

Harmless or not, most guys still find double chins unattractive. To help rid yourself of those extra folds—or at least hide them a little—experts offer these tips.

Drop 10. Or 15 or 20—pounds, that is. "The single best way to get rid of a double chin is to lose weight," Dr. Kotler says. "Lots of people come to my office wanting cosmetic surgery. But if they just take off some excess weight, the problem usually diminishes to the point where they don't need any more help."

The standard rules apply. Get regular aerobic exercise. Eat less fat. And avoid crash diets, which usually do more harm than good. And don't rely on miracle "spot-reducing" exercises for your neck. They won't remove the fat—and in some cases have caused dislocated jaws and severely strained neck muscles.

Stay loose. Nothing exposes a double chin more than a dress shirt that is too tight around the neck. "You start to look like a stuffed sausage," says G. Bruce Boyer, a New York City fashion consultant and author of *Eminently Suitable*. Swallow your pride and buy a bigger size. Boyer also suggests shirts with bigger collars, since they help keep things in proportion. And avoid spread, round and pin collars. They only accentuate your neck. With casual shirts, try open collars, and stay away from turtlenecks. The darker the color around the neckline, the better.

Know your knots. Silk ties are better than bulky knit or wool ones, Boyer says. And never use the oversize Windsor knot to tie them. A four-in-hand or half-Windsor knot produces a neater, smaller look that doesn't draw people's eyes to your neck.

Get cropped. Long hair—on your head or face—is no good. "Hair at or below your jawline is only going to make things worse," says Kathleen Walas, fashion and beauty director for New York City–based Avon Products. That means no shoulder-length hairstyles. Neatly trimmed moustaches and beards are okay.

Know the skinny on surgery. Cosmetic surgery is a last resort, Dr. Kotler says. But if you have tried everything else and can't shed your extra chin—and have about $4,500 to spare—you can have your neck "sculpted." The surgeon will make a small horizontal cut under your chin, then suck out the fat that has collected beneath the skin. Finally, he will make a vertical incision between the edges of the neck and jaw muscle and sew the edges together, tightening the muscle layer like a corset.

It's a relatively painless procedure that requires two Band-Aids to hide, Dr. Kotler says. Bruising is minimal, and within about ten days you won't see anything except your old single chin. "It's a common procedure," he says. "The technique has become very refined, and the results are quite good." The operation can be done under either general anesthesia or local anesthesia with sedation.

For an extra $500 or so, the surgeon can also add a chin implant. It's a piece of solid silicone that is slipped between your jawbone and the sheath of tissue that covers the bone. The implant gives you a more prominent jaw and further accentuates the angle between the jawline and neck, Dr. Kotler says. There is no addition to overall recovery time. It may have to be adjusted if you take one on the chin in a bar fight, but generally, implants tend to keep their positions. Surgeons use implants in about one-fourth of all double chin procedures, Dr. Kotler says.

DRINKING PROBLEMS

It's More Than Mud in Your Eye

He wakes up with a throbbing headache that tells him he drank far too much last night. Despite the pain, he manages to drag himself to work. But before long, he sneaks a swig from the bottle hidden in his desk to steady his nerves. For lunch, he gulps a martini—or two—to make it through the rest of the day. After work, he celebrates happy hour, which staggers on until last call. Then he weaves his way down the highway, hoping he won't get caught for drunk driving again. Once home, he nurses a nightcap until he passes out. Then he gets up the next morning and starts all over again.

That's the classic image of a man with an alcohol problem. But alcohol abuse has many subtle faces. It could be your golfing buddy, who keeps drinking despite pleas from his wife. Or your doctor, who drinks only on weekends. Or your neighbor, the life of the party. And yes, it could be you.

"An alcohol problem can strike anyone, at any time, from any walk of life. No one is immune from it," says Donald Damstra, M.D., an addiction medicine specialist and substance abuse consultant in Phoenix.

And no matter what you call it—alcoholism, drinking heavily or "that little problem"—abusing alcohol is a potent and sometimes deadly ager. It can destroy your liver, decimate your heart, dangerously elevate your blood pressure, sap your energy, ravage your stomach, shatter your sex life, short-circuit your brain, aggravate diabetes, lower your immunity, increase your cancer risk, trigger depression and stress, alienate your friends, destroy your career and end your marriage.

"When you see people who have been drinking heavily for a number of years, they tend to look bad. Some men in their forties can look like they're in their sixties. Their skin just looks old, their gait isn't good, they're overweight, and often they have lost bone mass—so they look like little old men a lot earlier than they should," says Frederic C. Blow, Ph.D., research director of the Alcohol Research Center at the University of Michigan in Ann Arbor.

Who Has a Drinking Problem?

Almost everyone who drinks has experienced a hangover or another torture that occurs after hoisting one too many. But after we recover from a few of those self-inflicted disasters, many of us learn to moderate our drinking.

"Drinking generally decreases as we age," Dr. Blow says. "It may be related to chronic diseases such as diabetes and high blood pressure or increased use of medications, or it could be that people just don't feel like drinking as much."

Maturity and a greater sense of responsibility contribute to the dip. Guys may also drink less as they get older because they find that alcohol has a greater effect. That's because as you tiptoe into your fifties and sixties, your body is gradually less able to handle alcohol. As a result, older men get drunker on less booze and may suffer greater negative consequences, Dr. Damstra says.

In fact, alcohol consumption in the United States is at its lowest level since 1967, according to the National Institute on Alcohol Abuse and Alcoholism. The average American drinks about 2½ gallons of alcohol each year. That's roughly the equivalent of 1½ 12-ounce cans of beer a day. That's within the range of one to two drinks a day that doctors believe can reduce your risk of heart disease. A standard alcoholic beverage is one 12-ounce beer, a 5-ounce glass of wine or a cocktail made with 1½ ounces (or one shot) of liquor.

But at least one in every ten guys downs three or more drinks a day and can be considered a heavy drinker, Dr. Damstra says. Problem drinking can lead to serious consequences, including drunk driving arrests, wife and child abuse and absenteeism at work, he says.

But how much or how often a guy drinks isn't conclusive evidence that he is among the 12 million American men who have serious drinking problems, Dr. Damstra says. An accountant who has a drink or two after work, for example, could have more problems with alcohol than an obnoxious drunk singing "Feelings" at a karaoke bar. A key measure, he says, is if booze is more important than anything else in your life, including your family and your health.

"There are some heavy drinkers who are not addicted to alcohol. These are the guys who quit drinking when their doctors tell them they have ulcers or other compelling reasons to stop. But if you're addicted to alcohol, you'll tell the doctor 'Take the ulcer out, Doc. I have to keep drinking,' " Dr. Damstra says. "When drinking causes serious negative consequences, no matter if they're physical, psychological, social, economic or spiritual, and the man continues to drink, then his drinking is out of control and is considered alcoholism."

Why some men have problems with alcohol and others don't is still being sorted out. Researchers believe that there is genetic predisposition, since men with family histories of alcoholism are more likely to become alcoholic. But predisposition doesn't mean a guy is doomed to be alcoholic, nor are men without family histories immune from drinking problems, says Norman Miller, M.D., associate professor of psychiatry at the University of Illinois College of Medicine in Chicago. Although the process is complex, some researchers speculate that a guy's risk for alcoholism depends on a combination of factors in addition to genes, including religious and moral attitudes, self-esteem, depression and peer pressure. But whatever the cause, the end result is an addiction that prematurely ages you in tragic and unnecessary ways.

Look Out Stomach, Here It Comes

When you quaff an ice-cold one after a long day at work, you're drinking one of the most unusual substances on earth. Alcohol is a source of empty calories. It is also a powerful drug that affects your judgment and emotions.

Is Alcohol Controlling Your Life?

So how do you know if you might have a drinking problem? Frederic C. Blow, Ph.D., research director of the Alcohol Research Center at the University of Michigan in Ann Arbor, suggests you ask yourself the following questions. Answer the questions yes or no, then follow the scoring at the end of the test.

1. Do you feel you are a normal drinker?
2. Have you ever awakened in the morning after drinking the night before and found that you could not remember a part of that evening?
3. Does your partner (or parents) ever worry or complain about your drinking?
4. Can you stop drinking after one or two drinks without a struggle?
5. Do you ever feel bad about your drinking?
6. Do friends or relatives think you are a normal drinker?
7. Are you always able to stop drinking when you want to?
8. Have you ever attended a meeting of Alcoholics Anonymous?
9. Have you gotten into fights when drinking?
10. Has drinking ever created problems between you and your partner?
11. Has your partner (or other family member) ever gone to anyone for help about your drinking?
12. Have you ever lost friends or girlfriends because of drinking?
13. Have you even gotten into trouble at work because of drinking?
14. Have you ever lost a job because of drinking?

Moderate drinking—two drinks a day for men—has some benefits, including lowering your heart disease risk. But in larger amounts, alcohol is a poison that affects every cell in the body, says Sheila Blume, M.D., medical director of the alcoholism, chemical dependency and compulsive gambling programs at South Oaks Hospital in Amityville, New York.

"Alcohol is a very tiny molecule carried in the bloodstream, and unlike other drugs, it's so small that it gets completely inside every cell. So its ability to do harm and mischief is endless," Dr. Blume says.

Alcohol, for example, can temporarily disrupt your sex life. "Alcohol is an aphrodisiac in moderate amounts. But if you become intoxicated, you may have difficulty getting or maintaining an erection," Dr. Damstra says.

15. Have you ever neglected your obligations, your family or your work for two or more days in a row because you were drinking?
16. Do you ever drink before noon?
17. Have you ever been told you have liver trouble? Cirrhosis?
18. Have you ever had delirium tremens (DTs) or severe shaking, heard voices or seen things that weren't there after heavy drinking?
19. Have you ever gone to anyone for help about your drinking?
20. Have you ever been in a hospital because of drinking?
21. Have you ever been a patient in a psychiatric hospital when drinking was part of the problem?
22. Have you ever been seen at a psychiatric or mental health clinic or gone to a doctor, social worker or clergy for help with a problem in which drinking had played a part?
23. Have you ever been arrested, even for a few hours, because of drunken behavior?
24. Have you ever been arrested for drunk driving or driving after drinking?

Scoring

If you answered yes to any of these questions, give yourself the following score: Questions 3, 5, 9 and 16 are worth one point each. Questions 8, 19 and 20 are worth five points each. All other questions are worth two points each. If you scored five or more points, you may have a drinking problem and should consider seeking counseling.

Drinking also can momentarily suppress production of growth hormone, which keeps our cells vigorous and active as we age, says Mary Ann Emanuele, M.D., professor of endocrinology at Loyola University Medical Center in Chicago. "Blood levels of growth hormone in normal adults fall after drinking, and that could be detrimental," Dr. Emanuele says. "Studies show that these changes do reverse after several hours. However, we don't know if continued heavy drinking can cause permanent suppression of the hormone."

When the Party Is Over

Researchers know that abusing alcohol can severely damage many organs, but heavy drinking doesn't affect every man in the same way. "The most serious consequences of drinking vary from individual to individual," Dr. Damstra says. "I've seen some alcoholics who drink prodigious amounts whose brains are fine, but their livers are shot. I've seen others who drink just as much, and their livers are great, but they have serious brain changes."

Alcohol abuse can cause blackouts, seizures, hallucinations and brain damage. Up to 70 percent of people entering alcohol treatment programs have difficulties with memory, problem solving and clear thinking.

Heavy drinking can cause confusion, slowed reaction time, blurred vision and loss of concentration and muscle coordination, all which can lead to injury and fatal accidents. Men and women who consume more than five drinks in one sitting are twice as likely to die from injuries as those who don't drink that much, according to researchers at the Centers for Disease Control and Prevention in Atlanta. The National Highway Traffic Safety Administration estimates that between 45 and 50 percent of all traffic fatalities in the United States each year are alcohol-related. And other statistics suggest that an estimated 22 percent of all deaths due to disease, accidents and homicides are alcohol-related.

Studies have shown that men with alcoholism have death rates up to six times higher than moderate drinkers or nondrinkers.

"Heavy drinkers die younger—there's no question about that," says Michael Criqui, M.D., professor of epidemiology at the University of California, San Diego, School of Medicine.

Why? One reason is that excess alcohol consumption generates free radicals, chemically unstable oxygen molecules that can damage the heart and liver and accelerate the aging process throughout the body, says Eric Rimm, Sc.D., a nutritional epidemiologist at the Harvard University School of Public Health in Boston.

Drinking heavily, for instance, severely damages a man's skin. "It causes rhinophyma—that famous big red nose, like W. C. Fields had. It causes blotchiness, puffiness and decreased skin tone, so a man who drinks heavily will look prematurely aged," Dr. Blume says.

In addition, studies have shown that people who consume three or more drinks a day have a 40 percent greater risk of developing high blood pressure, which has been linked to heart disease and stroke.

Excessive alcohol use can lead to cirrhosis, an incurable disease that stimulates the formation of scar tissue that destroys the liver. But if a man stops drinking, the progress of the disease is slowed, and his life can be prolonged. Heavy drinking also increases the risk of liver cancer.

"Alcohol is associated with some types of cancer, particularly in those parts of the body that come in direct contact with alcohol, such as the esophagus, throat and liver," Dr. Rimm says. "These types of cancer are usually rare, but among people who drink five or six drinks a day, they become less rare."

Some researchers believe that these cancers are more common in heavy drinkers because alcohol addiction suppresses the immune system and lowers the body's defenses against diseases such as cancer and AIDS.

Painful Talk Can Save Lives

It isn't easy telling a friend or a loved one that you are worried about his drinking. But it can be one of the most vital and rewarding conversations you'll ever have.

"If you're going to share your observations and thoughts about their drinking, you need to expect that it's going to be a painful discussion. But painful doesn't mean harmful," says William Clark, M.D., medical director of the Addiction Resource Center at MidCoast Hospital–Bath in Bath, Maine. "It's like surgery. It's painful when it's done, but it saves lives."

Don't label the person by saying "I think you are an alcoholic" or "You have a drinking problem," Dr. Clark suggests. This kind of statement will only increase the person's feelings of irritability, shame and anger.

Instead, use "I" messages that simply express your concerns and observations, says Sheila Blume, M.D., medical director of the alcoholism, chemical dependency and compulsive gambling programs at South Oaks Hospital in Amityville, New York. Say something like "I'm terrified because I know you've been driving under the influence a lot lately. That scares me. I don't want anything to happen to you, so maybe you could sit down with someone who knows more about these things than we do."

"If you enter the conversation respectfully and thoughtfully, they'll listen," Dr. Clark says.

Because alcohol impairs your judgment and reduces your inhibitions, you'll be more likely to engage in risky sexual behaviors that will increase your chance of getting AIDS and other sexually transmitted diseases. In addition, evidence from animal studies suggests that if you have AIDS and continue to drink, you increase damage to your immune system, reduce your body's vitamin and mineral levels and speed the progress of the disease, says Ronald R. Watson, Ph.D., director of the Alcohol Research Center at the University of Arizona in Tucson.

But if even you've drunk heavily for years, there is hope that you can still lead a long and healthy life if you quit. In an 11-year study of 234 alcoholic men, researchers at the University of California, San Diego, School of Medicine found that the men who quit drinking and stayed sober had death rates comparable to guys who didn't have drinking problems.

Starting Over

Acknowledging that you have a drinking problem is an important first step in a lifelong struggle to stay sober. "The sooner that alcoholism is recognized and treated, the less likely the disease will cause permanent damage," Dr. Damstra says. "Most alcoholics begin to feel better very quickly after they stop drinking. Many of the physical complications that are caused by excessive consumption begin to heal within two to three weeks."

High blood pressure, for instance, often returns to normal within a week or two, while stomach irritation and some types of liver damage are reversible within a month. But it can take more than a year to recover from some longtime effects of alcohol consumption, such as impaired memory and concentration. Other conditions, such as cirrhosis of the liver and damage to the pancreas, may be irreversible. Here are some tips to help you get a fresh start without alcohol.

Seek help. If you believe that alcohol is controlling your life, ask your doctor for help or contact an alcohol treatment program in your area. For confidential information, write to Alcoholics Anonymous, P.O. Box 459, Grand Central Station, New York, NY 10163.

Tell a friend. Some studies suggest that if the person with an alcohol problem goes public, it's easier for him to quit, Dr. Blow says. If you tell the people who are important to you—co-workers, family—that you're not going to drink anymore, it does two things. First, it reduces the amount of peer pressure that will be placed on you to drink. Second, it makes it easier for you to stick to the commitment, because you've made it out loud to the world.

Start sobriety at home. In the early phase of recovery, ask friends and family to not drink around you. Ask your partner to participate in your recovery by attending counseling sessions with you, Dr. Damstra says. If she refuses, she may have a problem, too, and you might have to decide if continuing the relationship is worth jeopardizing your recovery.

Say the three magic words. If you do go to a party or another gathering and are offered an alcoholic beverage, simply say "I don't drink" or ask for a soft drink, Dr. Blume says. No further explanation should be necessary. If the people around you continue to pressure you to drink, leave.

Find new pals. Hanging out with your old drinking buddies, even if you swear you won't drink, is a disaster waiting to happen, Dr. Damstra says. First, you need to get involved in a 12-step recovery program. Then find people who are interested in staying sober at your recovery group, church or gym.

Invest in fun. Get involved in activities that don't center around alcohol. Coach your son's soccer team, volunteer at a neighborhood school or get involved in a theater group, Dr. Damstra says. The more activities you do, the more you'll realize that being sober is more fun and rewarding than drinking.

Make no substitutions. Stay away from nonalcoholic beers and wines. "It will remind you of the taste of the real thing and, by association, make you crave alcohol," says Dr. Blume.

DRUG DEPENDENCY

Taking Back Control of Your Life

Forget the stereotype. The "typical" drug-dependent man doesn't live on the mean streets of America's inner cities. He lives right in your own neighborhood.

"Not everyone is in danger of becoming drug-dependent," says Joan Mathews Larson, Ph.D., director of the Health Recovery Center in Minneapolis and author of *Seven Weeks to Sobriety*. "But it cuts across all boundaries. You certainly don't have to be a poor urban youth to become hooked on drugs."

Drug use exacts a brutal toll. You could lose your money, your job, your friends, your spouse and your dignity. You could ravage your body by not eating or by eating in giant binges, by forsaking exercise or by letting your hygiene go. You could lose mental capacity. And you could even die.

"It doesn't have to be that way," Dr. Larson says. "But unless a person takes action, he will likely continue to deteriorate. People dependent on drugs can fall an awfully long way."

Filling the Void

Studies show how widespread the country's drug problem has become. A large-scale study of residents of five U.S. cities showed that as many as 1 in 14 American men either abuse or are dependent on drugs.

And drug dependency is horribly expensive. Figures from the University of California, San Francisco, show that use of illegal drugs in America costs nearly $7 billion a year in treatment, loss of productivity and other costs.

Why do people become drug-dependent, despite the risks? Because drugs make them feel good—at least at first. "Drugs fill a need in a person's life," Dr. Larson says. "Heroin, for instance, can help a person deal with his natural anxiety."

The relief, however, is always short-lived. Over time, drug use interferes with production of endorphins, your body's natural "feel-good" chemicals. "That means you have to use more drugs to make up the difference," says Adam Lewenberg, M.D., a New York City physician whose private practice includes addiction treatment. "It becomes a cycle where you crave the drug more and more and eventually become dependent on its use."

We're not just talking about cocaine, marijuana, heroin and other illegal drugs. Doctors and researchers have identified scores of over-the-counter and prescription drugs that can cause dependence, including cough syrups, anabolic steroids and anti-anxiety drugs in the benzodiazepine family, such as diazepam (Valium).

While anyone can become dependent on drugs, heredity can play a big role. In his book *The Good News about Drugs and Alcohol*, Mark S. Gold, M.D., estimates that one in ten people is genetically predisposed to becoming dependent on drugs. "There's no question that drug dependence, like alcoholism, can run in families," Dr. Larson says. "Unfortunately, we can't test for it. But if you know of alcoholics or drug-dependent people in your family, you have to be extra careful."

Alcohol abuse also increases your chances of becoming dependent on drugs. We've all heard about how alcohol is a "gateway drug," opening the door to further drug abuse. Well, here's the proof: The National Institute of Mental Health interviewed more than 20,000 American men and women over age 18 from five communities across the country. Researchers found that men who abuse alcohol run nearly six times the risk of abusing drugs as well.

The same study found that having a history of mental disorders also raises your risk. People with disorders such as depression could be 4.7 times more likely to abuse or become dependent on drugs. And those with anxiety problems such as panic disorder or obsessive-compulsive behavior are 2.5 times more likely to become dependent on or abuse drugs.

The most important thing to remember about drug dependency, Dr. Larson says, is that it can happen to anyone. "It's not something to be ashamed of. It doesn't mean you have a moral flaw or a character flaw," she says. "No one sets out to become hooked on drugs. But for a variety of reasons, many of them beyond a person's control, it just happens. And then you have to deal with it."

Stopping before You Start

Clearly, the best way to beat drug dependency is to avoid it in the first place. To help stay out of trouble, consider these tips.

Know the warning signs. "When thoughts of a drug fill your mind, you have a problem," Dr. Larson says. If you feel like you can't relax, be happy, get to sleep or do anything at all without first using a drug, it's probably time to seek help.

Other signs of trouble include lying to your doctor to refill a prescription, missing work because of drug binges or hangovers, raiding your savings to pay for drugs and consistently forsaking food, friendship or family to get high.

Shake your family tree. Look for signs of drug abuse in your family, because it may indicate that you're more prone to dependency. Include alcoholism in your search. And don't overlook things such as Grandpa's painkillers or Aunt Sophie's Valium.

"If you find signs of it in your family, be extra careful," Dr. Larson says. "Don't ever experiment with drugs, because it may take only once for you to get hooked."

Resolve conflicts. People use drugs to avoid dealing with problems such as anxiety, boredom, depression, frustration, bad relationships, pressure at work and unemployment. "Meet these problems head-on," Dr. Larson says. "Drinking or taking drugs to avoid them isn't going to solve anything. It's just going to add another layer—drug dependency—to the mix."

If you're bored, find a hobby or do some volunteer work. If you're having trouble at work or with your spouse, seek counseling. Whatever you do, don't turn to drugs for temporary comfort, no matter how appealing they sound.

Stick to the label. If your doctor gives you prescription drugs, particularly painkillers and tranquilizers, use them exactly the way you're told to. And never try to have them refilled unless the doctor says so. "Prescription drugs don't act differently in your body than illegal drugs," Dr. Lewenberg says. "In some ways they're more dangerous, because they're available and legal. People who wouldn't think of buying cocaine would not see the same problem in misusing a prescription drug. But they should."

When you're done taking a drug, throw away the bottle. If there's some left, don't shove it in the medicine closet, or you or someone else may be tempted to use it later, without a doctor's approval.

Just say no. It's trite. It's hackneyed. It was Nancy Reagan's claim to fame. But the phrase still rings true. Avoid illegal drugs. Because for some people, "recreational" drug use can quickly lead to dependency. "You can't become addicted to illegal drugs," Dr. Lewenberg says, "unless you use them."

When You Need Help

If you think you may already have developed a drug dependency, experts offer this advice.

Ask for help. "I'll say it again: Don't be ashamed," Dr. Larson says. "Tell a trusted friend. Tell your spouse. The sooner it's out in the open, the sooner you'll start dealing with it in constructive ways." You don't need to broadcast your problem to the world. But if there's even one person out there who knows and cares, you'll get the support you need to get back on the right track.

Find strength in numbers. Twelve-step groups are great aids to some men. You can find people with similar problems and hopes who can help you make it through the inevitable rough spots of recovery.

Start by looking for a local chapter of Alcoholics Anonymous, Cocaine Anonymous or Narcotics Anonymous. You can also call or write these groups for more information.

- Narcotics Anonymous, World Services Office, P.O. Box 9999, Van Nuys, CA 91409
- Cocaine Anonymous, 3740 Overland Avenue, Suite G, Los Angeles, CA 90034; 1-800-347-8998
- National Clearinghouse for Alcohol and Drug Information, P.O. Box 2345, Rockville, MD 20817-2345

Exercise in moderation. If you've been abusing drugs, you've been abusing your body, too. You may not have gotten any exercise for months, a factor that may only heighten depression or anxiety.

So start working out. Begin with moderate exercise; walking for about 20 minutes a day, at least three times a week, is best. Heavy-duty exercise isn't a good idea at first, according to Dr. Lewenberg. You're probably not in peak shape right now and could easily be injured or discouraged. And it's possible to become addicted to exercise, too, since it stimulates endorphin production. "It's not a bad trade, really—drugs for exercise," Dr. Lewenberg says. "But the idea is to bring your body back to normal slowly."

Eat right. Drugs can do some strange things to your appetite. People dependent on marijuana, for instance, are prone to overeating and obesity. And cocaine abuse can lead to malnutrition and even eating disorders such as anorexia nervosa. "When you're dependent on drugs, eating well is rarely a priority," Dr. Larson says.

Try to eat a balanced diet, whether you feel like eating or not. Replace sweets with fruits and vegetables. "Feeding your body and brain what it needs is a very necessary first step to recovery," Dr. Larson says.

Consider treatment. Inpatient and outpatient recovery centers offer people the chance to both detoxify their bodies and address the underlying causes of their drug dependencies. "Where there's addiction, there's depression," says Dr. Lewenberg. "It's not enough to go cold turkey and not deal with the other problems." Dr. Lewenberg's program has included nonaddicting drug therapy to handle depression and even electroacupuncture, which he says helps stimulate endorphin production and make medication more effective.

Many employers and insurance companies will cover the costs of recovery centers.

FATIGUE

How to Run on Full instead of Empty

Tom is an avid jogger. But lately, his running has left him feeling drained. He felt so exhausted the other day that after less than half his normal run, he stopped and limped home.

His friend Dick doesn't have any more energy than Tom does. Night after night, Dick wearily trudges home from work, so beat that he can barely lift his briefcase. Once he arrives, he plops down on the sofa, switches on the television and lies there until the wee hours.

Their friend Harry regularly gets a good eight hours of sleep. But every morning, Harry can barely wake up. One shower and many cups of coffee later, he still feels as weak as a kitten.

Every now and then, every Tom, Dick and Harry goes through a spell of fatigue. Usually, it's something he can take in stride. But sometimes an overwhelming bout of fatigue can knock a guy out for days, weeks or months.

Constant fatigue can make any guy look and feel like a worn-out, washed-up 100-year-old shadow of his former self.

"Fatigue's greatest impact is on human function and activity," says Lt. Col. Kurt Kroenke, M.D., associate professor of medicine at the Uniformed Services University of the Health Sciences in Bethesda, Maryland, and an expert on fatigue. "When you don't have the strength or energy to move, even simple tasks become difficult. You become sedentary, your productivity drops, your motivation suffers. For some, this persistent weariness can be so debilitating that they can't even get out of bed."

Fatigue can take a toll on your mind as well, experts agree. Thinking becomes difficult and confused. Decisions come slowly. Even your outlook on life turns gloomy.

The result is that fatigue can lead to poor work performance, less interaction with friends and family and less participation in the sports and activities you enjoy.

That's bad news if you're used to being an active man. But the good news is that with a little detective work, you can almost always get to the source of the problem and reclaim your vim and vigor.

What's Running You Down?

It's easy to shrug off a case of lethargy or poor stamina as just another sign that you're getting older or that you're coming down with something.

But for most of us, it's neither. "Most fatigue is not due to aging or to a serious medical problem," says Dr. Kroenke. "More often it's a signal that the body is getting too much or too little of something, and that's making you feel run-down." Most fatigue is caused by too much work, too much stress, too much weight, too much junk food and not enough exercise, doctors say.

"Most of us live and work in rapid, pressure-filled environments," explains Ralph LaForge, an exercise physiologist and instructor of health promotion and exercise science at the University of California, San Diego. "Much of the fatigue people experience is really due to the inability to pace themselves, to effectively stagger their workloads or to bring a sense of order to the chaos around them."

Just dealing with the pressures of everyday life takes a lot of energy, says Thomas Miller, Ph.D., professor of psychiatry at the University of Kentucky College of Medicine in Lexington. "One of the first things we look at whenever a patient complains of fatigue is stress. Whenever anyone has a hard time coping—with family problems, relationships, job pressure—there's usually a tremendous burnout factor, physically as well as emotionally."

Fatigue can also signal that you're not eating right, says Peter Miller, Ph.D., executive director of the Hilton Head Health Institute, a clinic in Hilton Head, South Carolina, that develops personal health programs. "The eating habits we established when we were younger are not suited for our middle years.

"Think of the body as a car and food as the fuel," he says. "When you're young, you can put almost any kind of gasoline in your tank. But as you get older, the body has a harder time running on that low-octane stuff. So you need to fill up with high-test fuel and in the proper amounts."

If you're an overeater, for example, you're going to be storing more fuel than you need in the form of fat. And lugging around that excess body weight can make anyone feel sluggish. At the other extreme, undereating can also cause fatigue by depriving you of sufficient calories to propel your body through the day. That's why many men who go on "crash" or very low calorie diets often find their energy levels crashing: They're like cars running on empty.

Your activity level also has a direct effect on whether you feel fatigued, says LaForge. Lack of exercise can easily create a pattern of inactivity that is difficult to break. "A body at rest tends to remain at rest," says LaForge. "Generally, the more active and fit you are, the more stamina and energy you'll have on a day-to-day basis. Letter carriers, for example, are always on their feet. Yet they complain of fatigue much less than office workers."

On the other hand, too much exercise can have a negative effect. "Overexertion can send your energy level crashing," says LaForge. That's because when we exercise, the body produces lactic acid, a substance that accumulates in our muscles, producing weakness and body aches. This accumulation usually doesn't pose a problem when we avoid working ourselves to exhaustion and we follow our workouts with proper rest, because then our bodies are able to get rid of the lactic acid.

But when we push our bodies during workouts and don't allow our muscles time to recover, lactic acid accumulates faster than we can get rid of it. And this can leave us feeling fatigued all the time.

Other factors that can make us tired all the time? Smoking, so-called recreational drugs, alcohol and inconsistent eating and sleeping patterns put enormous strain on the mind and body. Sometimes, experts agree, fatigue is your body's cry that your lifestyle is not one that supports a healthy body.

Recharge Your Batteries

Fatigue is a symptom of everything from the common cold to cancer. It's a symptom of hepatitis, diabetes, heart disease, tuberculosis, thyroid problems, Hodgkin's disease, multiple sclerosis, anemia, AIDS, anxiety and depression. And it's also a side effect of some medications used to treat these conditions.

But fatigue is rarely anything to worry about unless it's accompanied by other symptoms such as pain, swelling or fever or it lasts longer than a week. If your fatigue has lasted that long or you have other symptoms, see your doctor.

Otherwise, here are some tips to re-energize your life.

Slow your pace. "Fatigue is the price we pay for pushing ourselves beyond the point where our minds and bodies say no," says Dr. Kroenke. So think about where you might be pushing past your natural limits. Cut back on some activities. Don't work or exercise as hard, as fast or as long as you have been. Take frequent breaks. And make sure you get a good night's sleep every night—meaning you sleep well enough and long enough to wake up refreshed.

Avoid needless worrying. Agonizing over situations beyond your control only eats up personal energy, says Dr. Thomas Miller. Learn to let go of things you cannot change and focus your energies on those that you can.

Organize and prioritize. Does a list of tasks leave you feeling zapped before you even begin? Clear the clutter out of your life bit by bit, says LaForge. Start your day with a list of four or five tasks that you can definitely accomplish and work on them alone. The next day, try four or five more. What at first seemed like a mountain of work you couldn't climb then becomes a series of small hills that you can step over with ease.

Balance work with fun. All work and no play puts more stress on the mind and body than they can handle, says Dr. Thomas Miller. Mixing your daily schedule with a combination of social experiences and enjoyable activities provides a needed break in the action and relieves those stresses before they can drain your energy systems.

Take a hike. According to a study by Robert Thayer, Ph.D., professor of psychology at California State University, Long Beach, a brisk ten-minute walk causes a shift in mood that quickly raises energy levels and keeps them high for up to two hours. And an after-meal stroll can counteract the energy drop you experience after eating a big meal, adds Dr. Peter Miller. Digesting large meals increases blood and oxygen flow to the stomach and intestines, and this draws energy away from muscles and the brain. But a walk will keep blood and oxygen circulating evenly throughout the body.

Eat the right foods. A junk food diet high in sugar, fat and processed foods gives your body few or none of the basic vitamins, minerals and nutrients it needs to perform at normal levels. And sometimes just the slightest deficiency of any one nutrient is all it takes to send energy levels plummeting.

The answer, says Dr. Peter Miller, is to find a balance in both the amount and the types of food that you eat. "It's important to hit all the major food groups—fruits, vegetables, grains and cereals, dairy, nuts and meats—every day to guarantee that you're giving your body the right combination of fuel and basic nutrients to keep on running at peak levels," says Dr. Miller.

Ideally, every day you should be getting 60 percent (or more) of your calories from carbohydrate-rich foods such as pastas, breads, potatoes and beans, 25 percent (or less) of your calories from the fat found in foods such as canola oil, olive oil and peanut butter and 15 percent of your calories from protein-rich foods such as chicken and fish.

Focus on the carbs. Of the three energy-supplying nutrients—carbohydrates, fat and protein—carbohydrates pack the most fatigue-fighting punch. "Carbohydrates provide an efficient, long-lasting energy source," says Dr. Peter Miller. To produce an abundant reservoir of carbohydrate energy, add some of these foods to your plate whenever you sit down for a meal.

Eat four or five small meals. Skipping meals can leave your fuel reserves dangerously low, and digesting big meals can be an enormous energy drain. Unfortunately, the traditional three meals per day may contribute to the problem.

"Your body needs fuel in moderate doses throughout the day to keep performing at optimal levels," says Dr. Peter Miller. He recommends eating four or five small meals each day. "Reducing the amount of food you eat at any one time and spreading your calorie consumption more evenly over the day make more energy available to your body throughout the day," he says.

Snack wisely. When your stomach's growling and your energy's waning, the best pick-me-ups are of the natural variety, says Dr. Peter Miller. Fruits, raw vegetables, nuts and unbuttered popcorn—all which are low in energy-draining fat—are some excellent energizers.

Avoid the quick fix. Sugar-loaded foods such as candy and soda may zip up your energy level for a while, but they also cause your blood sugar levels to increase and then sharply drop. Unfortunately, the result is that your energy level will dip even lower than it was before, says Dr. Peter Miller.

Drink coffee. Studies at the Massachusetts Institute of Technology in

Do You Have
Chronic Fatigue Syndrome?

Chronic fatigue syndrome (CFS) is a rare, debilitating disorder that leaves its sufferers weak, exhausted and barely able to function for months or even decades.

The cause is still a mystery. "Because CFS usually appears after a flu or another illness, it was once thought to be caused by the Epstein-Barr virus," says Nelson Gantz, M.D., a member of the Centers for Disease Control and Prevention (CDC) Task Force on Chronic Fatigue Syndrome who is clinical professor of medicine at Pennsylvania State University College of Medicine in Hershey and chief of medicine and the Division of Infectious Diseases at Polyclinic Medical Center in Harrisburg, Pennsylvania. "Today, we're less sure of its origins. It probably doesn't have a single cause but is a combination of viral infections, allergies and psychological factors acting on the immune system."

There is no cure for the syndrome, says Dr. Gantz. Until one is found, people with the disease can find relief through a program of good nutrition, gentle exercise and rest developed with their personal physicians. In severe cases, nonsteroidal anti-inflammatory drugs and antidepressants are used to partially relieve symptoms, says Dr. Gantz.

How do you know if you have CFS? The CDC task force has developed a preliminary set of criteria. To be diagnosed as having CFS, you must have suffered from persistent fatigue for at least six months. The

Cambridge have discovered that the caffeine in a single cup of coffee can boost your energy level for up to six hours, researchers report. But don't overdo it.

Keep your whistle wet. Feeling run-down is often the first sign of dehydration, says Dr. Peter Miller. Drinking at least six glasses of water every day—more if you're active or trying to lose weight—will prevent this type of fatigue.

Avoid booze and pills. Regular use of alcohol, sleeping pills and tranquilizers will make any guy act like a zombie, says Dr. Kroenke. And believe it or not, stimulants and pep pills can take you from way, way up to way, way down after their immediate effects have worn off.

Check your medicine. Antihistamines and alcohol, found in many over-the-counter and prescription cold medications, can make you groggy, says Dr. Kroenke. Ask your doctor or pharmacist for a non-fatiguing alternative.

Explore alternative approaches. Many people fight fatigue by going be-

fatigue must not have existed previously, must persist despite bed rest and must cut your daily activity level in half for at least six months.

The existence of any other disease, infection, malignancy or condition that may produce similar symptoms, as well as the use of any drugs, medications or chemicals, must be ruled out by a physician. You must also have had 8 of these 11 symptoms for at least six months.

1. Mild fever or chills
2. Sore throat
3. Painful lymph nodes (glands on the sides of your neck)
4. Unexplained general muscle weakness
5. Muscle discomfort or pain
6. Fatigue of 24 hours or more after levels of exercise that used to be easily tolerated
7. Unusual headaches
8. Aches and pains (without swelling or redness) that travel from joint to joint
9. Any of these complaints: forgetfulness, excessive irritability, confusion, difficulty thinking, inability to concentrate, depression
10. Difficulty sleeping
11. Extremely swift development of these symptoms, from within a few hours to a few days

yond the traditional limits of Western science, says LaForge. Meditation, yoga and massage are just a few of the nontraditional options that practitioners say will energize, refresh and revive both body and mind.

Studies at Harvard Medical School in Boston show that taking a deep breath, exhaling, then sitting quietly for 20 minutes as you focus on a word that reflects your faith—*God*, *Allah*, *Krishna* or *shalom*, for example—will relax and re-energize both mind and body.

Check the Yellow Pages for organizations that teach these techniques. In many cases, you'll also find classes at your local YMCA.

Ask your doctor about supplements. In addition to a balanced diet, a multivitamin/mineral supplement should ensure that you're getting all the vitamins and minerals that you need, says Dr. Kroenke. Talk to your doctor about which one is right for you.

FOOT PROBLEMS

Sidestepping the Ache

The problems started long ago and innocently enough, with Mom and Dad cheering and steering you as you fumbled your way past the coffee table and La-Z-Boy chair on that maiden trek across the living room floor and into manhood. You were mobile. Going places. And the world was at your feet—quite literally.

But alas, that thrill of victory as a drooling toddler learning to walk paved the way for today's agony of the feet.

"The moment you begin to walk, you begin the process of wear and tear that could lead to future foot problems," says Glenn Gastwirth, D.P.M., deputy executive director for the American Podiatric Medical Association.

That's because each step—from running after fly balls in Little League to climbing the ladder of success at work—takes us one step closer to possible foot problems. Foot pain is not inevitable, but when our poor dogs are hounded with pain, it can hurt all over. "Bad feet can throw your posture out of whack, setting you up for possible knee pain, hip pain, back pain and neck pain," says Marc A. Brenner, D.P.M., a doctor of podiatric medicine in private practice in Glendale, New York.

Even our psyches gets their share of misery. "Debilitating foot problems make you feel older by robbing you of the vigor and energy you once had," says Dr. Gastwirth. "When your feet hurt, you can't perform your normal daily tasks, so you feel worse about yourself."

Tight Isn't Right

Part of the reason so many guys are bothered with foot problems—especially after age 40—is that our bellies aren't the only part of the body subject to middle-age spread. "What happens is that as we age, our feet become longer

134

and wider, a process called splaying," says Philip Sanfilippo, D.P.M., a podiatrist in private practice in San Francisco. "This occurs as the ligaments in our feet begin to collapse and the arches fall due to gravity and wear and tear. This flattens out our feet. Unfortunately, many people aren't aware of this process—which can occur in your thirties or forties—and they continue to wear the same size shoes they've always worn. And that causes the problem."

In other words, many of us are wearing tight shoes, which is a primary cause of corns, calluses, blisters and other foot problems. In fact, a 15-year study by Michael J. Coughlin, M.D., an orthopedic surgeon in private practice in Boise, Idaho, estimates that we spend an estimated $2 billion on conditions caused by tight shoes.

As if that weren't shocking enough, a study by the American Podiatric Medical Association found that one in five men knowingly buys and wears shoes that are too tight strictly for appearance' sake. "Granted, that's less than the number of women who will wear uncomfortable shoes because they look good, but it's still significant," says Dr. Gastwirth.

Teaching Old Dogs New Tricks

But don't give tight shoes all the blame. About the same time our feet begin to splay, the fat pads on the balls of our feet, which have cushioned our steps since toddlerhood, also begin to wear thin. It's "like the padding of a carpet," says Dr. Gastwirth. "When it's installed, it's nice and cushy. But after 20 years, that padding can get pretty worn."

Meanwhile, middle age also brings a loss of moisture in the skin of our feet, which can cause itching and make us more susceptible to athlete's foot and other fungi. And some men, especially smokers and those with Raynaud's disease, can suffer from circulatory problems that could result in a loss of sensation in the feet, particularly in cold weather.

So by the time we're in the prime of our lives, our feet can be well past their prime. Says Suzanne M. Levine, D.P.M., adjunct clinical instructor at New York College of Podiatric Medicine in New York City and author of *My Feet Are Killing Me*, "Any foot older than 25 is an aging foot."

But suffering isn't inevitable. With a little know-how, you can sidestep foot problems and recapture those glory days of walking that you had as a toddler—only with more grace and less drool. Here's how to get a toehold on common foot problems and give your soles a new lease on life.

Foot and Heel Pain: Support Yourself

There are several causes of those "unexplained" pains in your foot or heel, and most are the result of long-term use of your feet. They include fallen arches, Achilles tendon stiffness, plantar fasciitis, which is an inflammation in the bottom of the foot, and heel spurs, which are tiny growths of bone that may form from the constant pulling of ligaments through jumping, walking or running. "Usually, these problems result from overuse of your feet," says Richard Braver, D.P.M., sports podiatric physician for teams at Seton Hall University in South Orange, New Jersey, Fairleigh Dickinson University in Rutherford, New Jersey, and Montclair State College in Upper Montclair, New Jersey. No matter what the cause, here are the solutions.

Get some support. There's no getting around the deterioration of your feet's fat pads, but you can do something about the pain it causes on the soles of your feet. "Wearing high-quality, supportive, cushioning insoles in your shoes can certainly ease some of your discomfort," says Dr. Sanfilippo. These insoles are available at drugstores and sporting goods shops. If the pain is centered on your heel, a heel cup, also sold in these stores, can help prevent excess heel movement and ease pain. But perhaps more important than insoles and heel cups is wearing supportive shoes.

Stretch out your calf. For heel pain, some guys find relief by stretching the heel cord, or Achilles tendon, on the back of the foot, says Gilbert Wright, M.D., an orthopedic surgeon in private practice in Sacramento, California. Stand about three feet from a wall and place your hands on the wall. Lean toward the wall, bringing one leg forward and bending at the elbows. Your back leg should remain straight, with the heel on the floor, so you feel a gentle stretch.

Roll away pain. For heel spurs and plantar fasciitis, try massaging the bottom of your foot. "Roll your foot from heel to toe over a rolling pin, a golf ball or even a soup can," advises Dr. Braver. "This eases pain by stretching out the ligaments." Be sure the soup can is unopened.

Heat feet in the morning. "If you feel stiffness in your foot when you wake up, heat it to stimulate blood flow," says Dr. Braver. He recommends placing a warm compress or hot water bottle on the bottom of your foot for about 20 minutes.

Ice them in the evening. At nighttime, switch to ice. Suzanne M. Tanner, M.D., assistant professor in the Department of Orthopedics at the University of Colorado Sports Medicine Center in Denver, suggests placing an ice bag on your foot for 20 minutes, removing it for 20 minutes and then reapplying it for 20 minutes. Be sure to wrap the ice in a towel to prevent ice burns or frostbite.

Corns and Calluses: Here's the Rub

Corns are lumps of built-up dead skin that form on the bony areas of your feet, such as the toes. They're caused by friction, usually from shoes that are too tight. Calluses are bumps of skin that form on non-bony places for the same reasons. Both can make you feel as though you're walking on pebbles. Unless you have severe, constant pain—you'll need a doctor to help you over that—you can usually remedy these problems by yourself. And here's how.

Make sure the shoe fits. "If you have good-fitting shoes, you usually won't have corns and calluses," says Jan P. Silfverskiold, M.D., an orthopedic surgeon in private practice in Wheat Ridge, Colorado, who specializes in foot problems. To make sure your footwear fits, have both your feet measured for length and width each time you shop for shoes, advises Dr. Gastwirth. Be aware that the shape of your foot influences the best style of shoe to purchase. In general, the best styles for the corn-prone include sandals and running and walking shoes, which have roomy toe boxes.

Apply a moisturizer. Since corns and calluses result from too much friction, it's best to keep skin soft and well moisturized. Dr. Levine recommends that you apply a skin moisturizer to your feet immediately after each bath or shower. If your skin is already hardened with corns and calluses, scrape it with an emery board or a pumice stone anywhere from once a day to twice a week, adds Dr. Silfverskiold.

Go easy on the acid. Over-the-counter corn and callus removers (such as Dr. Scholl's) contain salicylic acid, which will erode lumpy lesions on your feet. But be careful: These medications should be applied only to the affected area, since they can burn healthy skin, says Dr. Levine. But don't use products containing salicylic acid if you have diabetes or poor circulation, cautions Dr. Levine. There are non-medicated cushions available (such as Dr. Scholl's Advanced Pain Relief Corn Cushions) that you can use to protect your corns.

Blisters and Bunions: The Big Hurts

Blisters are painful bubblelike rips in the skin that usually fill with fluid because of excessive friction. Bunions are bumps of bone and thickened skin at the side of your foot just below the base of your big or little toe. Tight shoes, arthritis and heredity can all lead to bunions, which can be accompanied by splaying of the foot and drifting of the big toe toward the little toe. As with corns and calluses, wearing properly fitting supportive shoes can prevent blisters and bunions. But if you already have either problem, here's how to fix it.

Pamper or pop 'em. Insoles, moleskin or even little balls of cotton stuffed between your toes can alleviate the immediate agony of blisters and prevent them from recurring. When blisters become too large for pads, however, you can pop them by pushing the fluid to one end of the "bubble" and pricking that area with a needle that's been sterilized with a flame or rubbing alcohol. After draining the liquid, repeat the procedure 12 hours later, and then again 12 hours after that, to ensure that you've removed all the liquid, advises Rodney Basler, M.D., a dermatologist and assistant professor of internal medicine at the University of Nebraska at Omaha. Don't pull off the skin, but if it has been torn off, wash the sore with hydrogen peroxide or soap and water and apply an antibiotic ointment.

Try a splint. Bunion pain can be relieved with a toe-straightening splint that's available at most pharmacies without a prescription. The most common version is a rubber plug that "pulls" the big toe away from the second toe, easing pain. While moleskin pads are often used by bunion sufferers, they're not as effective as these splints.

Athlete's Foot: Calming the Itch

This fungus, which leaves feet scaly, itchy, cracked and reddened, can be picked up just about anywhere—especially in warm, moist areas such as locker room floors (hence the name). Once you get it, athlete's foot is hard to get rid of, because it thrives in your shoes, but over-the-counter medications are the preferred course of action. Lotions are better than creams, since creams can trap moisture. Still, the best way to deal with athlete's foot is to avoid it. Here's how.

Sock it to 'em. Whenever you take off your socks, it's a good idea to rub one of them up and down the web of each toe, advises Dr. Basler. This helps keep feet desert-dry—and makes them an *un*welcome mat for athlete's foot. If sock rubbing isn't your style, you can use a hair dryer set on the low setting to dry those areas. If you have a problem with sweating after your feet have been dried, you can roll some antiperspirant on your feet after showering, he adds.

Be a shoe swapper. Try wearing different pairs of shoes as often as possible, says Dr. Basler. That's because shoes are full of moisture after a day of wear and need at least a day's "rest" to dry out. If you don't have enough pairs of shoes to go around, spray them with Lysol at the end of the day to help disinfect them.

Get cooking with baking soda. There are plenty of over-the-counter powders to prevent athlete's foot, but baking soda does essentially the same thing for a lot less money, says Dr. Levine. Just sprinkle it on dry daily to absorb excess moisture.

Ingrown Toenails: The Inside Story

All it takes is a teeny bit of nail to cause big-time pain. Once again, tight shoes can contribute to this problem by forcing the nail downward. If your nail is ingrown to the point that you're in constant agony, you may need a doctor to remove it. But here's how to avoid that anguish and keep nails trouble-free.

Cut nails straight across. Leave the half-moons for cloudy nights. The best way to cure an ingrown nail and prevent a new one from forming is to cut the nail straight across, not slightly curved or in a half-moon shape as most people do, says William Van Pelt, D.P.M., a Houston podiatrist and former president of the American Academy of Podiatric Sports Medicine. And don't cut it too short; it should be just over the crease of your nail fold. Be sure to soak your feet in warm water beforehand to make the cutting easier.

Take your piggies to market. There are several over-the-counter products that can soften an ingrown nail and the skin around it, thereby relieving pain. Dr. Levine recommends Dr. Scholl's ingrown toenail reliever and Outgro solution as two common brands. Make sure you follow the instructions carefully.

Avoid these products if you have diabetes or circulation problems because they contain powerful acids that could be dangerous for people with loss of sensation in their feet.

Nail Fungus: Avoidance Is Best

Nail fungus doesn't hurt. It won't harm your health. In fact, people won't even notice those thick, raggedy-looking toenails if you keep your shoes on. But this is one tough problem to cure. "There is a race among the drug companies for a cure for nail fungus, and so far, nobody's winning," says Dr. Braver, who tests foot products for one leading company. "If I knew the answer for curing nail fungus, I'd be a very rich man."

Some experts believe that nail fungus is often caused by an immune system problem and aggravated by moisture. So keeping your feet clean and dry is essential for holding nail fungus at bay. While curing it is difficult and needs a doctor's care, especially if your feet tend to be sweaty, here's how to avoid getting it in the first place.

Loosen up. "One way to prevent nail fungus is to make sure your shoes are big enough that toes have room to breathe," says Dr. Braver. "Runners, dancers and other athletes often get nail fungus because they get micro-trauma to their toes from their toes hitting the front of the shoes. If you can, wear looser shoes."

Apply an antiperspirant. Sweating makes matters worse, so prevent a potential problem by treating your feet like underarms—apply a daily dose of roll-on, says Dr. Braver. "There is a prescription product called Drysol made especially for this purpose. It's like using a much stronger underarm antiperspirant."

Foot Odor: The Big Smell

Even if you wash your feet, change your socks daily and make sure that nothing is growing in your shoes, your dogs can still smell bad enough to make those around you want to howl. If foot odor is your problem, here's how to fix it.

Have healthy feet. "Foot odor is usually related to a fungal infection; sweating feet and pimply or peeling skin are the usual warning signs," says Dr. Braver. "So treat foot odor as you would any fungus problem, with an antifungal lotion such as Lotrimin, which is available over the counter."

Spray away the smell. Other ways to kill the smell are to apply Lysol to your shoes and an antiperspirant to your feet, adds Dr. Braver.

Plantar Warts: A Powerful Punch

Like other warts, these ¼-inch nasties that form on the soles of your feet are caused by a virus, which is probably picked up walking barefoot. The problem with plantar warts, however, is that the pressure of walking flattens them until they are covered by calluses. When the calluses harden, you feel the plantar's punch, which is similar to walking on a pebble. "About 13 percent of all plantar warts disappear on their own, with no treatment," says Dr. Braver. "However, several strains of the wart virus have been known to spread rapidly." He advises aggressive treatment to get rid of the warts before this happens. Try these measures.

Eat your vegetables. "There is substantial evidence that vitamin A helps protect against warts," says Dr. Braver. While vitamin A in supplement form can be toxic, you can get this added protection by eating more yellow or orange vegetables and fruits such as carrots, squash, sweet potatoes, cantaloupe, apricots and nectarines as well as green leafy vegetables such as spinach.

Go commercial. Using an over-the-counter wart or corn remover (such as Occlusal) can rid you of plantar warts, says Dr. Braver. These products are available at drugstores.

Don't go barefoot. The best way to avoid plantar warts is to wear shoes or sandals, says Dr. Braver. "It's important to keep the soles of your feet covered, especially when you're around pools and other moist areas that are attractive to the virus." If a family member has a plantar wart, prevent it from spreading by keeping floors and showers clean and disinfected.

See a doctor. If you have tried the above measures for six weeks and notice little improvement, or if the problems are getting worse, see your podiatrist for care. Professional treatment may include freezing or burning the warts and traditional or laser surgical removal methods.

GOUT

Beating the Arthritis
That Prefers Men

If the word *gout* brings to mind the image of an old, scowling, overfed, Charles Laughton type cursing the world as his bandaged foot teeters precariously on a stool, you have a fairly good picture of both the condition and its effect.

For one thing, gout is a predominantly male condition. For another, it can be a hellish experience. "Gout has been described as a man's answer to labor pains," says Jeffrey R. Lisse, M.D., associate professor of medicine and director of the Division of Rheumatology at the University of Texas Medical Branch at Galveston. "The difference is that women eventually come out of labor; gout can linger."

Gout is a form of arthritis that strikes out of thin air. It can affect any joint but often begins by producing a deep, excruciating pain that leaves the big toe swollen, tender and red-hot.

Gout can make you feel old and crotchety. It can also be crippling. One Pearl Harbor–style sneak attack can put you out of commission for days and make getting around difficult for even longer. If the attacks become frequent, you can lose some of the function in the joint. And if the condition is allowed to progress untreated, it can disable a joint totally.

Even though gout is more common as we age, you don't have to be old to be shot down in flames. While most men experience their first attacks in their forties, bouts can occur much earlier. For years, it was thought to be the exclusive domain of royalty and the idle rich (who were paying the price for a life of excess). Today, we know that gout crosses all class and social lines. "The sedentary middle-aged guy who eats and drinks in abundance while his weight and blood pressure go up is a primary target for gout," says David Pisetsky, M.D., medical adviser for the Arthritis Foundation.

The Cause Is Crystal Clear

Your throbbing toe may come on like a bolt out of the blue, but chances are it was years in the making. Normally, your body produces a chemical called uric acid that's excreted through the urine. Some guys produce extremely high levels of this waste product or have trouble urinating it out. It has to go somewhere, and that somewhere can be the skin, the kidneys (where it can form stones) or other parts of the body, usually with little fanfare.

But when this excess uric acid beelines for your joints, watch out. "When uric acid collects in the joints, it forms long, needlelike crystals," says Christopher M. Wise, M.D., associate professor of internal medicine at the Virginia Commonwealth University Medical College of Virginia in Richmond. "These crystals irritate the joint and trigger an extremely violent response."

One reason for astronomical uric acid levels is diet. Certain foods—particularly rich and fatty ones—contain high amounts of purines, chemical substances that turn into uric acid in the blood. But you can't place all the blame on culinary excesses. Often it is an inherited tendency. It can also be related to certain conditions, such as kidney disease. And many medications can produce high uric acid levels.

Give Gout the Kick

Fortunately, there's a lot you can do to deal with gout and make sure it doesn't come back.

Raise your raging joint. During an attack, keep the affected joint elevated and at rest, says Dr. Lisse. Prop it up with some pillows so that it rests several inches above your torso, and try to move it as little as possible. This will drain fluids away from the joint and reduce the inflammation.

Chill out. Applying ice packs for 20 minutes at a time, several times a day, will lessen both pain and inflammation, says Dr. Lisse.

Reach for ibuprofen. When you need fast relief for the pain and swelling, the best over-the-counter product you can use is ibuprofen, says Dr. Pisetsky. The inflammation is the primary cause of the pain, and ibuprofen is a reliable pain-relieving anti-inflammatory. Aspirin, normally an effective pain reliever and anti-inflammatory, can actually raise uric acid levels, making the pain and inflammation worse.

Wet your whistle. Gout-producing uric acid is more likely to crystallize in your joints if you are dehydrated, says Dr. Lisse. Make sure you drink plenty of water every day. It will help the body flush out excess uric acid in your urine.

Lock up the liquor cabinet. Alcohol in the bloodstream causes uric acid levels to go through the roof and inhibits the body's ability to excrete these chemicals, says Dr. Wise. If you are a heavy or frequent drinker, you should either go on the wagon or reduce your consumption significantly. If your uric acid

Hold the Anchovies

Living high on the hog? Love to eat rich, fancy foods? Your expensive tastes may be not only socking it to your wallet but also stabbing you where it really hurts: your aching joints. "Some rich foods are sky-high in purines, compounds that your body turns into uric acid. And a uric acid overdose can trigger a gout attack," says Christopher M. Wise, M.D., associate professor of internal medicine at the Virginia Commonwealth University Medical College of Virginia in Richmond.

"Diet alone will probably not bring on a gout attack. But it's still worthwhile, if you're prone to gout, to limit your intake of high-purine foods," says Dr. Wise.

Here are foods to watch out for.

Foods with Extremely High Purine Levels (probably best to avoid)

Anchovies	Kidneys
Beer	Liver
Brain	Mussels
Fish roe	Sardines
Gravies	Sweetbreads
Heart	Wine
Herring	Yeast

Foods with Moderately High Purine Levels (limit to one daily serving)

Dry beans and peas	Seafood
Meats	Shellfish
Poultry	

levels are already high, one or two nights of debauchery could be enough to send levels into the danger zone.

Slim down. Overweight men run a greater risk of having higher uric acid levels and getting gout, says Dr. Wise.

Avoid crash diets. In general, losing weight is good. But if you lose too much weight too soon, or if you become malnourished, you can actually encourage gout, says Dr. Lisse.

Control your blood pressure—naturally. Because men with gout tend to have high blood pressure, doctors often recommend lowering your blood pressure to prevent future attacks, says Dr. Pisetsky. Unfortunately, certain drugs prescribed to lower blood pressure, such as diuretics, can actually raise uric acid levels. Along with treatment from your doctor, try other proven ways to control high blood pressure, such as losing weight, exercising and watching your intake of sodium, fats and cholesterol.

Get Thee to a Doctor

If you awake one morning in sheer agony, like your big toe is being stabbed with a rusty knife, you'll probably want to get medical help. Your doctor can prescribe medications to stop the inflammation, says Dr. Wise. Popular choices are a drug called colchicine and nonsteroidal anti-inflammatory drugs such asindomethacin (Indameth) and prescription-strength ibuprofen.

If your attacks are frequent or unusually severe, your doctor may prescribe medications to reduce the amount of uric acid in your system and to reverse the deposit of crystals in the joints, says Dr. Wise. Drugs such as allopurinol (Lopurin) and probenecid (Benemid) are very effective at preventing gout attacks, but they must be taken regularly.

GRAY HAIR

Finding Your True Colors

Those new gray hairs make you look so distinguished. You know, experienced. Wise.

That's what your mother says, anyway. But what's she supposed to tell her only son, her baby?

Lately, you've been toying with a few other words to describe your looks. Like grizzled. Paleozoic. Old. Gray hair may look great later in life—but to you, it's a little soon to be a silver fox.

"If you're going gray, I guarantee you're not happy about it," says Philip Kingsley, a hair care specialist based in New York City. "I have seen tens of thousands of people over the years, and none of them wants gray hair. It can really make people feel old before their time."

Pigment Loss: The Root of the Problem

If you're an average guy, you have about 100,000 hairs on your head. Up to now, every one of them has contained melanin, a pigment that gives your hair its color. But for reasons doctors don't know, the pigment cells near the roots of each hair are starting to call it a day. So when a black, brown or blond hair falls out, it's often replaced by a gray one.

A white one, actually. It's just like your old hair, except it has no color. It just looks gray because of the contrast with your other hair.

If you're looking for someone to blame, start with Dad or Aunt Gert or great-grandpa Joe. "There's a very strong hereditary link with gray hair," says Diana Bihova, M.D., clinical assistant professor of dermatology at New York University Medical Center in New York City. "If your family goes gray early, it's very likely you will, too."

One thing you shouldn't blame is stress. Dr. Bihova says that working tense

65-hour weeks won't give you gray hair—unless your stress is so bad that you deplete your store of some B vitamins. The evidence remains sketchy on this.

Overexposure to the sun might also cause hair to gray early, Dr. Bihova says—though the emphasis here is on *might*. The theory is that ultraviolet rays cause pigment cells on your scalp to work overtime, just as they do on your arms or legs when you get a tan. If they work too hard and burn out early, Dr. Bihova says, the result could be prematurely gray hair. Again, there's no concrete evidence, but Dr. Bihova still suggests wearing a hat or using hair products that contain sunscreen. "Let's just say it can't hurt," she says.

The average white male starts developing gray hair at age 34, while the typical black man gets about a ten-year reprieve. Japanese men start the earliest, between 30 and 34. Dr. Bihova says men usually start graying at the temples, then on the sides, the crown and finally the back of the neck. The process can go in fits and starts, with more gray hair growing in some years and less in others.

Eventually, the rule of 50 kicks in, and even the darkest-haired among us start to change. By age 50, Dr. Bihova explains, 50 percent of men will have gone 50 percent gray.

Generally, the hair on your head starts to change first, followed some time later by your beard, the hair on your chest, legs and eyebrows and, finally, your underarm and pubic hair. But again, everyone's different. You may end up with flecks of gray in your beard years before you see it on your head.

The good news in all this is that there's usually nothing physically wrong with getting gray hair. Studies show that people who go gray at an early age are usually not suffering from anything but a case of unwelcome genetics. "And at least you have hair to worry about," Dr. Bihova says. "Most men prefer gray hair to baldness anytime."

The bad news is that graying is irreversible. Scientists don't even know why pigment cells shut down, and they're not really close to finding a way to make your hair change color again.

Is It to Dye For?

So gray hair is on the way. You have two choices. You can accept it as an inescapable, even desirable, part of life. Or you can put it on hold for a while, using some form of hair dye until you're ready to show off the gray.

Here's some expert advice.

Feel the power. Clint Eastwood. Paul Newman. Even Julius Erving. None of these guys looks worried about going gray—and who wants to argue with them? Your initial reaction to gray might be shock. But before you color your hair, take stock of the situation. Does it really make you look old? Or does it add a little maturity? A little savvy? A little power?

"Some people grow to be quite comfortable with gray hair," Kingsley says. "The most important point to remember about gray hair, or hair in general, is

Follicle Fallacies: The Myths of Gray

There's a ton of folklore about gray hair—and precious few good, hard facts. While doctors might not know what causes gray, they do know a few things that won't.

Gray Hair Myth #1: You can go gray instantly because of a shocking event. It's physically impossible. Diana Bihova, M.D., clinical assistant professor of dermatology at New York University Medical Center in New York City, says existing hair won't turn gray. You get gray only when a colored hair falls out and is replaced by a gray one in the same follicle.

Gray Hair Myth #2: Your hair can return to its normal color after it has gone gray. Sorry. When a hair follicle starts producing gray hair, it rarely changes back. There are a few exceptions, Dr. Bihova says. Your hair could temporarily go gray if you have an endocrine gland disorder, are malnourished, suffer an injury or a disease of the nervous system or have an autoimmune disorder. Even then, hair may not return to its original color, she says.

Gray Hair Myth #3: If you pull one gray hair, two more will grow out. Nope. You go gray follicle by follicle. If you pull out a gray hair, it will be replaced by a gray hair in the same follicle. "You can't stop the process," Dr. Bihova says. "But pulling white hairs isn't going to speed it up, either."

that you have to be comfortable with it. If it makes you feel wise or dignified, that's fine."

Keep it short. If you do decide to stay gray, Kingsley suggests keeping your hair cut shport. "It's really simple," Kingsley says. "If you don't want gray hair or you're not sure about it, then short styles leave less gray to show."

Stay wet. Keep gray hair conditioned. It's not any dryer than other hair, but as you get older, your hair and scalp tend to dry out. To keep your gray in tip-top shape, Kingsley suggests using a conditioner each time you shampoo. And he suggests letting your hair air-dry once in a while, instead of using a blow dryer.

Set the tone. So you tried the gray look for a little while, and it's not for you—not yet, anyway. Well, maybe it's time to add some color. You won't be alone. In 1993, men spent $52.8 million on hair coloring products—most of it, Kingsley says, to cover up the gray.

"And there are lots more men who want to do something about it," he says.

"But a lot of them are afraid to take the first step, be it dyes or whatever."

Here are two hair-coloring choices.

Hit the highlights. This technique utilizes dye to subtly blend away the gray by coloring scattered strands of hair. Choose a color that's a couple of shades lighter than your natural hair.

Lighter dyes also help avoid unsightly gray roots.

Engage in a cover-up. The experts call this process color, meaning you're making all your hair one shade. If you opt for this, stay away from the darkest shades, which tend to make your hair look flat and unnatural. "Black colors don't really work well," Kingsley says. "All the hair is colored exactly the same, and you can instantly see that it's dyed."

There's also some question about whether dark hair dyes can cause cancer. Some studies have linked use of such dyes to increased risk of bone cancer and lymphoma.

The bottom line? "There isn't one yet," says Sheila Hoar Zahm, Ph.D., an epidemiologist at the National Cancer Institute in Rockville, Maryland. "The risk of getting cancer from hair dye isn't as high as getting lung cancer from smoking. But we definitely need to study the relationship further."

Just dye it. Kingsley says you should be wary of progressive dyes that promise to slowly hide your gray hair so that "no one will even notice." He says these products can give your hair an unnatural, yellowish green tint. They can also dry out your hair, making it unmanageable and brittle.

And once you start using them, it's hard to switch over to a regular dye. "That can turn your hair all sorts of colors that you would never want hair to be," Kingsley says.

Semipermanent dyes that wash out over several weeks offer somewhat better color but are not as good as permanent dyes. If you want to try a slow route to darker hair, Kingsley suggests doing it with increasingly darker permanent dyes.

HEARING LOSS

Silence Isn't Always Golden

Real men don't wear earplugs. At least that's what you thought. So for years, you worked at a noisy job, listened to loud rock 'n' roll and cut firewood with a shrill chain saw without so much as a flimsy piece of cotton in your ears.

But yesterday your wife asked you to go to the grocery store to get eggs, milk and boring jewels. Boring jewels?

"What?" you said. So she repeated herself a little louder, but you still didn't get it. What kind of power tools can you get at a grocery store? *"Orange juice!"* she finally screamed in exasperation. "Geez, you're getting to be more and more like a little old man every day."

You let it go, but deep down, you wonder if she's right. Is time catching up with you, even though you have a decade or two before retirement?

"Hearing loss is occurring at younger and younger ages and is more prevalent than is generally thought," says J. Gail Neely, M.D., professor and director of otology, neurotology and base of skull surgery at Washington University School of Medicine in St. Louis.

Overall, about 13 million men have significant hearing impairment, and at least 4.2 million of those men are under age 45, according to the American Speech-Language-Hearing Association. In a survey of 2,731 people with hearing impairment, nearly 57 percent said they first noticed the problem before age 40, says Laurel E. Glass, M.D., Ph.D., professor emeritus and former director of the Center on Deafness at the University of California, San Francisco, School of Medicine.

The toll of that hearing loss is enormous, doctors say. It can lead to social isolation, limit your job prospects, complicate your sex life, rob you of your self-esteem and make you feel as if life's parade is passing you by.

The Five-Minute Hearing Test

Suddenly, everyone around you mumbles, mutters or whispers. Could it be that you have a hearing problem? To find out, take this quiz prepared by the American Academy of Otolaryngology–Head and Neck Surgery. Your choices are almost always (A), half the time (H), occasionally (O) and never (N).

1. I have a problem hearing over the phone.
2. I have trouble following conversation when two or more people are talking at the same time.
3. People complain that I turn the TV volume too high.
4. I have to strain to understand conversations.
5. I miss hearing some common sounds, such as the phone or doorbell ringing.
6. I have trouble hearing conversations in a noisy background, such as at a party.
7. I get confused about where sounds come from.
8. I misunderstand some words in a sentence and need to ask people to repeat themselves.
9. I especially have trouble understanding the speech of women and children.
10. I have worked in noisy environments (on assembly lines, with jack-hammers, near jet engines and so on).
11. I hear fine—if people just speak clearly.
12. People get annoyed because I misunderstand what they say.
13. I misunderstand what others are saying and make inappropriate responses.
14. I avoid social activities because I cannot hear well and fear I'll reply improperly.

To be answered by a family member or friend:

15. Do you think this person has a hearing loss?

Scoring

Give yourself three points for each "almost always," two points for every "half the time," one point for every "occasionally" and no points for every "never."

0 to 5. Your hearing is fine.

6 to 9. The academy suggests that you see an ear, nose and throat specialist.

10 and above. The academy strongly recommends that you see an ear, nose and throat specialist.

Hear Ye, Hear Ye

Before looking at why men have hearing problems, it's important to understand how your ears work. When your best friend tells you about his date Saturday night, the sound of his voice enters your ear canal and strikes the eardrum, a cone-shaped elastic membrane stretched across the end of the canal. As the eardrum vibrates, it causes tiny bones in the middle ear to move back and forth. These movements trigger small waves of fluid in the inner ear that ripple through a small shaped organ called the cochlea. Inside the cochlea, 30,000 hairlike cells transmit impulses to the auditory nerve, which carries the sounds to the brain. There they are interpreted as the funniest story you've ever heard, and you laugh.

Some hearing loss is a natural part of aging, says Debra Busacco, Ph.D., audiologist and coordinator of the Lifelong Learning Institute at Gallaudet University in Washington, D.C., the world's only liberal arts university for the deaf. The eardrum stiffens with age, reducing its ability to vibrate. Age-related changes to the bones in the middle ear, such as the degeneration of joints and calcium deposits in those joints, cause the middle ear system to become stiffer, resulting in less effective transmission of sound. Over time, irreplaceable hair cells in the inner ear are damaged by a combination of aging, noise exposure, medication, decreased blood supply to the ear and infection. And once the hair cells are damaged, the auditory nerve becomes less efficient. But most of those changes don't occur until a man is in his late forties and early fifties.

If symptoms of hearing loss appear at an earlier age, the cause could be something as simple as excessive earwax or the very rare side effect of a medication. It can also be caused by a shattered eardrum, a head injury, high blood pressure, ear infection, meningitis or a tumor. Some types of hearing loss run in families, such as otosclerosis, a disease that causes excessive bone deposits in the middle ear and prevents it from conducting sounds to the inner ear, says John House, M.D., associate clinical professor of otolaryngology at the University of Southern California in Los Angeles.

But the most common cause of hearing loss in adults under age 50 is excessive noise exposure, says Susan Rezen, Ph.D., professor of audiology at Worchester State College in Worcester, Massachusetts, and author of *Coping with Hearing Loss.*

"There are no continuous loud sounds such as rock concerts or jackhammers in nature. Our ears were designed to be sensitive, so our ancestors could have heard a twig snap, which might have meant food or danger was nearby. So when you go into a noisy environment, you're putting yourself into an environment that your ears simply weren't designed to handle," says Flash Gordon, M.D., a primary care physician in San Rafael, California, and co-founder of Hearing Education and Awareness for Rockers (HEAR), a San Francisco–based nonprofit organization that encourages high-decibel musicians and fans to turn down the volume and wear earplugs.

Sudden loud noises close to the ear, such as firecrackers or gunshots, can cause immediate hearing loss. But usually, noise-induced hearing loss happens gradually, over years. In general, the longer you expose yourself to sounds louder than 85 decibels, whether it's a rock concert or a leaf blower, the more likely you are to harm the inner ear and damage your hearing, Dr. Rezen says.

How Loud Is Loud?

Decibels are how hearing experts measure sound intensity (sound pressure), beginning with the softest sound a person can hear in a laboratory setting, which is 0 decibels. Using this system, 20 decibels is 10 times more intense than 0, 40 decibels is 100 times more intense, 60 decibels is 1,000 times more intense, and so on.

So how loud is 85 decibels? That's about the same amount of noise as a vacuum cleaner, a food blender or a power lawn mower. In contrast, a normal conversation is about 65 decibels. Noise levels at some rock concerts may exceed nearly 140 decibels, a level that can cause rapid and irreparable hearing damage in some sensitive ears. Even symphony orchestras can generate sounds louder than 110 decibels, which can cause ear discomfort and pain in some people.

In fact, just one two-hour rock concert can potentially age a guy's hearing by nearly two years if he doesn't wear ear protection, according to calculations by Daniel Johnson, Ph.D., an engineer who tests hearing protectors for the military at Kirtland Air Force Base in Albuquerque, New Mexico. Based on that, he estimates that after 50 concerts, the same guy could have a decline in hearing similar to a man 12 years older who hasn't been exposed to high noise levels. In addition, if a 30-year-old guy who doesn't wear earplugs began working eight hours a day near machinery that produces noise averaging 95 decibels, by age 40 he could have the high-frequency hearing loss of a 60-year-old.

Louder Isn't Better

But of course, most of us have gone to loud concerts, stood by passing trains or worked near noisy equipment such as chain saws. So what exactly are those noises doing to your hearing?

Try this the next time you go to a rock concert or a loud event, Dr. Gordon suggests. Before you leave your car, tune to a talk radio station and turn down the volume to where you can just barely understand all the words. Then after the concert but before starting your engine, turn on the radio. Chances are the voices that were understandable before the concert won't be then.

That's what doctors call a temporary hearing threshold shift. Basically, it means that the noise has overstimulated the hair cells in your inner ear. As a result, the hair cells aren't functioning as efficiently as they usually do, so sounds have to be louder for you to hear them, Dr. Neely says. Researchers at the University of Manitoba in Manitoba, Winnipeg, for example, tested the hearing of 11 men before and after a 2½-hour rock concert. For most of the guys, the threshold of their ability to hear was ten or more decibels higher after the concert than before.

That may not sound like much, but for several hours you'd probably have difficulty hearing rustling leaves or whispered conversation. Fortunately, your hearing would return to normal within 24 hours.

But a temporary threshold shift is a warning sign that your hearing is at risk if you continue to expose yourself to loud sounds. Some people never experience temporary threshold shifts and mistakenly assume that they are immune to the dangers of loud noise, Dr. Neely says. In truth, repeated exposure to loud noises can gradually kill off hair cells and permanently damage your ability to hear, particularly high-frequency sounds such as the consonants *sh*, *ch*, *t*, *f*, *h* and *s*, which are frequently used in conversation.

"If you miss hearing those high-frequency sounds, the remaining part of a word won't make sense to you," Dr. Neely says. "You literally won't know if people around you are talking about fish or tin cans. That can be very confusing and frustrating."

Protecting Your Ears

Although most of us will suffer some hearing loss due to aging, you can keep your hearing sharp well into your golden years if you protect your ears from noise now. "Imagine that your hearing is a big barrel of sand," Dr. Gordon says. "Either you can empty it out gradually with a teaspoon, so it will last a long time, or you can use a shovel and run out of it a lot sooner." Here are some ways to prevent hearing loss.

Turn it down. You probably can't do much about traffic noise, jackhammers and many other sources of excessive sound. But you can turn down the volume on your stereo, says Stephen Painton, Ph.D., an audiologist at the University of Oklahoma Health Sciences Center in Oklahoma City. Some sound systems can produce noise equal to the loudest rock concerts. As a general rule, you shouldn't be able to hear your stereo from outside your home when your door is closed. If you can, it's too loud. The same rule applies to your car radio. If you use headphones or a personal stereo, someone standing next to you shouldn't be able to hear the sound.

If you have to shout, get out. If you have to raise your voice to be heard by someone standing a foot or two away from you, that's a clear warning that the noise level may be dangerous, and you should get away from it as soon as possible or wear ear protection, Dr. House says.

Keep plugs handy. Stuffing cotton or pieces of crumpled tissue into your ears does virtually nothing to minimize damage to your hearing. Instead, get in the habit of carrying earplugs with you, Dr. Busacco says. Most earplugs are small and will fit in your pocket. That way, she says, you'll be prepared for unexpected noise. The foam rubber types are good because they're inexpensive and available over the counter at most drugstores and they can be quickly rolled up and placed in your ears. Look for the noise reduction rating on the side of the box, Dr. Painton says. This will tell you how many decibels of sound the earplugs will muffle. Buy plugs that have a rating of at least 15; they'll reduce noise by 15 decibels and slash the chances that your hearing will be damaged. If you want better protection, an audiologist can design a pair of custom-made plugs for about $80 that reduce noise by about 35 decibels, Dr. Busacco says.

Take time-outs. The longer you expose yourself to loud sounds without a break, the more likely you are to cause permanent damage to your hearing, even if you're wearing earplugs. So give your ears a 5- or 10-minute break from noise every 30 minutes, Dr. Gordon says. "It's like putting your head underwater for 20 minutes. You can do it if you hold your breath for a minute at a time, then take a 10-second break. But if you'd try to do it in two 10-minute segments, you'd be dead. If you give your ears an occasional break, they can rest and recover from the excessive work that loud noise makes them do."

Spread out the noise. Placing several loud appliances or power tools near each other will compound your noise problem. So if your TV set is in the same room as your dishwasher, for example, you might be tempted to turn up the TV volume excessively when you do a load of dishes. Instead, move the television into a quieter room, says Lt. Col. Richard Danielson, Ph.D., supervisor of audiology in the Army Audiology and Speech Center at Walter Reed Army Medical Center in Washington, D.C.

Swab the deck, not your ears. Attempting to clean wax out of your ears with a cotton swab, matchstick or anything else smaller than an aircraft carrier does more harm than good, Dr. House says. Earwax is actually good for you. It repels water and helps keep dust away from your sensitive eardrum. Sticking small objects in your ear pushes the wax farther into your ear and can cause infection. "The best thing to do about earwax inside the ear canal is leave it alone," Dr. House says. If it becomes bothersome, see your physician or get an over-the-counter earwax removal kit that contains drops that will soften the wax and allow it to flow naturally out of your ear.

Muzzle your medication. Taking six to eight aspirin a day can cause ringing in your ears and temporary hearing loss, Dr. Gordon says. Antibiotics such as gentamicin, streptomycin and tobramycin can also damage your hearing, says Barry E. Hirsch, M.D., a neurotologist at the University of Pittsburgh School of Medicine. If you are taking any drug and develop hearing problems, tell your doctor.

Stop smoking. Smoking reduces blood flow to the ears and may interfere with the natural healing of small blood vessels that occurs after exposure to loud noise, Dr. House says. In a study of 2,348 workers exposed to noise at an aerospace factory, researchers at the University of Southern California School of Medicine found that smokers had greater hearing loss than nonsmokers. So if you smoke, quit.

Slash the java. Like nicotine, caffeine cuts blood flow to the ears, increasing your chances of hearing loss, Dr. House says. Drink no more than two eight-ounce cups of coffee or tea a day. If possible, drink decaffeinated brews.

Balance your diet. The same fatty and cholesterol-laden foods that are bad for your heart also endanger your ears, Dr. House says. Both high blood pressure and fatty deposits in your arteries can reduce blood flow to the ears and gradually strangle your hearing. So eat a balanced daily diet that includes at least five servings of fruits and vegetables, six servings of breads and grains and no more than one three-ounce serving (about the size of your wallet) of lean red meat, poultry or fish.

Exercise. Walk, run, swim or do any other aerobic exercise for 20 minutes a day, three times a week, Dr. House suggests. It will stimulate blood circulation, lower your blood pressure and help keep your ears in peak condition.

Making the Best of It

The average person waits five to seven years to seek help for a hearing problem. Those can be years of unnecessary social isolation and frustration, Dr. Busacco says. The earlier you seek help, the sooner the problem can be diagnosed and treated. "People are a lot more self-conscious about their hearing than they are about their vision," Dr. Hirsch says. "It's often an issue of vanity. Wearing a hearing aid somehow implies aging, while wearing glasses doesn't."

If you suspect that you have a hearing problem, particularly if you have ringing in your ears or develop a sudden sensitivity to loud noises that didn't bother you in the past, see your doctor or a physician who specializes in diseases of the ear, nose and throat. Some hearing problems such as Ménière's disease, a disorder that causes ringing in the ears and dizziness, can be treated with prescription medication or surgery. Other conditions, such as perforated eardrums and otosclerosis, may be corrected with surgery.

Even if the loss can't be fully corrected, powerful but inconspicuous hearing aids—some small enough to fit inside the ear canal—are available to help you get back in touch with the world. Prices range from about $550 for a basic hearing aid to more than $2,500 for top-of-the-line computerized models. An audiologist, a professional trained to fit hearing aids, can help you choose one that fits your needs.

Here's how to recognize if you have a hearing loss and how to cope with it.

Tune in to your turn signal. Sure, it's annoying when you drive down the road and realize that your turn signal has been on for miles, but it could also be a clue that you have a hearing problem. If you flip on your turn signal and can't hear the accompanying clicking sound in your car, it's time to get your hearing checked by an audiologist or doctor, Dr. Painton says.

Don't be shy about it. If you have difficulty hearing or understanding people, tell them, says Philip Zazove, M.D., assistant professor of family medicine at the University of Michigan Medical School in Ann Arbor who has had profound hearing loss since birth. Simply saying "I don't hear as well as I used to," "Could you repeat that?" and "Talk a little slower" can prevent a lot of mis-

The Noisy Sounds of Silence

The supersonic blast of rock 'n' roll reverberated in your ears as you danced the night away at the hottest club in town. But since then, you've heard a less welcome sound—a relentless ringing in your ears that has sapped your energy, disrupted your sleep and nearly driven you insane.

You could be one of the 3.6 million American men who endure chronic tinnitus, a baffling ear problem that causes annoying ringing, humming or buzzing in the ears, says Christopher Linstrom, M.D., director of otology and neurotology at the New York Eye and Ear Infirmary in New York City. Tinnitus can be a symptom of everything from excessive earwax to high blood pressure to heart disease. Both tinnitus and hyperacusis—an extreme sensitivity to sounds—can also be signs of noise-induced hearing loss caused by damage to the hair cells in the inner ear that conduct sound to the auditory nerve and brain. In fact, 95 percent of men who have tinnitus also have some hearing loss, says John House, M.D., associate clinical professor of otolaryngology at the University of Southern California in Los Angeles.

Hyperacusis causes individual hair cells, each of which is normally stimulated only by certain frequencies, to react to the same range of sounds. As a result, more and more hair cells vibrate in unison, and that

understandings, frustration and anger, he says. If necessary, ask the person to repeat himself, or if you have trouble with a key word, have him write it on a piece of paper.

Find a quiet spot. If you really want to talk to an interesting woman at a party, move away from the middle of the room and into a quieter corner. Not only is that more intimate, you can concentrate on what she's saying and don't have to compete with laughter, music and other background noise, Dr. Zazove says. At home, consider turning off the television, radio or other noisy appliances before you try to listen to someone.

Light up your sex life. Hearing loss can cause havoc in the bedroom. Those whispered sweet nothings you used to enjoy so much when you were making love are often the first casualty. Leave in your hearing aid if there is any possibility of sex, or ask your partner to leave on the light so that you can see well enough to lip-read, Dr. Rezen suggests. Talk about what you want sexually before you go into the bedroom. If necessary, develop your own secret code, such as "Two taps on the back means kiss me."

can make the quietest noises seem loud and jarring. When this damage occurs, sounds that are quite tolerable to many people can be painful to you, says Lt. Col. Richard Danielson, Ph.D., supervisor of audiology in the Army Audiology and Speech Center at Walter Reed Army Medical Center in Washington, D.C.

In some cases, tinnitus can be treated with drugs or surgery, particularly if it's caused by excessive fluid in the middle ear, high blood pressure, a partially blocked artery in the neck or allergies. But in most instances, there is no cure for either tinnitus or hyperacusis, Dr. Linstrom says.

Once tinnitus or hyperacusis is diagnosed, you should avoid loud noises and wear earplugs to prevent more hearing damage that can make these conditions worse. Masking devices that produce pleasant sounds such as raindrops or ocean waves can help men with tinnitus drown out the ringing their ears, Dr. Linstrom says. Caffeine and nicotine aggravate the symptoms, so quit smoking and avoid coffee, tea and chocolate, he says. Some medications such as aspirin, antibiotics and anti-cancer drugs can also cause tinnitus. A hearing aid might help, because the better you hear, the less noticeable the ringing may be, Dr. House says.

If you suspect that you have tinnitus, see your doctor or write to the American Tinnitus Association, P.O. Box 5, Portland OR 97207.

"If you don't plan, you may lose the opportunity altogether," she says.

Laugh it off. A good sense of humor is vital if you have a hearing problem, particularly during sex, says Rick Ledbetter, a 45-year-old songwriter in North Hollywood, California, who has had severe hearing loss for about five years. He recalls, for example, a night when things didn't go smoothly. "We finally arrived in bed together, and she tenderly reached up to caress my ears with her hands. That caused feedback in my hearing aids. *Screech.* It was a case of instant wilt, if you know what I mean. But we had a good laugh about it and went on from there."

Do your homework. If you're attending an important business meeting or conference, get there early and try to nab a front row seat facing the person who you think will do most of the talking, Dr. Zazove says. If possible, tell the speaker about your hearing loss and ask him to avoid turning away from you. Maintain eye contact with the speaker. Try to get a written summary of the topic or agenda, so you'll be prepared for words or phases that might come up. That way, if you do miss a few words, you'll have a better chance of filling them in accurately.

HEART ATTACK

Something You Can Live Without

Every so often you hear a story about some young man cut down in his prime by a heart attack. And you wonder "Can it happen to me?"

It's an unsettling question—one that makes you feel like an old man worried about his vitality and mortality. In most cases, however, heart attacks spare younger men. In fact, experts say that only 12 percent of heart attacks occur in men ages 44 and under.

As uncommon as heart attacks may be, that doesn't mean you need not be concerned about having one. In fact, as men get older, the possibility of a heart attack can become a worrisome fact of life.

Few things can age you as rapidly as a heart attack. It can strike like lightning, though the stage may have been set with years of fatty deposits forming on your coronary arteries.

Inner Chaos

By definition, a heart attack is a reduction or blockage of blood flow in a coronary artery that causes potentially life-threatening damage to the heart. Nearly one million men have heart attacks each year, often visited by the crushing chest pain, heavy sweating and shortness of breath that are signs of a sudden clot in the coronary artery and its effect on the heart. One-third of these heart attacks are fatal. Four in five heart attack deaths occur in those ages 65 and older.

As you age, your heart and the blood vessels that nourish it begin to show and feel their age, even without the dramatic intrusion of a heart attack. The heart will gradually start to pump a little less efficiently, and the walls of the arteries will become a little stiffer and less flexible.

But a heart attack is something different. In minutes or hours, it can take a devastating toll upon your heart, as though you were adding 20 or 30 years to your age overnight. As the supply of blood to your heart is impaired, the heart cells can become severely injured. The longer this blood flow is interfered with, the greater the chance of irreversible damage, producing cell death and the demise of part of your heart muscle.

But there's good news, too. Most heart attacks are preventable if you adopt lifestyle habits that can slow the buildup of fatty deposits in your coronary arteries. Yes, there are exceptions to this rule. On rare occasions, for example, stress might set off a heart attack, even in a young person without heavily clogged blood vessels. "Coronary arteries can go into spasm in stressful situations, which can reduce the blood flow to the heart," says James Martin, M.D., a family physician with the Institute for Urban Family Health at Beth Israel Medical Center in New York City. "If the spasm lasts long enough—for about seven to ten minutes—you can have a heart attack."

But don't panic. That type of scenario is extremely rare. Whether you ever have a heart attack is, in most cases, much within your control.

Fight the Good Fight

So where do you begin? Here are some crucial strategies to keep in mind.

Know the score. "It's important to know where you stand," advises Richard Helfant, M.D., vice chairman of medicine and director of the Cardiology Training Program at the University of California, Irvine, Medical Center. That means being aware of the risk factors that may increase your chances of having heart problems, he says. As a man, you risk getting heart problems earlier than your wife or sister just by virtue of your sex. If close relatives have had heart attacks at early ages—less than 55—you also need to be extra cautious. And if you have conditions that increase your risk that you can change or control—high blood pressure, an elevated blood cholesterol level, diabetes or cigarette smoking—you need to attack them before they attack your heart. Talk to your doctor about how to do that.

Toe the line. No one is asking you to be a fanatic—to swear off red meat for good or train for the next Boston Marathon. But if you live a reasonably careful, energetic lifestyle, you can keep your heart beating with the vigor of a man much younger, with less worry about the Big One.

Two tips in particular are worth re-emphasizing here, since they serve as the foundation of any program for creating a safe haven for your heart.

Get active. If you're one of those people who feel more comfortable with TV remote control devices in their hands than with tennis rackets or basketballs, it's time for a change of heart. Regular exercise, such as brisk walking for just 20 minutes at least three times a week or some laps in the pool, can turn that pump in your chest into a mean machine.

"Exercise is beneficial for your heart in a number of ways," says Stephen

Havas, M.D., associate professor of epidemiology and preventive medicine at the University of Maryland School of Medicine in Baltimore. "It can boost your HDL (high-density lipoprotein) cholesterol, which is the protective component of your blood cholesterol level. It also can modestly decrease your blood pressure and help you control your weight." It can help keep your heart fit and conditioned, too, just as it gets the other muscles in your body into shape.

Eat like every bite counts. It's not a magic bullet, but proper diet can be the heart and soul of any personalized cardiac care program. Research shows that the best way to keep your heart out of danger is to slash the fat and cholesterol in your diet, says Fredric J. Pashkow, M.D., medical director of the Cardiac Health Improvement and Rehabilitation Program at the Cleveland Clinic Foundation in Cleveland. That means when it comes to menu planning, choose fish more often than steak, skim milk more frequently than whole milk, egg whites rather than whole eggs and low-fat frozen yogurt instead of ice cream. Keep your daily dietary fat intake to 25 percent or less of your total calories.

After You've Been Struck

Prevention may sound good, but what if you've already endured a heart attack? Well, count your blessings that you survived it—and then make a commitment to some health habits that might keep you from going through it a second time and that might put you on the fast track to a zestful, healthful life. If you've bought into the belief that a heart attack will permanently impair your mobility, activity level, job function or sex life, it's time to dispel those myths. Despite your heart attack, your best years can still be ahead of you.

"With lifestyle changes, you may be able to reduce your risk of having another heart attack," says Dr. Helfant. "These changes will also allow you to take control of your health and live a purposeful, meaningful life while protecting yourself to the maximum degree possible."

So what kind of action should you take? The recommendations may sound familiar, but here's the specific impact they can have when a heart attack is part of your medical history.

Eat healthfully. After something as major as a heart attack, you might think the damage that has been done to your heart makes simple measures such as healthier eating about as helpful as applying a Band-Aid to your chest. But when researchers at the National Heart, Lung and Blood Institute conducted an analysis of studies of heart attack survivors, they found that people could significantly decrease their chances of having another heart attack by reducing their high blood cholesterol readings. Various studies have shown that declines in blood cholesterol levels of 10 percent cut the risk of having a second heart attack by between 12 and 19 percent. A key to lowering blood cholesterol is cutting back on saturated fat (the kind found in animal products and tropical oils) and dietary cholesterol (found in most animal products).

Make your moves. In many programs for heart attack recovery, physical activity is the center of attention, often beginning at very modest levels even while patients are still hospitalized. Most cardiac rehabilitation programs recommend exercising for 15 to 30 minutes at least three times a week.

"People who have done no exercise in the past would certainly be better off doing even a little bit now," says Peter Wood, Ph.D., professor of medicine emeritus and associate director of the Stanford University Center for Research in Disease Prevention in Palo Alto, California. By gradually increasing the amount of physical activity you do—with your doctor's guidance—your heart will reap even more benefits, Dr. Wood says. And perhaps you'll avoid another ambulance ride to the emergency room.

Pop an aspirin. In this age of high-powered, high-priced medications, can a simple aspirin make you the picture of health? An American Heart Association team of researchers analyzed six studies in which people were given aspirin after heart attacks. This inexpensive white pill reduced the death rate from heart disease between 5 and 42 percent and cut the rate of subsequent nonfatal heart attacks between 12 and 57 percent.

One other piece of good news: You needn't go overboard on aspirin dosages. "A baby aspirin a day is all that's necessary," says Dr. Helfant. Nevertheless, some people should probably stay away from aspirin completely, despite its potential benefits. "If you have a bleeding disorder or an ulcer, for example, taking aspirin is not a good idea," says Julie Buring, Sc.D., associate professor of ambulatory care and prevention at Harvard Medical School in Boston. She suggests talking with your doctor before taking aspirin.

HEART DISEASE

You Can Make the Beat Go On and On...

You're a man, and you're getting older. When it comes to heart health, this is a serious combination.

Increased age and being male are two of the leading risk factors for heart disease—that is, they are among the characteristics (along with smoking, excess weight and others) that can increase your chances of developing problems. Simply by virtue of your gender and your age, you run a greater chance of developing heart disease than either a woman or a younger man.

Naturally, heart disease is something we can all do without. In its minor form, angina, heart disease can knock the youthfulness out of a man by winding him and giving him chest pains after every exertion. At its worst, heart disease kills. Heart attack is the number one killer of men in the United States, claiming more than 250,000 male lives a year.

That may sound grim. But there's no need to resign yourself to a life of worry. True, you can't change your age, your sex or any inherited tendency toward heart disease. But that doesn't mean there are no other influences you can alter. In fact, there is a lot you can do to keep heart disease at bay.

Committing to Change

Heart disease doesn't happen overnight. Most heart disease results from a narrowing of the coronary arteries, known as atherosclerosis, over decades. What makes arteries narrow? Largely, it's the way we Americans live our lives. In some other countries, where lifestyles are simpler, arteries are healthy and wide open, even in the very elderly.

The encouraging news for American men is pretty straightforward: Progres-

162

If the Worst Happens

Sometimes even the most conscientious efforts at prevention just aren't enough. If you start to feel the warning signs of a heart attack—such as pressure or squeezing sensations in the chest, pain shooting into the shoulders, arms or neck or shortness of breath and nausea—you need to react quickly.

As the American Heart Association warns, "Delay can be deadly!"

Clot-dissolving drugs called thrombolytics are administered in the emergency room and can restore blood flow, thus minimizing damage to the heart muscle. But time is crucial. "The later you come in to the emergency room, the less likely a thrombolytic is going to be effective," says Gerald Pohost, M.D., director of the Division of Cardiovascular Disease at the University of Alabama School of Medicine in Birmingham. "The first two hours are the best time, but as time passes, the success of these drugs diminishes."

---

sion of heart disease can be slowed, and in some cases reversed, without drugs or surgery. But don't think you have to go to extremes or have a will of steel to do so. "Moderate changes go a long way," says Richard Helfant, M.D., vice chairman of medicine and director of the Cardiology Training Program at the University of California, Irvine, Medical Center. "You don't have to be a fanatic or be perfect to make a difference in your health."

Let's look at some strategies that can keep your heart pulsating and pounding as though it inherited an extra decade or two of life.

Say good-bye to cigarettes. Okay, maybe you've smoked for years and even tried to quit with no luck. But a lot of ex-smokers successfully stopped only after their second, third or even sixth attempts. So don't give up.

Why not? The American Heart Association reports that when you smoke, your blood vessels constrict. That places extra strain on your heart. But that isn't all. Cigarette smoke also forces your heart to beat more rapidly and raises your blood pressure. According to the American Heart Association, cigarettes directly cause nearly one-fifth of all deaths from heart disease.

Cut your cholesterol. Everyone needs at least some of this substance in his body for essential body functions to take place. But the truth is that your own liver produces all the cholesterol your body requires.

So if your diet leans too heavily on high-fat, high-cholesterol foods, your total blood cholesterol readings are likely to go up. A total cholesterol of below 200 milligrams per deciliter of blood, or mg/dl, is what you need to shoot for.

Get up to 240 or above, and you're at a perilous level that will double your chances of heart disease.

By making some leaner food choices, however, you can get yourself on a heart-healthy track—perhaps even reversing atherosclerosis.

When Dean Ornish, M.D., president and director of the Preventive Medicine Research Institute in Sausalito, California, put people on a comprehensive lifestyle program that included a very low fat diet, moderate exercise, smoking cessation and stress management training, 82 percent of them experienced a significant regression of the fatty deposits that had clogged their coronary arteries after one year.

But don't think that to prevent heart disease you need to adopt a deprivation diet that's just a step above a hunger strike. "No one ever got a heart attack from a steak or a piece of pie," says Dr. Helfant. "We're talking about an overall change in lifestyle and not worrying about an occasional slip." The trick is to limit fat intake to no more than 25 percent of calories over the long term.

Tip the triglyceride scale. As if cholesterol weren't enough to worry about, you and your doctor should keep tabs on your triglycerides, too. They are a type of fat in the bloodstream, and though they appear to play a role in heart disease, their exact role in that process is still not as clear as the link between cholesterol and heart problems.

Many experts say that a triglyceride level above 200 mg/dl should serve as a warning flag. What's one of the best ways to temper your triglycerides? Regular exercise, says Peter Wood, Ph.D., professor of medicine emeritus and associate director of the Stanford University Center for Research in Disease Prevention in Palo Alto, California.

Sweat a little. Sure, it's tempting to toss out the jogging shoes and spend every weekend planted like Gibraltar in front of the television, with your activity limited to punching the buttons on the remote control. If that's your idea of Shangri-la, you're not alone—but you are paying a price. In fact, almost 60 percent of American men don't exercise, a lifestyle choice that greatly increases their risk of heart attack.

Exercise can do more than just get you some fresh air and make you feel more invigorated. "It strengthens the heart muscle," says Dr. Wood. "With regular exercise, the heart becomes a more efficient pump. As a result, the heart rate becomes slower for a given amount of effort." Each beat is more efficient, he says, and so the heart doesn't need to work as hard as it would if you were out of shape.

Even moderate amounts of exercise are better than none. In fact, John J. Duncan, Ph.D., chief of clinical applications at the Cooper Institute for Aerobics Research in Dallas, found that while overall fitness improved when exercisers walked at faster rather than more moderate paces, even leisurely strolls raised levels of HDL (high-density lipoprotein) cholesterol, the good kind, by 6 percent. You don't need to push yourself to the point of exhaustion to reap the benefits of physical activity.

Trim your gut. In a country that seems obsessed with slogans like "Thin is in," a lot of us could never be mistaken for being undernourished. About 15 million American men are a bit more than pleasantly plump (approximately 20 percent or more over their desirable weights). It's a little like playing Russian roulette with their hearts. Data from the Framingham Heart Study indicate that men who weigh more than 30 percent over their desirable weights double their chances of heart disease.

So whether or not you consider flab to be unattractive, it's clearly hazardous to your health. "If you're obese, the heart has to work harder to move nutrients to the additional cells in your body," says James Martin, M.D., family physician with the Institute for Urban Family Health at Beth Israel Medical Center in New York City. That extra strain on the heart can be particularly worrisome if you already have other risk factors that can contribute to heart disease, such as high cholesterol or high blood pressure. (Being overweight also adds to the likelihood that you will have high cholesterol and high blood pressure.) Set some goals for shedding that stockiness by relying more on low-fat foods and getting more exercise.

Pump iron. The typical loss of muscle that occurs as we age can also increase the risk of heart disease, says Brent M. Egan, M.D., associate professor of pharmacology and medicine at the Medical University of South Carolina in Charleston. Unfortunately, when muscle is replaced by fat, you can end up with

Are You an Apple or a Pear?

In the fruit basket, pears tend to age somewhat faster than apples. But when it comes to your heart—and "pear" and "apple" are describing different body shapes—the pear definitely ages slower.

Unfortunately, most obese men tend to be shaped like apples (with their extra weight tucked into the midsection) rather than pears (with the fat around their hips). Studies clearly show that an apple shape creates a higher risk of heart attack (as well as of diabetes, stroke and high blood pressure).

Why is a beer belly so malicious? No one really knows for sure. One theory is that abdominal fat is more easily converted into cholesterol.

No matter what the cause turns out to be, however, experts advise you to trim the size of your own "apple" by losing a few of those extra pounds. Here's a guideline to keep in mind: To cut your risk, your waist measurement should not be more than 90 percent of your hip measurement.

an increased risk of heart disease, similar to that of an obese person, even if your weight stays the same. The easiest way to combat this, suggests Dr. Egan, is to add some muscle-building exercise to your routine.

Consider aspirin. It may not be the fountain of youth, but the drug that can keep your heart vital may be as close as the medicine cabinet in your bathroom. Aspirin, the tiny white pill that has been relied on a zillion times to zap headaches and other mild pain problems, appears to be a heart saver as well.

The Physicians' Health Study at Harvard Medical School in Boston, involving more than 22,000 healthy male doctors ages 40 to 84, found that those who popped one adult aspirin (325 milligrams) every other day slashed their chances of a first heart attack by 44 percent. But particularly if you're prone to bleeding problems, consult your doctor before self-prescribing aspirin, since it's a medication that discourages blood clotting in your body.

Comfort your hostile heart. For nearly four decades, heart experts have been hanging the scarlet A on people who are hard-driving, competitive and often hostile. These Type A personalities, say the experts, are much more likely to be mauled by life's stresses, with their hearts suffering hurricane-like beatings and batterings like outclassed street fighters.

So what's the antidote to Type A? First, it's important to acknowledge that your hard-driving personality may be hazardous to your health. Although psychotherapy generally isn't necessary, you can probably benefit from some relaxation exercises and some counseling on time management. Also, try hitting the health club on a regular basis.

A study by Jon M. Gerrard, M.D., Ph.D., and his colleagues at the University of Manitoba in Winnipeg examined both Type A's and non–Type A's (called Type B's), specifically looking at their levels of thromboxane, a clot-promoting chemical that can help provoke a heart attack. Sure enough, the physically fit Type A's had thromboxane levels similar to the calmer Type B's, suggesting that exercise may excise the corrupting chemicals that can wreak havoc on your heart.

Sip the spirits. You've probably heard a lot about the downside of drinking too much alcohol, from cirrhosis of the liver to cancer to auto accidents to a life-threatening heart condition called cardiomyopathy that can weaken your heart muscle. As a result, you might find it surprising that in moderation, alcohol can be a heart healer.

The reason: A drink or two a day can raise your level of HDL cholesterol, the type that picks up and carries the bad LDL (low-density lipoprotein) cholesterol out of your body. Studies have shown that mild alcohol consumption—a 5-ounce glass of wine, a 12-ounce beer or one cocktail containing 1½ ounces (or one shot) of hard liquor per day—can cut your risk of a heart attack by about 40 percent compared with teetotalers.

Get your vitamins. For decades, mainstream doctors have considered vitamin supplements just a small step away from quackery. But not anymore. It's hard not to be impressed with a study involving nearly 40,000 men, conducted by researchers at the Harvard University School of Public Health in Boston, that concluded that men who took vitamin E supplements of at least 100 IU per day for two years had a 37 percent reduced risk of heart attack or advanced heart disease. (The Recommended Dietary Allowance for adult men is ten milligrams alpha-tocopherol equivalents, or 15 IU.)

What's the secret of vitamin E? The vitamin is an antioxidant, meaning that it protects cells from malicious molecules called free radicals that trigger a process called oxidation, which can contribute to the clogging of arteries.

"I'm giving vitamin E to my patients in standard doses that do not pose risks," says Marianne J. Legato, M.D., associate professor of clinical medicine at Columbia University College of Physicians and Surgeons in New York City. She advises daily supplements of 400 IU of vitamin E, along with 1,500 milligrams of vitamin C and 6 milligrams of beta-carotene, both of which are also antioxidants. She also advises 1,500 milligrams of calcium, which studies have shown can help protect your heart.

Deflate your blood pressure. High blood pressure is called the silent killer, quietly doing sinister work that puts so much extra strain on the heart and arteries that it can ultimately provoke a heart attack (not to mention a stroke or kidney failure).

But by pulling the plug on your high blood pressure—which you can do by reducing sodium in your diet, losing weight, exercising and (if necessary) taking one of many available medications—you can give your heart a breather. Here are some comforting statistics: For each one-point decline you can achieve in your diastolic blood pressure (the bottom number), you can cut your risk of a heart attack by 2 to 3 percent. And with proper therapy, it's not uncommon for people with high blood pressure to lower their diastolic readings by 20 points or more.

A Multitude of Treatments

The good thing about heart disease—surely the only good thing—is that it most often gives you warning signs before striking hard. The most common warning sign is angina, chest pain caused by inadequate blood flow to the heart. Should you experience angina, your doctor might prescribe nitroglycerin to relax the blood vessels and allow the heart to get more blood. Or for chronic angina, he might suggest other medications, such as beta-blockers, calcium channel blockers or ACE (angiotensin-converting enzyme) inhibitors.

"The choice of drugs will depend on your own particular situation," says Dr. Martin. "If you have high blood pressure as well as heart disease, there may be a single drug that can help both of these conditions. If you have heart failure in addition to heart disease—that is, if your heart isn't pumping as efficiently as possible—an ACE inhibitor is a good choice. Some patients do need to be placed on more than one medication. So it's an individualized decision."

If the blockage of your coronary arteries has become severe, then your doctor might recommend an open heart operation (coronary bypass surgery) or angioplasty. In angioplasty, a tiny balloon-tipped catheter is guided into the coronary arteries, where the balloon is inflated to flatten the fatty deposits that are causing the obstruction.

Although angioplasty successfully opens the arteries in up to 90 percent of people, these arteries can become clogged again, sometimes within months of the procedure. At that time, angioplasty needs to be repeated, or the doctor may suggest bypass surgery instead.

In a bypass operation, healthy blood vessels (often transplanted from the leg or the chest) are grafted onto the heart to bypass the obstructed portions of the coronary arteries. Although it is a more serious procedure, its benefits tend to last longer. Dr. Legato says that surgery is usually chosen for so-called three-vessel disease, in which three or more of the major coronary arteries are obstructed, severely interfering with blood flow to the heart.

If you wind up opting for either medication or surgery, it is still important—perhaps doubly so—to maintain a healthy, active, low-fat lifestyle.

HEMOCHROMATOSIS

Ironing Out a Deadly Problem

You're a tough guy. Never miss a day of work. You play through pain on the softball field and the basketball court. But lately, your joints are stiff, and you feel as worn out as your favorite old shirt. Some jokers have even suggested you're rusting from the inside out.

That is exactly what's happening to the 1 in 200 American men who has hemochromatosis, a genetic disease that causes the body to horde excessive amounts of iron, which then attacks organs such as the liver, heart and pancreas. It may be one of life's most insidious and catastrophic agers. Unless it's detected and treated early, the disease can also lead to arthritis, diabetes, cancer, even premature death.

"Hemochromatosis can certainly slow you down prematurely. If it causes fatigue, you can feel like you're 80 when you're only 40," says Jerome L. Sullivan, M.D., Ph.D., a pathologist and director of clinical laboratories at the Veterans Affairs Medical Center in Charleston, South Carolina.

It's All in the Family

Hemochromatosis occurs when a man inherits a pair of abnormal genes from his mother and father. Once considered a rare ailment, it is now believed to be one of the most common inherited diseases, afflicting more people than cystic fibrosis, Huntington's disease and muscular dystrophy combined, according to Randall Lauffer, Ph.D., assistant professor at Harvard Medical School in Boston and author of *Iron and Your Heart*. About 500,000 men in the United States may have the disease.

What happens when you have it? Normally, you store small amounts of iron in your body and stop absorbing it when you have enough in reserve. If you have hemochromatosis, however, your body doesn't know when it has enough iron. So you keep absorbing the mineral—often to the point where you can actually set off metal detectors. Symptoms of hemochromatosis can appear at any age. It has been detected in children as young as age 2 and in men as old as 101.

Once iron is in your body, it's there to stay—unless you bleed. Iron is a major component of red blood cells, says William H. Crosby, M.D., director of hematology at Chapman Cancer Center in Joplin, Missouri. If you have hemochromatosis and you don't lose iron through bleeding, your body will cram the mineral into every major organ to the point that some men with the disease have up to 100 times more iron concentrated in their livers, 15 times more iron in their hearts and 5 times more iron in their kidneys than an average person.

In excess amounts, iron generates free radicals, chemically unstable oxygen molecules that can damage the heart and liver and accelerate the aging process throughout the body, Dr. Lauffer says.

"That excess iron is a true poison and can increase your risk of cancer," says Sylvia Bottomley, M.D., a hematologist at the University of Oklahoma Health Sciences Center in Oklahoma City.

Men with hemochromatosis, for example, are 200 times more likely to develop liver cancer than an average person. In addition, excess iron can lead to cirrhosis, an incurable ailment that causes scar tissue and eventually destroys the liver, Dr. Sullivan says.

Excess iron also interferes with the pumping ability of the heart and leads to a form of heart disease called congestive cardiomyopathy, which causes enlargement of the heart muscle. This condition is 300 times more fatal among men with hemochromatosis than among the population at large.

Hemochromatosis can also turn the skin bronze and damage the pituitary gland, causing lowered sex drive, impotence and infertility.

Fortunately, some complications of hemochromatosis, including heart disease, are reversible if the disease is diagnosed and treated early. But hemochromatosis often does much of its damage before symptoms appear.

"It's an insidious disease. It comes on gradually. It's like being a lobster in the pot. You're cooked before you realize you're in the pot and water is boiling," Dr. Sullivan says.

Even when symptoms are present, hemochromatosis often eludes detection because it has no standard pattern of onset.

"It really hits a lot of different organs, so the first symptom may be different in different people," Dr. Sullivan says. "There really isn't a reliable initial symptom of it. The classic findings are heart disease, diabetes, cirrhosis, fatigue and bronzing of the skin. But I've met a woman whose first symptom was just hip pain. It's really unpredictable and very confusing."

Doctors are often confounded by the disease. Some may treat the complications, such as diabetes or arthritis, without realizing that hemochromatosis is the underlying cause, Dr. Crosby says. In some cases, men with hemochromatosis end up seeing several physicians before getting proper diagnoses.

Getting the Iron Out

Once it has been diagnosed, hemochromatosis is treated by removing blood. Bleeding works because a pint of blood contains about 200 milligrams of iron and because it forces the bone marrow to draw on the body's iron stores in order to replenish removed red blood cells with new ones.

Depending on the amount of excess iron, a man may need to have bleedings, called phlebotomies, once or twice a week for up to three years to get his iron stores down to normal levels. After that, he will need to have a pint of blood removed every three or four months for the rest of his life in order to prevent new iron buildup, Dr. Bottomley says.

Men who have phlebotomies early, before damage to their vital organs is widespread, can have normal life expectancies, Dr. Crosby says. Skin color usually returns to normal, and fatigue and heart disease are often relieved. In addition, bleeding can sometimes alleviate the symptoms of diabetes and correct liver function.

"If you need 150 phlebotomies to get rid of iron in your body, you can see it's going to be an arduous road, but it's very doable," Dr. Bottomley says. "When you start having phlebotomies, you're not going to feel better tomorrow, but you should within in a few months."

For more information, contact the Iron Overload Disease Association, 433 Westwind Drive, North Palm Beach, FL 33408, or the Hemochromatosis Foundation, P.O. Box 8569, Albany, NY 12208. In addition, here are a few things that can make this disease easier to live with.

Get tested. By the time symptoms show up, there may be permanent damage to your vital organs. So detecting hemochromatosis early is critical, particularly if you have a parent or sibling who has the disease, says Margit Krikker, M.D., founder and president of the Hemochromatosis Foundation. Ask your doctor to do the blood test called transferrin saturation index, which shows how much iron is in your blood.

Stay away from supplements. Never take iron supplements without your doctor's permission, Dr. Sullivan advises. Some men assume that when they feel worn down, they have anemia. But hemochromatosis can also cause fatigue, and taking supplements could make your symptoms worse.

Eat a healthy diet. While avoiding iron-rich foods may seem sensible, it isn't that practical or wise, says Dr. Krikker. That's because many iron-laden foods such as potatoes, broccoli and tuna have other indispensable nutrients. Other important foods are fortified with iron, such as cereals and grains.

Keep in mind that iron is actually a small part of your diet and that you store it very slowly, says Dr. Krikker. It's the total accumulation of it over the years that causes problems. Once you begin having phlebotomies, many of those problems should be behind you.

So eating a balanced diet that includes poultry, fish, grains, fruits, vegetables and dairy products such as cheese and milk is still your best bet.

HIGH BLOOD PRESSURE

Stopping the Silent Thief of Youth

Next time you trot onto the court for a game of five-on-five basketball, take a good look at the guys on your team.

If it's a typical bunch of trash-talkin', burger-eatin', couch-sittin' American males, the odds are good that at least one of you has high blood pressure.

Here's the worst part. Even if it's you, you won't be likely to know. You'll just keep working, eating, sleeping, playing. And high blood pressure (also called hypertension), one of life's quietest health hazards, will just keep aging you.

"There really aren't any noticeable outward signs. But if you have hypertension, it is doing damage," says Patrick Mulrow, M.D., chairman of the Department of Medicine at the Medical College of Ohio at Toledo and chairman of the American Heart Association's Council for High Blood Pressure Research. Yet symptoms or no, the damage is being done. High blood pressure is directly linked to the deaths of nearly 14,000 American men each year—and it contributes to the deaths of untold thousands more.

It can make you 12 times more likely to suffer a stroke, 6 times more likely to suffer a heart attack and 5 times more likely to die of congestive heart failure. It's also a major risk factor for kidney failure. And even though it affects 64 million Americans—including 38 percent of black men and 33 percent of white men between the ages of 18 and 74—nearly 50 percent of all guys with high blood pressure aren't aware of it.

"We could save lives if people discovered they have high blood pressure and then took measures to control it," Dr. Mulrow says. In many instances, it's just a matter of going to the doctor and having your blood pressure checked once or twice a year, cutting back on salt and fat and breaking a sweat a few times a week. That's really a small price to pay, Dr. Mulrow says, considering that it could add years to your life.

172

Hyper-What?

If we have to keep reminding you to control your blood pressure, then maybe it's already too high. That's because high blood pressure may weaken your memory.

A study of 100 adults found that people with higher blood pressure scored lower in a process called short-term memory retrieval. That means it took longer for them to remember whether a number shown to them had been part of an original set of numbers that they had seen earlier.

No one is certain why high blood pressure fogs your memory. It may be related to the way blood circulates in the brain or to a reduction in the amount of oxygen that reaches the brain. "Whatever the mechanism, this is just another reason to keep your blood pressure under healthy control," says David J. Madden, Ph.D., professor in the Department of Psychiatry at Duke University Medical Center in Durham, North Carolina.

Pressure Packers

Doctors take two measures when they check your blood pressure. The first is called the systolic reading. It indicates how hard your heart pumps to push blood through your arteries. The second measure, called the diastolic reading, shows how much resistance your arteries put up to the blood flow. Blood pressure is measured in millimeters of mercury, or mm Hg, and a reading of about 120 mm Hg systolic and 80 mm Hg diastolic is considered healthy. You read it simply as 120/80.

Everyone's blood pressure varies widely throughout the day. Generally, it will rise when we're exercising and drop when we're asleep. But when your baseline, or resting, reading creeps up to 140/90, you have borderline high blood pressure. That means your heart is working too hard to pump blood, either because your arteries have stiffened or narrowed with plaque or because you have too much blood in your system due to water retention or other problems. The result of the extra stress can be heart disease or dangerous blood clots that can cause stroke or heart attack.

A man's blood pressure usually rises with age. A combination of factors causes this, including less physical activity, extra body weight and a number of hormonal changes, according to Robert DiBianco, M.D., director of cardiology research at the Washington Adventist Hospital in Takoma Park, Maryland.

About one in five men between the ages of 35 and 44 has high blood pressure. That figure doubles between the ages of 45 and 54. About half of all men between the ages of 55 and 64 have it. And between the ages of 65 and 74, about three in every five men have at least borderline high blood pressure. Until age 55, men are at greater risk of high blood pressure than women; after that, the percentage of women with high blood pressure is higher than that of men. Experts think hormonal changes play a role in the later development of high blood pressure in women.

In 90 to 95 percent of cases, Dr. Mulrow says, the exact cause of high blood pressure is unknown. But researchers have identified a number of risk factors that may increase your risk of developing high blood pressure. Family history is one. If several members of your immediate family have high blood pressure, you're more likely to develop it. Obesity is another major factor. Studies show that 60 percent of people with high blood pressure are overweight.

The amount of sodium in the foods we eat is also a big contributor to high blood pressure, experts say. Sodium makes many of us retain water, Dr. Mulrow says, which increases the volume of blood in our bodies and makes our hearts work harder to pump it. There's also evidence that sodium in some way damages the linings of blood vessels, making scarring and clogged arteries more likely.

The vast majority of our sodium intake is from the salt in our foods. Table salt, for instance, is about 40 percent sodium. After analyzing dozens of studies on sodium and high blood pressure, one British research team found that cutting salt by 3,000 milligrams per day—that's a little less than a teaspoon's worth—could prevent 26 percent of all strokes and 15 percent of heart attacks caused by blood clots.

Some people are more sensitive than others to the effects of salt or, more specifically, of sodium, Dr. DiBianco says. "Maybe you can eat a lot of salt, process and get rid of it quickly and not have to worry about it," he says. But maybe not. There's no reliable test for salt sensitivity. If you are overweight, don't get a lot of exercise or have a family history of high blood pressure or diabetes, Dr. DiBianco says you're probably more at risk and need to limit your salt intake.

Psychological factors can also play a role in high blood pressure. A 20-year study of 1,123 American adults found that severe anxiety and worry make middle-aged men twice as likely to develop high blood pressure. Data for this study came from the famous Framingham Heart Study, which tracked the health of more than 5,200 adult residents of Framingham, Massachusetts. Job stress may lead to high blood pressure, too. A study of 129 working adults found that men with high-pressure jobs—positions with lots of responsibility but little decision-making power—showed bigger increases in blood pressure during the workday than those with less demanding jobs. While everyone's blood pressure rose at work, the high-stress men had jumps of six points in systolic pressure and four points in diastolic pressure compared with their less stressed co-workers. Anger may play a role in high blood pressure as well, Dr. Mulrow says, though the evidence is sketchy and sometimes contradictory.

Scientists have found that the combination of too much sodium and high stress can create a powerful pressure problem. A study of 32 students at the Johns Hopkins University School of Medicine in Baltimore showed that people who ate high-sodium diets and faced high-stress conditions for a two-week period saw their systolic blood pressure readings jump more than 6 points. The high-sodium, low-stress people, by comparison, saw increases of just 0.6 point,

How Low Can You Go?

Here's the only rule you need to know about blood pressure: the lower, the better.

"It doesn't really matter how low your reading is, even if it's something very, very low, like 85 systolic. As long as you're not feeling any ill effects from it, that's just fine. In fact, you should feel good knowing you're in a low-risk group," says Robert DiBianco, M.D., director of cardiology research at the Washington Adventist Hospital in Takoma Park, Maryland.

The landmark Framingham Heart Study, which took a decades-long look at the health of more than 5,200 residents of Framingham, Massachusetts, found that people with systolic blood pressure readings below 120 mm Hg (millimeters of mercury) had the least chance of suffering heart attacks. The risk rose steadily with increased pressure. People with the highest readings, 170 mm Hg or above, were over three times more likely to die of heart attacks than those at or below 120 mm Hg.

Still, there are a couple of problems to watch for with low blood pressure. As people age, they're more likely to suffer from a form of temporary low blood pressure called orthostatic hypotension—the sensation you get when you hop out of bed and suddenly feel weak, like the room is spinning or the lights are dimmed. "If you have ever fainted from that, or if it happens more than very, very rarely, you should see a doctor," Dr. DiBianco says. The problem could be caused by mild dehydration, a reaction to medication, fever, illness or heat exhaustion, he says.

For some people, especially the elderly and people with diabetes or heart disease and possibly those being treated for high blood pressure, readings that fall too low may be a particular risk. If you fit in one of these groups, consult your doctor, Dr. DiBianco says.

and the low-sodium, high-stress people showed increases of just 0.1 point.

Then there's alcohol. Scientists have long known that excess drinking can contribute to high blood pressure. But a study from the Research Institute on Alcoholism in Buffalo, New York, shows that how often you drink may be as important as how much you drink. Researchers looked at 1,635 residents of Erie County, New York, and found that people who drank every day had systolic readings 6.6 points higher and diastolic readings 4.7 points higher than people who drank only once a week. But the study found no significant relationship between blood pressure and the total amount of alcohol consumed.

Slowing the Flow

Lots of prescription drugs help reduce high blood pressure. Diuretics flush excess fluids from your system. Beta-blockers reduce the heart rate and the heart's total output of blood. Vasodilators widen your arteries and allow easier blood flow. Sympathetic nerve inhibitors also prevent blood vessels from constricting.

But drugs should be a last resort. They can cause fatigue and inhibit your sex life, among other problems. The trick is to avoid high blood pressure in the first place—and the tips below will get you started. Even if you already have mild high blood pressure, the advice could reduce your dependence on drugs and maybe even help you control things naturally.

Check it. There's only one way to know for sure if you have high blood pressure: Have your doctor check your blood pressure. Once a year should be sufficient, unless your doctor orders more tests. It's a quick, painless procedure. The doctor puts an inflatable cuff around your arm and checks your pulse with a stethoscope. If you show a borderline high reading, the doctor may order several retests over a couple of weeks or months.

You can even find do-it-yourself blood pressure monitors in pharmacies, grocery stores and shopping malls. These can give you a rough estimate of your blood pressure, but Dr. Mulrow warns that the machines aren't a substitute for an annual doctor's visit. Some machines are not well calibrated and provide grossly inaccurate results. Too many external factors—have you been walking, or are you wearing a thick sleeve?—can interfere.

Lose it. If you're overweight, even moderate weight loss may help lower your blood pressure, says Marvin Moser, M.D., clinical professor of medicine at Yale University School of Medicine in New Haven, Connecticut, and senior adviser to the National High Blood Pressure Education Program. In some cases, he says, weight loss of 10 to 15 pounds may be enough to lower slightly elevated blood pressure to normal and help you avoid medication.

A nationwide study of 362 overweight men, ages 30 to 54, showed how well weight loss can work. Over a 12-month period, the men on a weight loss program lost an average of 12 pounds. Their systolic readings fell an average of 6 points, while diastolic readings fell 6.4 points.

Move it. Exercise, combined with a low-fat diet, is the best way to lose weight and keep your arteries clog-free. Research shows that people who don't exercise are 35 to 50 percent more likely to develop high blood pressure. And the American College of Sports Medicine says that regular aerobic training can reduce systolic and diastolic blood pressure by as much as ten points.

You don't have to be Mr. Endurance to reap the benefits, either. In fact, some studies have found that lower-intensity workouts such as walking are as good or better at lowering blood pressure than running or other heavy-duty aerobic activities. Many experts recommend working out at least three times a week for 20 minutes a pop.

Shake it off. Remember that not everyone is sensitive to the effects of sodium. But until doctors can reliably tell who is or isn't, it's a good idea to limit your intake. "It certainly isn't going to hurt anyone to cut down on salt and probably will be of real value if you're successful," Dr. DiBianco says.

Cut salt from your diet wherever you can. Most of us are eating about 2½ times more than we should. Swearing off the table shaker will have some effect. But research shows that three-fourths of all the salt we eat comes from processed foods such as cheese, soup, bread, baked goods and snacks.

"You have to read labels," Dr. Mulrow says. Check for sodium content, and shoot for a daily total of about 2,400 milligrams. When shopping, look for labels that say "low sodium." That means the products contain no more than 140 milligrams of sodium per serving. And spend some extra time in the produce aisle. Almost every fruit and vegetable is naturally low in sodium.

Be careful when you eat out, too. You'll be surprised how fast sodium can add up. A hamburger from your favorite fast-food restaurant, for instance, may give you almost half a day's total.

Power up on potassium. Studies have shown that eating 3,500 milligrams of potassium can help counteract sodium and keep blood volume—and blood pressure—down. And it's easy to get enough. A baked potato packs 838 milligrams of potassium all by itself, and one cup of spinach has 800 milligrams. Other potassium-packed foods include bananas, orange juice, corn, cabbage and broccoli. Check with your doctor before taking potassium supplements. Too much may aggravate kidney problems.

Meet your magnesium needs. Researchers seem to have found a link between low magnesium intake and high blood pressure. But just how much magnesium you need to combat high blood pressure remains unclear. For now, Dr. DiBianco says, your best bet is to get the Recommended Dietary Allowance (RDA) of about 350 milligrams.

Unfortunately, America's intake of magnesium has been dropping for a century, since we started processing foods and robbing them of their trace elements. Good sources of magnesium include nuts, spinach, lima beans, peas and seafood. But don't overdo it by taking supplements; Dr. Mulrow says too much magnesium can give you a nasty case of diarrhea.

Keep up your calcium. The link between calcium intake and blood pressure is controversial. Some studies show that extra calcium can lower blood pressure, while others show that it has no effect.

But experts aren't yet convinced that large doses of calcium are going to help. Dr. Mulrow says getting the RDA of 800 milligrams per day—three eight-ounce glasses of skim milk provide more than enough—and keeping your other risk factors under control is the best advice for now. Other calcium sources include low-fat cheeses, canned salmon and other canned fish with bones. If you want to take calcium supplements, see your doctor, since too much calcium can cause other problems, such as kidney stones.

Fill up with fiber. A Swedish study of 32 people with mild high blood pressure found that taking a seven-gram tablet of fiber each day helps lower diastolic blood pressure by five points. No one is sure why; perhaps it's because of weight loss due to people being fuller and eating less or because they eat less sodium. Whatever the reason, seven extra grams of fiber is easy to find. There's almost that much in a bowl of high-fiber cereal.

Drink in moderation. "A little alcohol isn't going to hurt," Dr. Mulrow says. "But drinking every day, and drinking to excess, could mean trouble." For guys fighting high blood pressure, three ounces of alcohol a week seems to be about the limit. A 12-year study of 1,455 men, with a mean age of 47, showed that both systolic and diastolic pressure readings begin to rise steadily after that. That means six 12-ounce beers, six 4-ounce glasses of wine or six cocktails containing 1 ounce of hard liquor each week.

Stop smoking. Smoking markedly increases your risk of developing a stroke or blood vessel damage from high blood pressure, says Dr. Mulrow. When you smoke, it encourages your body to deposit cholesterol within your coronary arteries. This decreases the size of your vessels and forces your heart to work harder. "Anyone with high blood pressure should stop smoking immediately," advises Dr. Mulrow.

IMPOTENCE

Living Well Shrinks Your Risk

The woman of your dreams stands before you in a sizzling red teddy. She leans over, kisses you passionately and beckons you toward the bedroom.

Your pulse quickens, your breath speeds up, all systems are go. But then faster than you can say "Mission impossible," your rocket launcher transforms into a mass of quivering Jell-O.

Oops. You've heard that it happens to every guy at one time or another, so you try to shrug it off. But you can't, and even though you strain to achieve it, getting an erection seems more difficult than hauling a 1,000-pound piano up three flights of stairs.

While it's annoying, an occasional inability to get or maintain an erection shouldn't worry you too much, doctors say.

"As you age, it takes longer to get an erection and more physical and psychological stimulation to maintain it," says Roger Crenshaw, M.D., a psychiatrist and sex therapist in private practice in La Jolla, California. "It's the guy who notices that his erection is fluctuating and worries about it who will become psychologically impotent, because he isn't accepting that his body is aging."

While you're in your twenties, you never think twice about getting an erection. But by the time you creep toward 40, the sexual comings and goings of your penis are less predictable. Certainly, that can be scary and depressing for any guy, because it raises the possibility that he will join the estimated ten million American men whom doctors consider impotent, meaning they can't get or sustain erections sufficient for intercourse 75 percent of the time. "I've seen men who've coped better with the loss of a leg than with impotence," Dr. Crenshaw says.

But in reality, few men in their thirties and forties are impotent, and there are many things you can do to make sure that you won't ever be. Even if you are impotent, in many cases it can be cured.

179

Keeping Up

Doctors, who once considered impotence almost exclusively a psychological problem, now believe that at least seven in ten cases of impotence have physical causes, including diabetes, thyroid disorders, atherosclerosis or injury to the penis. Medication, alcohol consumption, smoking and psychological factors such as depression, stress and performance anxiety can compound the problem.

What it boils down to is that anything that disrupts blood flow to your penis will shrivel your chances of getting an erection, says John Mulcahy, M.D., professor of urology at the Indiana University Medical Center in Indianapolis.

But if you take care of yourself, you can remain ready, willing and able to have sex into old age, says Joseph Khoury, M.D., a urologist in private practice in Bethesda, Maryland.

"Theoretically, there is no reason for your potency to change as you age," says Dr. Khoury, who knows men in their eighties who still have sex three times a week. The one thing they have in common: They took care of themselves better than most men.

Here's a few ways to keep your private parts in good working order.

Cut out the smoke signals. Smoking accelerates the formation of blockages in the heart's arteries, and there's every reason to believe that it does the same to the vessels that supply blood to the penis. In fact, smoking is now considered a major factor in erection problems, with the first signs of harm appearing by age 40. So if you smoke, quit, Dr. Crenshaw advises.

Run, don't walk, to the gym. The fitter you are, the more sex you'll have, and the better it will be, says a study published in the *Archives of Sexual Behavior*. In the study, conducted at the University of California, San Diego, 78 healthy but inactive men began aerobic exercise three to five days a week for an hour each time. Another group simply walked at a moderate pace three to five days a week. During the study, each man kept a diary of sexual activity. The results showed that the sex lives of the aerobic exercisers significantly improved. Meanwhile, the sex lives of the walkers changed very little.

It doesn't matter which type of aerobic exercise you choose, as long as you do it a minimum of three times each week and stick with it for at least 20 minutes per session. Running, swimming and rowing are good choices, Dr. Crenshaw says.

Nix the fat. When it comes to diet, the bottom line is limiting your fat intake. Again, logic says that what's good for the arteries supplying blood flow to the heart will also be good for those supplying blood to the penis.

Dr. Khoury believes that a high-potency diet should be low in fat, with about 20 percent of its calories from fat. If you eat 2,500 calories a day, that would be about 50 grams of fat. To get started in the right direction, read food labels, look for low-fat and nonfat products, avoid fried foods, switch to skim milk and eat at least five half-cup servings of fruits and vegetables every day, along with one three-ounce serving (about the size of a deck of cards) of fish, poultry or lean red meat.

Trim your waistline. Excess pounds can actually make important inches of the penis disappear. Informal studies of overweight men by Dr. Mulcahy show that up to a point, an overweight man will regain one inch of his penis for every 35 pounds of weight lost. Not a bad incentive for someone who's really heavy. But more practically, keeping your weight down will reduce the risk of high blood pressure and diabetes, both of which impair the ability to have an erection.

Watch your drug use. Hundreds of drugs can cause impotence as a side effect, including diuretics, high blood pressure medications, some antidepressants and antipsychotics. Ask your doctor or pharmacist if medication could be causing your problem.

Go light on the booze. Alcohol is a depressant that slows down reflexes, including sexual ones. Besides impairing immediate performance, alcohol,

It Happened One Night . . .

So what exactly do you say to a naked woman when she says yes but your penis says no?

"Don't apologize," says Herb Goldberg, Ph.D., a clinical psychologist in Los Angeles and author of *The Inner Male*. "If you treat it casually, perhaps the woman will treat it casually also, if she cares about you."

Find other ways to please her, says Marty Klein, Ph.D., a licensed marriage counselor and sex therapist in Palo Alto, California, and author of *Ask Me Anything: A Sex Therapist Answers the Most Important Questions for the '90s*. "I'd shrug, tell my partner 'Well, it looks like we're not going to have intercourse tonight, but we're still going to have great sex, don't worry.' Then I'd use my hands, mouth, nose, elbows—anything to have great sex."

Afterward, don't dwell on it. It could trigger performance anxiety, which makes a recurrence more likely. "Once a guy starts thinking rather than feeling, he can say good-bye to his erection," says Roger Crenshaw, M.D., a psychiatrist and sex therapist in private practice in La Jolla, California.

To relieve the pressure, Dr. Crenshaw suggests that you not have intercourse the next few times you sleep with a woman. Instead, keep following Dr. Klein's advice to kiss, hug and do other things you enjoy and satisfy your partner.

when consumed excessively for too long, can have a direct effect on the testicles, decreasing production of the male hormone testosterone and upsetting the
delicate balance of hormones and brain chemicals required to get an erection.
Limit yourself to two beers or glasses of wine a day, suggests Saul Rosenthal,
M.D., director of the Sexual Therapy Clinic of San Antonio in San Antonio,
Texas, and author of *Sex over 40*. If you're having sexual difficulty, stop drinking
for three months to see if that helps, he advises.

Be on guard. Penile fracture is an all too common cause of impotence, says
Irwin Goldstein, M.D., professor of urology at Boston University School of
Medicine. "Fracturing the penis breaks the fibrous lining that contains the
pressure that allows you to have an erection. It literally cracks like the wall of
tire that goes over a curb too fast," he says. The most vulnerable position is
when the woman is top, because the penis can slip out of her vagina and she can
slam her pelvis down on it. Abnormal bending during sex, bicycling accidents
and blows to the crotch can also damage the penis and testicles.

Erasing the Mind Games

So you're eating right and exercising and you don't smoke, but you still
have an occasional erection problem. Then the difficulty could be anger, stress
or some other psychological cause, Dr. Crenshaw says. Here are some tips for
coping with these problems.

Look at your relationship. Often your sexual relationship reflects what is
going on with your partner outside of bed. "If your relationship with the woman
is unhealthy, impotence could be your body's way of giving you an early
warning that something is wrong, and you should try to interpret your body's
signals in order to understand the meaning of your response," says Herb Goldberg, Ph.D., a clinical psychologist in Los Angeles and author of *The Inner Male*.

Leave your anger at the door. Anger can inhibit sexual arousal, says
Domeena Renshaw, M.D., director of the Sexual Dysfunction Clinic at Loyola
University of Chicago Stritch School of Medicine in Maywood. A classic example of this is a fellow who had a vicious argument with his ex-wife over an
upcoming weekend visit with his three-year-old son. The conversation stayed
in his mind the entire evening.

"My girlfriend was dressed to kill, and she was in the mood," he says. "But
all I could think about was how to strangle my ex-wife. Nothing was happening
below the belt."

Talk about your anger and frustration with your partner outside the bedroom. Letting it fester will only put a clamp on your erections.

Get real. There's no point in trying to compete with the 20-year-old you.
You are bound to have a bit less spontaneity in your sex life than you had back
then, if only because you have more on your mind, greater responsibilities,
richer interests, a fuller schedule and more stress, says Jack Jaffe, M.D., director
of the Potency Recovery Center in Van Nuys, California. The way to avoid psy-

chological problems that could interfere with your performance is to not wait for the magic moment. "You've got to make it happen," he says. "That may mean setting a date, sitting down to discuss what your needs are, whatever it takes."

What the Doctor Can Do

Even if you have a recurrent impotence problem, there's plenty a urologist or sex therapist can do for you. If you have a psychological problem, then counseling can help. If it's a physical problem, there are several treatment options, including drugs and penile implants.

Yohimbine hydrochloride (Yocon), a prescription drug derived from the bark of the African yohimbe tree, helps relieve impotence in about one in three men. It takes up to eight weeks to work, however, and its side effects include nausea, dizziness and irritability.

Your doctor might suggest self-injections of drugs such as papaverine and prostaglandin (Prostin VR) directly into the penis. The injections cause blood vessels in the penis to dilate, and you get an erection that can last up to three hours, even if you ejaculate. Sure, sticking a needle in your favorite body part doesn't sound thrilling. But it's less painful than a bee sting. On the downside, if the injection-induced erection lasts more than four hours, it could permanently damage the penis. Only 1 in 100 men who use penile injections ever faces this problem. However, if you still have an erection after three hours, take a 30-milligram decongestant tablet that contains pseudoephedrine (such as Sudafed severe cold formula). This will constrict blood vessels and deflate your penis, Dr. Crenshaw says. If your erection doesn't fade within an hour after taking the pill, contact your doctor or go to a hospital emergency room immediately.

You could also try a vacuum device that fits over the penis. A pump then removes air from the plastic vacuum tube. That creates negative pressure in the chamber, which draws blood into the penis and causes an erection. Most men who use this device then place rubber rings around the base of the penis to keep the blood from escaping.

"If a man is anxious about getting an erection, he can put on the device, pump the vacuum and have an erection within a minute," Dr. Crenshaw says. "It relieves his anxiety and saves him a lot of time and money in therapy."

The rings must be removed within 20 to 30 minutes, however, or you could bruise the penis.

Inflatable or semi-rigid implants can be surgically inserted in the penis to create erections. But up to 50 percent of these devices fail within five years, and corrective surgery is often necessary.

INFERTILITY

Ready, Willing but Unable— For Now

For years, Scott Read faithfully used birth control to prevent an unwelcome visit from the stork. But when he married in 1982 and both he and his wife, Karen, wanted children, he faced an altogether different and painful surprise.

"We wanted to have kids, but we tried and tried and couldn't make it happen," says Scott, a 36-year-old hotel executive in San Francisco and the adoptive father of a six-year-old daughter. "It was frustrating. I would find myself thinking about a couple of friends I had in high school who jumped into the back of car and made love once, and boom, the girl was pregnant. Yet here were two people like us who were ready to have kids, and it wouldn't happen."

Scott and Karen's story is typical of the 10 to 15 percent of American couples who struggle with infertility. These couples watch months turn into years and hope melt into disappointment. Sex becomes a chore, and each month they don't conceive makes them feel a little more over the hill.

"Infertility is devastating. One of the major aspects of a man's sense of youthfulness is his ability to reproduce. There's nothing more devastating to a man than struggling with the realization that he can't conceive a child. Psychologically, it can damage his self-esteem and make him feel like he is really getting old and decrepit," says Reed C. Moskowitz, M.D., founder and medical director of the Stress Disorders Medical Services at New York University Medical Center in New York City and author of *Your Healing Mind*.

What's Wrong?

More than likely, you learned the ABCs of making babies in a high school sex education class. You probably remember your teacher droning on about how

184

normally during intercourse a man ejaculates millions of sperm into the woman's vagina and these sperm travel up into the fallopian tubes. There, if you happen to have sex during the one or two days a month when a woman's egg is released from the ovary and is traveling down one of the tubes, the sperm and the egg meet. If one of the sperm penetrates the egg, fertilization occurs, and pregnancy begins. If conditions are ideal and you and your partner don't use contraception, there is a one in five chance of pregnancy each month.

But your teacher probably didn't tell you what could go wrong. Infertility is usually diagnosed after a couple has tried unsuccessfully to conceive for 12 months or more. Infertility can occur even if you've had children in the past. About 40 to 50 percent of the time, doctors determine that the woman has problems in her reproductive tract. In another 40 percent, they can pinpoint that the man is the cause of the problem. Sometimes both the man and the woman have difficulties that are interfering with pregnancy. Ten percent of the time, doctors can't determine the cause.

Most of the time, if the guy is the problem, either he has a low sperm count or the sperm he does have aren't very motile, meaning they have a hard time swimming to meet the egg in the fallopian tubes. Some men, like Scott Read, have both problems.

"Men can have low sperm counts for a number of reasons," says Donald I. Galen, M.D., director of the In Vitro Fertilization and Reproduction Medical Division at San Ramon Regional Medical Center in San Ramon, California. "Smoking, alcohol abuse, drugs, exposure to chemicals and radiation, childhood diseases such as mumps and trauma to sexual organs can reduce sperm counts in any man."

A varicocele—a varicose vein in the scrotum—could also lower your sperm count, says Fred Licciardi, M.D., assistant professor of obstetrics and gynecology at New York University School of Medicine in New York City. The testicles need to be about 2°F cooler than the rest of your body in order to produce sperm. But a varicocele elevates the temperature in the testicles and kills sperm.

Other causes of male infertility include blockage of the vas deferens (the tubes that carry sperm from the testicles to the penis), testicular cancer, infection, trauma and antibodies that attach to your sperm, inhibiting their movement and making them vulnerable to destruction by white blood cells. Antibodies may show up as a result of infection or trauma to the testicles.

Our Clocks Are Ticking, Too

Although we've all heard about men in their seventies who father children, for most of us having kids gets more difficult, because our fertility gradually drops as we get older, Dr. Galen says.

"Infertility occurs in less than 1 percent of couples in their teens," says Sherman Silber, M.D., a fertility specialist at St. Luke's Hospital in St. Louis and author of *How to Get Pregnant with the New Technology*. "In the twenties, it

When the Subject Is Infertility

While you and your partner try and try again to conceive, your dream of coaching your own kid in Little League is fading, and your sex life has become about as exciting as frozen waffles.

Then one day your frustration leads to an explosion, followed by a raging argument.

No matter how caring you are, the strain that infertility places on your relationship can be enormous. Fortunately, you can alleviate the tension if you maintain good communication and use this problem to strengthen your bond rather than tear it apart, says Reed C. Moskowitz, M.D., founder and medical director of the Stress Disorders Medical Services at New York University Medical Center in New York City and author of *Your Healing Mind*.

"Accept that it is not you or she that has the problem. As a couple, you have a problem together. It affects both of you," Dr. Moskowitz says. "It's irrelevant who has the physical difficulty. Remember that both of you have the psychological pain because both of you want that little darling."

So maintaining as loving and nurturing a relationship as you possibly can is a powerful healer, says Vicki Rachlin, Ph.D., psychologist and co-director of the Womankind Counseling Center in Concord, New Hampshire.

"One of the most helpful things I've ever heard a man do in this situation is to point out to his wife the value of their relationship together and the positive things in their lives that they have aside from a child. It's important to stress that the positive quality of life can continue even if they don't find an answer to the infertility," Dr. Rachlin says.

---

rises to 13 to 15 percent and climbs steadily until 35, when it takes a dramatic turn upward. Twenty-five percent of couples between the ages of 35 and 40 are infertile, and after 40, nearly 50 percent will not be able to conceive."

So although a couple is considered infertile only after one year, couples older than 35 who have tried unsuccessfully to conceive for six months should seek medical help, doctors say. That's because the older you get, the less time you have to overcome infertility.

"After six months, come in and at least get some testing started," Dr. Licciardi suggests. "It doesn't mean you have to do anything at that point, but at least you'll get rolling with the diagnostic process."

Where to Start

Overcoming male infertility often requires the help of a urologist or reproductive endocrinologist, who, after testing your sperm, may suggest fertility
drugs or high-tech wizardry (more on that later). But there are some natural
ways you can try to boost your chances of having a child. Here's how.

Up your C, men. Low vitamin C levels may cause sperm to clump together, rendering as many as 16 percent of all men infertile. And some studies
have shown that daily vitamin C supplements improve fertility in male
smokers. "Vitamin C is an antioxidant that stabilizes cell membranes and may
have a helpful effect on sperm," says Larry Lipschultz, M.D., professor of
urology at Baylor College of Medicine in Houston. "It's not going to hurt anybody to take 1,000 to 1,500 milligrams of it a day." Citrus fruits, watermelon,
honeydew melon, canteloupe, strawberries and vegetables such as broccoli,
tomatoes and brussels sprouts are good dietary sources of vitamin C.

Searching for the Cause

It's been a year, and your spouse still isn't pregnant. It's time to see
your physician. Here's what will happen.

First, your doctor will review your medical history and order a complete physical. If this doesn't identify the problem, both of you will undergo diagnostic tests.

For you, that means a semen analysis. You'll likely be asked to masturbate into a small cup at home and to take the sample to the doctor as
soon as possible, or your doctor may ask you to do it in his office. At
least three specimens should be obtained at intervals of two to four
weeks, since sperm counts can vary. A semen analysis costs $50 to
$125. Here are some things your doctor will be looking for.

Sperm count. Twenty million to 200 million per cubic centimeter is
normal.

Motility. This test, graded from none to excellent, rates sperm activity. If they don't move, they can't get to the egg. It's that simple.

Morphology. This tells your doctor the shape of your sperm. They
can be micro (too small) to macro (too large). Like Goldilocks, you
hope yours are just right.

pH. Semen should be slightly alkaline—7.0 to 8.5.

Viscosity. Semen should pour easily.

Volume. Two to five cubic centimeters (½ to 1 teaspoon) is normal.

A Day in the Life of a Sperm

Imagine you're one of the 200 million sperm that an average guy ejaculates during intercourse. Here's the odyssey you face. First, you must find the natural mucus stream that helps carry you out of the woman's vagina and through her cervix.

Once you get past the cervix, you wiggle through the uterus until you get to the fallopian tubes. Since only one egg is produced each month and travels down one of the tubes, you face the important choice of going left or right. One path leads to oblivion, but if your partner is ovulating, the other leads to the egg. You have only one shot at this, since your strength is waning. Once you make your choice, you're now swimming against the current, because cells on the walls of the tube are gently pushing the egg toward the uterus.

Some sperm get disoriented and start swimming in aimless circles. But you're like a missile homing in on its target, and your trajectory remains true. Finally, you reach the egg. You're one of about 300 survivors of a microscopic journey that has lasted just a few hours. Yet as triumphant as that feels, you must still penetrate the egg. You and the remaining sperm surround the egg and begin relentlessly banging against its outer covering. Overall, there's only a 1 in 300 chance that one of you will break through and fertilize the egg. Will you be the lucky one? Who knows. But the odds of an individual sperm surviving this journey from beginning to end are a little better than a person's chances of being struck by lightning but less than getting a cab on a rainy winter night in the theater district of New York City.

Soothe your stress. Although doctors don't know why excessive amounts of stress lower sperm counts, practicing stress reduction techniques such as biofeedback or progressive muscle relaxation can help, Dr. Moskowitz says.

Make sure you're turned on. Men who are really aroused when they make love ejaculate higher amounts of semen and have more potent sperm, says Niels H. Lauersen, M.D., Ph.D., a founding member of the New York Society of Reproductive Medicine in New York City and author of *Getting Pregnant*. Allow at least 20 minutes for foreplay, he suggests.

Keep a lid on it. Avoid having sex for two to five days before your spouse is expected to ovulate, Dr. Lauersen says. It will increase your sperm count, and you'll ejaculate a higher percentage of healthy sperm.

Ease up on extreme exercise. Men who exercise excessively may be reducing their sperm counts due to the heat that builds up around the testicles during strenuous activity, says Mary Jane De Souza, Ph.D., an exercise physiologist at the University of Connecticut Health Center in Farmington. In studies there, researchers found that runners who trained more than 65 miles a week had lower sperm counts and more immature sperm cells than men who ran less than 35 miles weekly.

However, moderate aerobic exercise such as walking or swimming, three times a week, 20 minutes a session, shouldn't affect sperm production, says Eli Reshef, M.D., a reproductive endocrinologist at the University of Oklahoma Health Sciences Center in Oklahoma City.

Be a boxer. Although it's not as effective as was once believed, switching from bikini briefs to boxer shorts may increase your sperm production, because your testicles will be cooler. "It may have some basis in fact, but we simply don't see tremendous differences in sperm production when we switch men to boxer shorts," says Dr. Galen. Still, if you'd like to try it, it couldn't hurt, he adds.

Shed a few pounds. If you're overweight, losing a few pounds might increase your fertility. "If you're overweight, fatty tissue can surround the testicles, increase temperature in that area and kill off sperm," Dr. Lipschultz says.

Analyze your antibiotics. Although antibiotics play a minor role in infertility, some types have been shown to affect sperm quality by decreasing their count and motility, or their ability to "swim." The names of these groups are nitrofurans, such as nitrofurazone, and macrolides, such as erythromycin. Ask for penicillin (Beepen VK) or quinolones, such as cinoxacin (Cinobac), instead.

Turn down the sauna. Sitting in saunas, hot tubs or even baths that are hotter than body temperature for prolonged periods of time can decrease sperm production, says Wolfram Nolten, M.D., associate professor of endocrinology at the University of Wisconsin–Madison Center for Health Studies. Spend no more than 15 minutes a day in a hot tub or sauna, and lower the temperature to 98°F.

Put a cap on lubricants. Jellies and other lubricants may make sex easier, but they can impair sperm motility, even if they don't contain spermicides, Dr. Nolten says.

Whack the weed habit. If you smoke, your chances of becoming a papa may literally be going up in smoke, Dr. Galen says. Smoking has been linked to sluggish sperm and low counts, and in addition, findings suggest a 64 percent increase in miscarriages when both partners smoke or when just the man smokes.

Limit your liquor. Excessive amounts of alcohol can lower sperm counts. "Drink in moderation," Dr. Galen says. "I'd say no more than one or two alcoholic drinks a day."

Don't go to pot. Long-term use of marijuana and other illegal drugs results in a low sperm count and sperm that exhibit abnormal patterns of development, according to Dr. Galen.

High-Tech Conception

Okay, so you've tried everything natural, and you're still not a father. Don't give up hope yet. In most cases, experts can pinpoint and treat infertility problems with dramatic advances in drugs and surgery. In fact, more than half the couples seeking such treatment will conceive. RESOLVE, a support group for infertile couples, can refer you to a specialist in your area. Write to 1310 Broadway, Somerville, MA 02144-1731.

So what will a doctor do? After thorough testing, he may prescribe fertility drugs such as clomiphene (Clomid) to stimulate more sperm production. If you have a varicocele or blockage of the vas deferens, he may recommend corrective surgery.

In some cases, such as when a man develops sperm antibodies or doesn't respond to fertility drugs, doctors will suggest one of the many high-tech fertilization methods. They're costly, and there's no guarantee they'll work, which is why couples, including Scott and Karen Read, choose adoption.

Here's a sample of some of the most successful high-tech options.

Artificial insemination. Semen is deposited directly into the vagina or uterus. If the man's sperm are of poor quality, the couple could consider donor sperm.

In vitro fertilization (IVF). Eggs are surgically removed from a woman's ovaries, transferred to a petri dish and mixed with her partner's sperm for fertilization. After a two-day incubation, usually a few fertilized eggs (or embryos) are placed into the uterus.

Gamete intrafallopian transfer (GIFT). Eggs and sperm (gametes) are inserted into the fallopian tube, where, it is hoped, fertilization will take place.

Zygote intrafallopian transfer (ZIFT). As in IVF, eggs and sperm are combined in a petri dish and incubated for two days. But rather than being placed into the uterus, the embryo, or zygote, is placed into the fallopian tube. From there it will travel a natural course down the tube and into the womb for implantation. The advantage of this procedure over GIFT is that you know fertilization has taken place.

Zona drilling. In this technique, a surgeon uses chemicals, a laser beam or a needle to open part of the outer layer of the egg, or zona pellucida, so that sperm have a better chance of penetration.

Microinjection. In this procedure, which is in the experimental stage, a thin needle is used to insert a single sperm into an egg.

INJURIES AND ACCIDENTS

Learning the Hard Way

The 36-year-old right fielder arrived at the baseball field for a company softball tournament.

Both teams knew they were the best in the company; both were hot to prove it.

By the fourth inning, the right fielder's team was losing, and every play counted. Then a batter for the opposing team hit a long drive deep into right field. Realizing that the ball would fly over his head, the fielder pivoted to move back and get in place.

He never made it. His spikes dug into the grass, holding his foot and lower leg pointed at home plate while the rest of him headed in the opposite direction. The ligament in the knee that holds the upper and lower leg bones together snapped like an overstretched rubber band.

Nothing is more likely to make you feel like your body is 110 years old than an injury that lands you on your back or confines you to a chair. But whether the injury is caused by a traffic accident, a fall or a tricky move in a game of softball, just about everyone is at risk for an injury at one time or another.

According to the National Safety Council, injuries kill about 83,000 Americans every year, primarily through traffic accidents or falls. Despite what you might think, the risk isn't reserved for the elderly. In fact, more than half of all accidental deaths occur among men and women between the ages of 25 and 44.

But most of us won't die from injuries or accidents; we'll be temporarily sidelined. And for people between the ages of 25 and 44, the usual cause is a strained or torn muscle from a sports injury.

The Trouble with Weekends

Sports injuries result in 6,000 deaths a year. Nonfatal injuries in recreational activities such as baseball and softball, basketball, football and bicycling put more than two million people in the emergency room every year. Add to that the mammoth numbers of strains and sprains that are treated in locker rooms, plus injuries from dozens of other sports, and you can understand why the National Safety Council estimates that the total number of sports injuries exceeds three million each year.

Although these huge numbers do include adolescents in team sports, they also include a surprising number of adults. Informal games of basketball involving players between the ages of 25 and 64, for example, account for more than 24 percent of all basketball-related injuries that are treated in emergency rooms every year.

People between the ages of 25 and 64 also make up more than 74 percent of all emergency room visits for scuba-diving injuries, 68 percent for squash, racquetball and paddleball injuries, 51 percent for horseback-riding injuries, 45 percent for fishing injuries, 44 percent for tennis injuries, 42 percent for volleyball injuries and 40 percent for weight-lifting injuries.

Why are so many people in this age group getting hurt? "By age 25, people have become 'weekend athletes,' " explains Stephen J. Nicholas, M.D., associate team physician for the New York Jets and associate director of the Nicholas Institute of Sports Medicine and Athletic Injuries at Lenox Hill Hospital in New York City. "They're getting more involved with work, and social demands begin to take precedence over physical well-being. They taper off activities in which they play basketball or run three times a week.

"It's like putting your body in a cast and taking it out only on weekends," says Dr. Nicholas. "The muscles get short, weak and stiff. And they're no longer able to function at their optimal levels."

But the mind still thinks that the body is in peak condition, he adds. So when you play on the weekend, the mind still pushes the body the way it used to when you were playing several times a week.

The result? The mind pushes, the muscles fatigue, the mind pushes more, and the muscles cramp, strain, then pull to the point where they can actually tear, says Dr. Nicholas.

Getting on the Side of Caution

It's difficult to rein in your mind once you're going for that extra mile, hit or point. Here's how to help your body keep up—and reduce your risk of injury.

Take a high school exam. If you're over age 25 and participating in weekend sports, schedule a physical exam with a family physician who does the local high school's team physicals, says Rosemary Agostini, M.D., a staff physician at the Virginia Mason Sports Clinic and clinical associate professor at the University of Washington, both in Seattle.

Ask him to give you the same type of physical that he gives the local football or basketball team, including a review of any previous sports injuries. Combined with a "weekend warrior" approach to sports, old injuries have a way of coming back to haunt you—sometimes on a chronic basis, says Dr. Agostini. A physician can evaluate the likelihood of that happening and make specific suggestions to avoid reinjury.

Turn in your shoes every 500 miles. Shoes need to provide good support and shock absorption to prevent injuries, says Dr. Agostini. Replace them every six months or 500 miles, whichever comes first.

Make midweek moves. "You'll be able to minimize injuries if you go on a regular exercise program—one that involves 30 or 40 minutes every day or at least three or four times a week," says Dr. Nicholas. The key is that your body not be allowed five or six days in a row in which to stiffen up.

Loosen hams and quads. Begin your exercise program with at least 25 minutes of stretching every time you work out, Dr. Nicholas says. The muscles in the back and front of your thighs—the hamstrings and quadriceps—plus those in the lower back are the most important to loosen up.

"These usually don't get any stretching during the day unless you specifically set out to do it," says Dr. Nicholas.

Make your body work. After you stretch, do any aerobic exercise—shooting baskets, running, jumping rope—that accelerates your heart rate and keeps you breathing hard for 20 minutes, says Dr. Nicholas.

Lift. Strengthen your muscles by lifting at least a minimal amount of weight, says Dr. Nicholas. Get an athletic trainer to review your doctor's recommendations regarding any old injuries, then ask him to prescribe the specific weights and number of repetitions you should do. And don't forget to stretch before your workout.

Buddy up. "I was talking to a friend of mine the other day, and we admitted that as we get older, there's always something that gets in the way of exercise," says Dr. Nicholas. "You have to meet someone for a drink, or you're trying to deal with a mortgage, a patient or the kids."

But if you arrange to meet friends for a game of basketball instead of a drink or you take your kids to the ice rink instead of a movie, you're much more likely to get the extra exercise you need to stay loose and injury-free.

When You Make a Mistake

No matter how carefully you keep your body in shape, every once in a while you're going to pull or strain something when you twist the wrong way, intensify your exercise program or simply fall over your own two feet.

So here's what Dr. Nicholas advises for a pulled or strained ligament, tendon or muscle.

Apply RICE. *RICE* may be the sports world's most important acronym. It means *r*est, *i*ce, *c*ompression and *e*levation. And that's exactly what you should do for any new injury, says Dr. Nicholas. The idea is to minimize the amount of inflammation that occurs. It's inflammation that produces the swelling that causes the pain, which can then limit your movement.

"Put ice on the injury for three or four days," Dr. Nicholas says. "Apply it for 20 minutes of every hour you're awake." Wrap an elastic bandage around the injured area afterward, then elevate the injured muscle.

Take ibuprofen. "I also tell people to take Advil if they don't have any stomach problems," says Dr. Nicholas. That also reduces inflammation. Just follow package directions.

Use wet heat. Once you have RICE'd yourself for three or four days, it's time to work on getting your normal function back and preventing the injured area from becoming a chronic problem, says Dr. Nicholas.

The difficulty is that after three or four days, dried blood from torn or traumatized muscle fibers is sitting at the injured site.

"We need to get it out of the area," says Dr. Nicholas. "So we start what we call the wet heat program. We wrap a warm, wet towel around the injured area, put plastic—the kind of plastic bag you get at the dry cleaner's—around the towel to provide insulation, then put a heating pad on top.

"We leave it that way for about an hour and a half, three times a day, being careful not to burn the skin," he adds. "It will liquefy the dried blood in the injured area, bring the blood to the surface and help the body absorb it.

"It also helps with the healing process by loosening up the muscles."

Restretch the injured muscle. Once a muscle has been injured, both it and the surrounding muscles have contracted into shorter lengths, says Dr. Nicholas. So before you can resume your normal workouts, you have to restretch the muscles until they achieve their normal resting lengths. Ask an athletic trainer which stretches he suggests for your particular injury.

"If you don't achieve that resting length, you're more subject to chronic pulls that can occur again and again," says Dr. Nicholas.

Falling Down on the Job

Sports injuries may be costly in terms of time, pain and aggravation, but falls are more likely to kill. And not just older people. Nearly 1,100 men and women between the ages of 25 and 44 fell to their deaths in one year.

While falls that occur in the home are most likely to involve older folks with failing eyesight or wearing floppy footwear, falls by people between the ages of 25 and 44 are more likely to happen on the job, says researcher John Britt, R.N., state injury prevention program coordinator at Harborview Hospital in Seattle.

People fall when they're moving from one height to another on everything from stairs and stages to ladders and girders, according to safety experts at the Occupational Safety and Health Administration (OSHA) in Washington, D.C. Railings may stop unexpectedly before the last step, movable sets may not be clamped into place on stages, safety ropes may be torn or frayed on ladders, tools may inadvertently be left on girders.

Want to make sure you're not the next one to go bottoms up at work? Here's how Britt says you can reduce your risk.

Find the fall guy. Every company has a person whose job it is to make detailed reports of accidents to insurance companies, safety committees and workers' compensation, says Britt. Find that person, then ask when and where every injury took place during the past 12 months. Then make sure you don't fall into the same traps that others did.

Take a good look. People tend to pay attention to the little things and ignore huge ones, says OSHA. They see the tiny X-Acto blade that might slice their fingers in the art room but not the pool of ink on the floor that can cause them to fall into the moving parts of a press.

Try to make the invisible visible. Walk into any room at your workplace, stand in a corner and look for anything that can trip you or hurt you in any way. Then either report the hazard to management or take care of it yourself.

Wear safety gear. If your company suggests you wear nonskid soles, boots or other special footwear designed to keep you from falling on the job, do it.

Be a Road Scholar

Many of the men and women who survive the ten million or so traffic accidents in the United States each year can no longer expect friends and co-workers to automatically extend their sympathies.

Instead, says Britt, their accident recitals are just as likely to be met with the question "Were you wearing your seat belt?" or "Did you stop by the bar before you drove home?"

"There's been a subtle shift in public opinion about motor vehicle accidents in the past couple of years," Britt explains. People used to feel sorry for accident victims. But today—partly due to national safety programs and citizen groups such as Mothers Against Drunk Driving—there's more of a sense that accidents are preventable.

What can you do? Here are three safety strategies that Britt sees as key to preventing—or surviving—motor vehicle accidents.

Banish booze. Safety studies indicate that between 40 and 50 percent of all fatal accidents involve drunk drivers, says Britt. Alcohol is most likely to be involved in fatal crashes with adult male drivers between the ages of 20 and 55. And the more violent the crash, the more likely that a drunk was driving. So don't drink before you drive.

Stay alert on Fridays and Saturdays. One-third of all fatal crashes occur between 6:00 P.M. and 6:00 A.M. on Fridays and Saturdays, researchers report. Stay particularly alert during those times.

Use lap/shoulder belts. Many people simply won't wear safety belts in the mistaken belief that they have less chance of injury if they're "free" to get out of the car quickly. Unfortunately, these are the people who are least likely to get out of their vehicles at all. A study by the National Highway Traffic Safety Administration indicates that when they're worn correctly, lap/shoulder belts reduce the odds of death in a crash by 45 percent.

MEMORY

Revving Up Your Recall

Spark plugs. Oil. Fuel filter. Fan belt. Simple. You don't even need to make a list.

So you hop in the Honda and head for Parts Palace. And you're cruising the aisles, buying spark plugs, oil, an oil filter and—wait a minute, did you need an oil filter? Or was it a fuel filter? Yeah, that's it. A fuel filter and floor mats. Floor mats? Floor mats??

Stuff like this is happening way too often these days. You're forgetting appointments, phone numbers and clients' names. And even when you remember to pick up Junior after soccer practice, sometimes you forget where practice is.

Years ago you could memorize entire baseball rosters, player by player, homer by homer, season by season. Now you can't even remember the name of the guy you met on the softball field 15 minutes ago.

Talk about feeling old.

"There's no doubt: When you forget things, it makes you feel like your mind is slipping away on you," says Douglas Herrmann, Ph.D., a memory researcher at the National Center for Health Statistics in Washington, D.C., and author of *Super Memory*. But don't despair. While you may need a little tune-up, your memory probably isn't ready for the junkyard. "In all likelihood, you're not losing your memory," Dr. Herrmann says. "With a little focus and a little work, your memory will be just as good as it was in your teens and twenties—maybe even better."

The Matter's Still Gray

When it comes to memories, all doctors really know is that people store them in their brains. Somehow. Somewhere. The mechanics of the process are still pretty much a mystery. One theory holds that people may keep memories in three-dimensional or holographic form, using networks of brain cells and

GLAD You Can Remember

You have to buy *g*as, pick up the *l*aundry, get some *a*pples and make a bank *d*eposit. To remember the list, try forming a word using the first letter of each item—in this case, GLAD. It's called mnemonics, according to Francis Pirozzolo, M.D., a neuropsychologist at the Baylor College of Medicine in Houston. If you convert information into a familiar form, such as a simple word, you're more likely to remember It, he says.

electrochemical reactions to gain access to the system. Researchers do know that you can reach the same memory through a number of different paths. Smells can trigger a memory, as can a familiar sight, word or phrase.

Most scientists break down memory into three parts. First is the working memory, also called the scratch-pad memory. Dr. Herrmann says people use this to recall phone numbers or other information they need for a very short period of time—usually about a minute. Then it's usually just forgotten.

The mid-range, or intermediate, memory keeps all the information you've consciously and unconsciously absorbed within the past few hours or days. Eventually, you either forget that stuff because it's not important (what did you have for breakfast three days ago?) or transfer it to long-term memory. There you store permanent recollections, such as important addresses and names, the Pledge of Allegiance and memories of childhood Christmas mornings.

For years, studies kept showing that scratch-pad and mid-range memories start declining relatively early in life—even in your forties. But the research was flawed, Dr. Herrmann says. New evidence shows that you probably won't suffer serious memory loss until well into your sixties or seventies, he says.

So why are you forgetting things more than you used to? Stress could be one reason. "Your ability to concentrate and make decisions, along with short-term memory, may be one of the first areas of mental functioning hit by stress," says Paul J. Rosch, M.D., president of the American Institute of Stress in Yonkers, New York. And try not to worry about forgetting things; Dr. Herrmann says anxiety about memory makes it even harder to remember.

High blood pressure can also be a culprit. Studies of men in their thirties and forties show that guys with high blood pressure are consistently slower when trying to remember things stored in short-term memory. Researchers notice this effect even in men with mild cases of high blood pressure.

Then there's just plain old sensory overload. When life is pulling you like taffy, Dr. Herrmann says, you're less likely to concentrate on details. "And the less you pay attention, the less you're going to remember," he says.

For most men, memory loss never becomes a serious problem. But some diseases, most notably Alzheimer's, can blow your memory to bits. If you forget significant appointments at work, can't recall the names of family members or good friends or become severely disoriented or confused, see a doctor, advises Francis Pirozzolo, M.D., a neuropsychologist at Baylor College of Medicine in Houston. It's a sign that you could be experiencing something more than normal memory loss.

Hold That Thought

Okay. It's been about three minutes. What were those items you needed at Parts Palace?

If you can't remember, your memory may need some minor adjustments. Experts offer these tips.

Jog your mind. Regular physical exercise may give you a memory boost. In one study, people who took a nine-week water aerobics class scored better on general memory tests than a similar non-exercising group. "The aerobic exercise may have increased oxygen efficiency to the brain," says the co-author of the study, Richard Gordin, Ph.D., professor in the Department of Health, Physical Education and Recreation at Utah State University in Logan.

Dr. Gordin stresses that the results are preliminary. But other studies report similar findings. And then there are the added benefits of lower risk for heart disease and stroke and all the other helpful side effects of exercise.

Pay attention. This is the most basic—and most forgotten—memory aid. Don't expect to memorize a client's product line while you're talking to another client long distance. Don't expect to remember a person's name if you're

Tune Out

Are you sometimes forced to remember information amid the continual chaos at home or work? Practice will help. Turn on the television, volume high, and try to concentrate on something else for a few minutes, such as reading a book or memorizing a phone number. This will help you learn to overcome the background noise and pay attention, says Douglas Herrmann, Ph.D., a memory researcher at the National Center for Health Statistics in Washington, D.C., and author of *Super Memory*. You could also try watching two televisions at once. That forces you to pay attention only to important information and helps you hone your concentration.

Be a Slow Learner

You'll remember information longer if you absorb it gradually rather than all at once, according to Harry P. Bahrick, Ph.D., professor of psychology at Ohio Wesleyan University in Delaware, Ohio. In an eight-year study, he found that people who practiced their Spanish vocabulary once a month remembered four times more words than people who practiced daily. Dr. Bahrick says the principle works for physical skills, too. "If I was learning how to golf, I'd practice an hour a week for seven weeks rather than an hour a day for seven days," he says.

thinking about Monday Night Football when you make your introductions.

"It's simple," Dr. Herrmann says. "Focus, focus, focus. If it doesn't register in your brain initially, you have no chance of remembering it." So when there's key information to recall, drop what you're doing and spend a couple of minutes concentrating. Then move to the next task at hand.

Dream on. A good night's sleep will do wonders for your memory. Research shows that people who are awakened during dream sleep fail to process memories from the day before and thus forget more. Dr. Herrmann also says that regular sleep allows your entire body to recharge, making you more alert and more attentive to detail. "And avoid sleeping pills," he says. "You don't get the same quality sleep, and you're less likely to remember things during the following day."

One more hint: If you're studying or working into the night, go to sleep as soon as you're done. Going out afterward for a drink or a cup of coffee, or staying up to watch the news, makes it harder to remember the information the next day.

Don't try to remember everything. Man has invented telephone books, address books, computer files, pencils, pens and those little yellow sticky pads—all to help us remember things. Use them. "Why spend time trying to memorize giant shopping lists when you can just write them down?" Dr. Pirozzolo asks. "If you are a busy person with a lot to remember, making lists frees up your memory to recall more important items."

Mind your minerals. There's nothing better for your memory than a balanced, healthy diet with lots of fruits and vegetables, Dr. Herrmann says. There's also some evidence that keeping up your intake of the mineral zinc and the trace mineral boron can revive your memory, according to James G. Penland, Ph.D., research psychologist with the U.S. Department of Agriculture's Grand Forks Human Nutrition Research Center in Grand Forks, North Dakota.

Byte Off What You Can Chew

Computers remember information in small pieces, or bytes. That's the best way for you to do it, too, according to Francis Pirozzolo, M.D., a neuropsychologist at the Baylor College of Medicine in Houston.

The process is called chunking. Since your mind remembers items in groups of five to nine, break down lists into segments of that size. It's much easier to remember five groups of 5 items than it is to remember a list of 25 items, Dr. Pirozzolo says. And if you can group similar things together—fruits on one list, paper products on another—you'll do even better.

One study showed that men on low-zinc diets scored lower on short-term memory than they did when they got their Recommended Dietary Allowance of 15 milligrams. A half-dozen steamed oysters gives you a whopping 76.4 milligrams of zinc. Meat is also a good source of zinc—but remember: Make it lean.

The same held true for boron, which your body needs in tiny amounts. Men who ate high-boron diets of 3.25 milligrams per day scored significantly higher on tests of attention and memory. That's the same amount you'll find in three apples. Other good boron sources include prunes, dates, raisins and peanuts.

Dr. Penland points out that these studies show that you're better off with recommended levels of boron and zinc than you are with low levels. But it doesn't mean that taking high doses of the two will improve memory further.

Can the coffee. Caffeine is a proven memory killer, Dr. Herrmann says. More than one cup during the workday is probably going to overstimulate you and make it harder to concentrate. "It's an out-and-out myth that coffee helps you remember. It may keep you awake, but by wrecking your sleep you'll remember even less," Dr. Herrmann says.

Smoking causes the same problem with overstimulation, Dr. Herrmann says. And alcohol, even one drink, reduces the ability of individual brain cells to process and store information. Long-term drinking also kills brain cells, Dr. Herrmann says.

Don't believe the hype. Avoid pills or powders that advertise themselves as "miracle memory boosters." They don't work, according to Thomas H. Crook, Ph.D., a clinical psychologist and president of Memory Assessment Clinics, based in Bethesda, Maryland. There has been promising research into memory enhancement drugs, but Dr. Crook says nothing on the market today will help. "They're really just nutritional supplements masquerading as cures," he says. "They're just a big waste of money."

Metabolism Changes

No Excuse to Go to Pot

Your body is like a machine, and food is the fuel that keeps it chugging. It has always taken a lot of food to fill your tank and run your motor, right? Not so long ago, you could down a cheeseburger, hot dog, fries and a milk shake—all in one sitting—and still have room for a big hunk of chocolate cake.

Try that now, and what's the first thing you think about? Probably your waistline.

Today, being a lean, mean machine isn't so easy. You may even be eating less than you did way back when. But now the pounds are piling on, your belt needs to be let out a few notches, and your get-up-and-go seems to have just gotten up and gone.

That's because your body is playing by a new set of rules. Your metabolism—how your body converts food into energy and then burns that energy as calories—is slowing down. This is a natural process that begins at about age 30. From then on, your body burns energy about 2 to 4 percent slower every ten years. So fewer calories are burned, and more are stored as fat. You can see that if you do nothing to counter this trend, you'll become heavier and less energetic. And you'll put yourself at greater risk for serious health problems such as high blood pressure and heart disease. Hardly a recipe for a youthful life.

Why the slowdown? "Metabolism changes are a direct response to changes in body composition," says Robert Kushner, M.D., director of the Nutrition and Weight Control Clinic at the University of Chicago. "As we age, we tend to lose muscle and gain fat. Since muscle burns a lot of energy, our energy needs diminish as we lose muscle, and our metabolism slows."

Unfortunately, we bring a lot of this upon ourselves. "The major cause of this muscle loss is inactivity," says Eric T. Poehlman, Ph.D., associate professor of medicine in the University of Maryland at Baltimore Department of Medicine. "The more inactive we become with age, the less lean muscle we have. The less lean muscle we have, the more inactive we become. Over the years, the two feed on each other, and our metabolism plummets."

What Are Your Calorie Requirements?

If you knew how much energy your body burns in a day, you'd know how many calories you need to maintain, lose or gain weight. Here's a handy formula to get you started on balancing your energy equation.

First, multiply your weight by 11. This is your basal metabolic rate, the minimum number of calories you need to keep your system running.

Next, determine your activity level and multiply your basal metabolic rate by the appropriate percentage below. This gives you the additional calories you require for the day.

Sedentary activity refers to the time you spend sitting around the house watching television, reading your favorite magazine or talking on the phone. Light activity includes things such as housework, cooking and a stroll around the block after dinner. Moderate activity includes swimming or walking at a brisk pace while able to talk without gasping for breath. Strenuous activity includes heart-pounding exercise such as running or aerobics.

Activity Level	Percent
Sedentary	30–50
Light	55–65
Moderate	65–70
Strenuous	75–100

Add these two numbers together, and you have your total calorie needs for the day. So if you're a 190-pound man whose daily activity level is on the low end of the moderate scale, you would need 3,449 calories.

$$190 \times 11 = 2{,}090$$
$$2{,}090 \times 0.65 = 1{,}359$$
$$2{,}090 + 1{,}359 = 3{,}449$$

This figure is only an estimate, however. Your metabolism can be measured more accurately by an exercise physiologist or a physician specializing in weight loss and metabolism.

Unless you have thyroid disease, which can play havoc with how your body burns energy, you can get your metabolism cranked up again by making some lifestyle changes. But first, here's what's going on inside.

Overfueled and Underactive

To keep running, the body needs energy, which it burns in the form of calories. Add up all the energy needed to power the activities in a resting body—everything from breathing and digestion to the activity of nerve cells during thinking—and you have your basal metabolic rate, the minimum energy requirement to stay alive. For most men, this is around 1,800 calories per day.

A man's total calorie needs consist of his basal metabolic rate plus the additional energy he expends on physical tasks. This means, of course, that two men may have the same basal metabolic rate but burn very different amounts of calories every day. For example, an active 165-pound man can easily burn about 3,200 calories per day, while a sedentary 165-pound type can barely burn 2,500.

Which takes us to the punch line of this brief lesson in calories—the metabolic formula for not gaining weight. Calories in must equal calories out. The calories that aren't "out" are, sorry to say, stored in your body as fat. But if you burn more calories than you take in, stored fat is burned, and you lose weight.

So the way to not gain weight as you get older is simple: Cut back on calories. Pretend you like rice cakes. You know the routine. But there's a small problem. Your body doesn't know you're on a diet; it thinks you're starving to death. So instead of burning fat, your metabolism goes into famine mode, trying to preserve your fat stores.

"Very low caloric dieting can decrease your basal metabolic rate by 15 to 30 percent, making weight loss even more difficult," says Dr. Kushner. A very low calorie diet is one that consists of fewer than 600 calories a day. Because your body is trying to save you by keeping your fat level intact, it chooses another source of fuel: muscle. You've heard the phrase "Diets don't work." Now you know why.

Okay, dieting isn't the answer. So what can you do when your age causes your body's metabolism to shift into a lower, slower gear?

Exercise.

Aerobic exercise—walking, riding a stationary bike, aerobic dancing, any activity that boosts your heart rate for 20 minutes or more—is the best way to burn calories. And the benefits of exercise just keep going and going. Exercise sets your metabolism at a higher rate, so calories are incinerated for hours after you've stopped.

But the best way to boost your metabolism is to participate in an aerobic activity and a regular period of a strength training, such as weight lifting. "The major reason one person burns 1 calorie per minute and another burns 1.5 is that the second person has more muscle mass, and muscle is an extremely energy-hungry tissue," says Dr. Poehlman. "Strength-building exercises such as weight lifting will add muscle mass at any age. And the more you do such exercises, the better for your metabolism."

The Male Advantage

Men are much more efficient calorie burners than most women, a fact that the women in our lives won't let us forget. Over the same amount of time and with the same amount of physical activity, a typical man will lose more pounds than a typical woman.

Men burn calories faster for two reasons. One, we are usually heavier to begin with and are burning more calories all the time. Two, guys have a greater proportion of fat-burning muscle. As a result, the average woman's basal metabolic rate is 5 to 10 percent lower than the average man's.

The male anatomy has another advantage. Men are more likely to put on fat around the gut, while women will develop it in the thighs and buttocks. Some experts believe that the fat cells in the gut are more metabolically active; thus, men can shed that fat easier than women. However, the drawback is that belly fat has a far higher association with heart disease, stroke and high blood pressure than hip and thigh fat.

We might have some advantages over women on the metabolism front, but none of us is going to get a free ride. Here are some tips to keep your metabolism revving at peak levels.

Pick up the pace. An easy way to burn more calories in the same amount of time is to put a little more speed into your current aerobic workout. Suppose you're a walker who covers a mile in about 15 minutes (about four miles per hour), burning roughly 365 calories per hour (or about 90 calories per mile). If you bump up your speed to a 12-minute mile (five miles per hour), your calorie burn increases to about 585 for the same hour. That's a bonus of 27 calories a mile. That extra calorie burn each day can translate to a weight loss of about 15 pounds in less than a year.

Go longer. If you're already working out at your top speed, don't go any faster, but try to go longer. "Just like a car, your body will burn more fuel—in this case, fat—the longer it is engaged in an activity," says Dr. Kushner.

Work your arms and legs. Exercises that vigorously use both arms and legs are better fat burners than those that involve only your legs. "Cross-country skiing rates highest in lab tests for burning the most calories per minute because you're using your legs, upper body and even your torso," says Wayne Westcott, Ph.D., strength-training consultant for the International Association of Fitness Professionals. Stationary rowers and bikes with moving hand levers also rate high.

Start your day with breakfast. Experts say your body burns calories at a slower rate as you sleep. Breakfast acts as your metabolism's wake-up call, kicking it into the calorie-burning mode. If you don't eat something in the morning, you may ultimately burn fewer calories during the day. And it's more likely that when you do eat, you'll grab the first high-fat snack you see.

Spread out your meals. Eating small meals throughout the day instead of your standard three squares may be better for fat burning. After you eat, your body releases the hormone insulin, which causes your body to store fat. The larger the meal, the more insulin your body releases. But smaller, more frequent meals keep insulin levels lower and more stable. The less insulin you have in your blood, the more fat you burn, and the less you store.

Don't skip meals. Skipping meals and then eating one big meal at night can be a triple whammy, says Dr. Kushner. First, it puts you into a slow burn mode during the day. Second, the big meal provides an energy overload: The body can metabolize only so much food at one time, so the excess is likely to become fat. Third, most of the metabolizing will take place while you sleep—when your metabolic rate is at its lowest.

Exercise after you eat. A moderate workout right after a meal gives you a fat-burning bonus. A brisk three-mile walk on an empty stomach burns about 300 calories. But walking on a full stomach will burn about 345 calories. That's because eating gives your metabolism a boost; add exercise, and your metabolism gets a double boost and burns even more calories.

Stay away from stimulants. Caffeine, alcohol and other stimulants may raise your metabolic rate, but once they're out of your system, your metabolism crashes back to normal or below. The wise move, says Dr. Poehlman, is to avoid any artificial means of raising your metabolism unless it's prescribed by a doctor.

Spice up your life. Keeping an eye on your metabolism doesn't mean you have to give up tasty foods. In fact, hot, spicy foods such as mustard and chili may even shift your metabolism into high gear for a short period. In a study by British researchers, spicy food was shown to increase basal metabolic rate by an average of 25 percent.

Have your thyroid checked. While thyroid disease is more common in women than in men, an overactive or underactive thyroid can affect your metabolism. An underactive thyroid causes the body to burn energy at a slower rate than normal, and an overactive thyroid has the opposite effect. Your doctor can run tests to see if your thyroid is out of whack. If you have a thyroid hormone deficiency, it can often be controlled with prescription drugs.

MIDLIFE CRISIS

A Time to Turn Despair into Hope

At age 10, you were indestructible. At 20, you were invincible. At 30, you were incredible. But at 40, you suddenly feel insignificant.

You find yourself questioning your career choices, re-evaluating your commitments to your friends and family, worrying about fading sexual drive and mourning the passage of your youth.

Welcome to your midlife crisis—that uncomfortable time when you no longer feel secure about your life as it is but you can't look backward without regret or forward without foreboding.

"There are three wake-up calls in midlife. First, you realize that you're not going to live forever. Second, you realize you're never going to be president of the company, or if you are president of the company, you're not enjoying it as much as you thought you would. Finally, you realize your family life doesn't look like 'Ozzie and Harriet' or 'Father Knows Best,' " says Ross Goldstein, Ph.D., a San Francisco psychologist and author of *Fortysomething: Claiming the Power and Passion of Your Midlife Years*. "That's the drumbeat of midlife, and the question is, what do you do about it?"

How you cope with those realizations can literally make you feel older or younger than your years, says Leonard Felder, Ph.D., a psychologist in Los Angeles and author of *A Fresh Start: How to Let Go of Emotional Baggage and Enjoy Your Life Again*.

"Some people become more discouraged because they realize that they've set some goals they're having trouble following through on or made choices they're not comfortable living with," Dr. Felder says. "But many men who go through a midlife crisis get motivated to do what they've always wanted to, and that gives them more energy and a greater sense of being alive."

Beyond the Myths

Although most of us will experience some degree of anxiety and upheaval between the ages of 30 and 60, the average middle-aged man doesn't suddenly dye his hair, buy a fire engine–red sports car, change careers and dump his wife for a woman half his age. (Some do, but they're the minority.) Instead of being a complete overhaul, midlife is usually more like a minor tune-up, says Gilbert Brim, Ph.D., a social psychologist and director of the John D. and Catherine T. MacArthur Foundation Research Network on Successful Midlife Development, headquartered in Vero Beach, Florida.

So instead of buying a Ferrari, a typical guy in his forties may make subtle changes, such as coaching a Little League team, beginning a fitness program to take better care of his aging body or getting his finances in order for the first time, Dr. Goldstein says.

"Most people look at midlife challenges as an opportunity," Dr. Brim says. "They tell us things like 'Yeah, I got fired, but that wasn't a crisis. It was a chance to get a better job' or 'Yes, my mother died, and I miss her, but it was a release of a burden.' "

In fact, only about 10 percent of men really go through what we view as a midlife crisis, Dr. Brim says in his book *Ambition: How We Manage Success and Failure throughout Our Lives*. And researchers suspect that as few as half of them suffer severe psychological symptoms such as confusion, anxiety, suicidal thoughts, substance abuse and doubts about career and family choices. And of those men, most have had difficulty handling stress and trauma throughout their lives.

"If you had chronic troubles on the job or in your relationships earlier in your life, you're more likely to have trouble dealing with midlife events," Dr. Brim says.

Some psychologists even see similarities between adolescence and midlife. "At both times, everything gets tossed in the air, and you find yourself rebelling against the phase of your life that just occurred. So if you're 16, you don't want to be treated like a 12-year-old. If you are 40 and want to take a leading role in the business, you don't want to be treated like a junior partner. In both instances, you want a new relationship with the people around you," says Edward Monte, Ph.D., director of the Couple and Family Therapy Program at the Crozer Chester Medical Center in Upland, Pennsylvania.

What Triggers It

Some researchers believe that midlife crisis is exacerbated by hormonal changes that produce the so-called male menopause. Alternatively, other researchers take the point of view that there are a multitude of factors that may contribute to a midlife crisis.

More likely, a midlife crisis has psychological roots and no single cause, they

Midlife Crisis: The Telltale Signs

Are you on a collision course with a midlife crisis? To help you find out, we asked Ross Goldstein, Ph.D., a San Francisco psychologist and author of *Fortysomething: Claiming the Power and Passion of Your Midlife Years*, to develop this test. Answer the following statements yes or no. Scoring follows.

1. My future looks as positive now as it always has.
2. My life is as rewarding to me as I expected it to be.
3. Security is becoming more important to me.
4. Sometimes I feel excitement is missing in my life.
5. I am more flexible in my values today than I was ten years ago.
6. I get angry about the struggle to find "satisfaction" in life.
7. It feels like time is running out on me.
8. I wish there was an effective way of making all of the tension and stress go away.
9. I am more sure of who I am today than ever before.
10. Balancing my work and family is becoming more difficult.
11. Sometimes I feel exhausted from the struggle of "making it."
12. I have a hard time accepting that I am as old as I am.
13. I miss the excitement and adventure of my earlier years.
14. My work is as satisfying as it has always been.
15. I am more aware of my health as I grow older.

Give yourself two points for each "yes" to questions 3, 4, 6, 7, 8, 10, 11, 12, 13 and 15 and two points for each "no" answer to questions 1, 2, 5, 9 and 14. Total your score.

0 to 8. Your life is running smoothly. Your philosophy: If it isn't broke, why fix it?

10 to 16. Occasionally, you yearn for a day at the beach, but in general, you feel secure and comfortable with your life. Your outlook: You're ready to make a few minor midlife course adjustments, but you don't yearn to sail off to Tahiti with your secretary.

18 or more. Who is that old guy in the mirror, and why is he still working at a job that seems as grueling as watching an IRS agent audit his tax return? Your dilemma: how to make significant changes in your life without sacrificing the best of what you have. Career counseling may help.

say. In fact, at least 40 common stressful midlife events, including death of a parent, divorce and job change, can combine to unleash a crisis, Dr. Brim says. But however it occurs, it does change how you see yourself and the world, Dr. Felder says.

"Somewhere between ages 40 and 50, men begin to see life differently," Dr. Felder says. "Instead of seeing the years since birth, they begin to consider how many years they have left. They develop a real sense of time urgency. That can be extremely depressing or highly motivating."

Damage Control

A midlife transition doesn't occur overnight, and navigating through it can take you years, Dr. Monte says. But if you prepare yourself, you can sail through just fine.

"You can come through midlife feeling better about yourself, more alive and younger in some ways," Dr. Goldstein says. "Midlife is an opportunity to have a new beginning. It's a chance to pursue some of the dreams, passions and hopes you didn't have time to explore at earlier points in your life."

Here are a few ways to avoid a crisis and help you make a smooth mid life transition.

Rediscover the wonder years. What did you like to do as a child? If you had a favorite book when you were young, reread it. If you liked to play baseball, go to a Little League game, or get a ball and play catch with someone.

"It may sound silly, but it has a real psychological purpose," says Susan Olson, Ph.D., director of psychological services at the Southwest Bariatric Nutrition Center in Tempe, Arizona. "Doing these childlike things will help you realize that you really don't have to mourn your youth, because it's still within you to a certain extent. Once you realize that, your energy levels will literally surge."

Get a little help from your friends. Contact your best friend from high school or college, Dr. Olson suggests. "It will rekindle old feelings and bring perspective to your current life," she says. "It may help you realize that you're mourning a time that wasn't as ideal as you once believed."

Do lunch. Take at least one person who has been through a midlife crisis to lunch. Ask him which of the urges he resisted and which ones he followed through on and why, Dr. Felder recommends. It may give you some insight into your own situation.

Keep a half-full glass. Think positive, because being older can be neat, says Stanley Teitelbaum, Ph.D., a clinical psychologist in private practice in New York City. Instead of concentrating on lost vigor or sex appeal, consider what you have now that you didn't have at 20, such as a prosperous career, a good marriage, a supportive family or independence. "Life really does begin at 40 for many people. Yes, you're older, but the things you have now may outweigh or counteract the things you had in the past," he says. "So even if you're less sexually active, your sex life may be better because you're not ejaculating as quickly and you're pleasing your partner much more."

Switch gears. One good way to be a leader, help others and build your self-esteem is to become a role model to someone younger—say, a colleague at work. "A man who was captain of his high school baseball team probably can't play the game as well now that he's in his forties. But he can still get gratification out of the game by coaching a youth baseball team," Dr. Teitelbaum says. "Instead of being the star of the show, why not get satisfaction from helping others shine in the spotlight?"

Share your feelings. Men who express their feelings will do better during midlife than those who clam up. In fact, if you can't articulate what you want from your relationship, you're likely to destroy it, Dr. Monte says.

Arrange a time each week to discuss your feelings in a non-threatening way. If, for example, you lust after other women, you might say "I love you, and I'm attracted to a co-worker. It doesn't mean I love you less, but maybe it means something is missing in our relationship. Can we talk about it?" "The key is to discuss the topic in a way that doesn't cause either of you to panic and think your relationship is doomed," Dr. Monte says.

Celebrate the years. So your 40th birthday is approaching, and you dread it. Don't, Dr. Goldstein says. Instead, embrace the moment. Rituals such as birthdays, anniversaries and class reunions help us unleash feelings and reflect on who we are and where we're going in life. Use these natural pauses to rest, observe the vista, chart or correct your course and move on, he suggests. It's also an excellent time to share feelings and seek the support of family and friends.

Don't panic. "Making impulsive decisions during the midlife almost always ends up creating a bigger mess and, in some cases, disaster," Dr. Felder says. "If you think you need to resolve these midlife issues in the next two weeks, you're not going to get happy solutions. You need a plan that will allow you six months or a year to experiment with new options and that has room in it for you to stumble and fall at least a couple of times."

To get started, take a sheet of paper and divide it into three columns, Dr. Olson suggests. In the first column, list the goals you had as a child, such as "I want to be a spy." In the second column, write down which of those goals you should abandon, such as "I'll never be police commissioner." In the last column, list new goals that you'd like to accomplish in the next five years, such as "I'd like to save enough money that I could quit my job as a detective and start my own home security business."

MIGRAINES

Heading Off
Trigger-Happy Headaches

It's quitting time—and not a second too soon. The boss rode you all week about the Dinkman project, and your brain is aching from the abuse.

Throb-throb.

To top it off, you'll be late for Jerry's party. There's no time to cook, so you swing by your favorite Chinese restaurant for a pint of take-out chow mein.

Throb-throb.

Par-ty! You grab a glass of red wine, dance like a madman, wolf down a dozen Vienna sausages and argue about Johnny Unitas (clearly a better quarterback than Namath) until 3:00 A.M. You say your good-byes, drive home, fall into bed and sleep until noon.

THROB-THROB-THROB-THROB-THROB.

And you wake up with a migraine—the headache to end all headaches.

Eighteen million Americans tangle regularly with these mammoth headaches. For men, the peak years to get them are between ages 30 and 45. So just when you reach your most productive years, you find yourself battling crushing pain, curled up in a dark room for hours, longing for those days when you could eat or drink anything, pull two all-nighters a week and never pay the piper.

"Migraines are painful, unwelcome and often debilitating," says Seymour Diamond, M.D., director of the Diamond Headache Clinic in Chicago and executive director of the National Headache Foundation. "The pain lasts for hours, even days, and people aren't able to do much at all until it goes away."

211

Stop the Stress—And Stop the Pain

That pounding between your ears may be telling you something: Relax.

The National Headache Foundation reports that about 50 percent of migraines occur immediately after a period of unusual stress. To combat stress, doctors can prescribe hypnosis, biofeedback (where you're wired to a monitor and taught how to relax parts of your body) and other relaxation techniques, according to the foundation's executive director, Seymour Diamond, M.D., who is also director of the Diamond Headache Clinic in Chicago.

If you're looking for a way to beat stress, Dr. Diamond suggests this at-home relaxation exercise, which should take four to five minutes to complete.

Settle into a chair. Let all your muscles go loose and heavy.

1. Frown and furrow. Wrinkle up your forehead, then smooth it out. Picture your entire forehead and scalp becoming smoother as the relaxation increases.

Now frown, crease your brows and study the tension. Let go of the tension again. Smooth out your forehead once more.

2. Close and clench. Now close your eyes tighter and tighter. Feel the tension, then relax your eyes. Keep your eyes closed gently, comfortably, and notice the relaxation.

Now clench your teeth. Study the tension throughout the jaw, then relax.

3. Rock and roll. Press your head as far back as it can go, and feel the tension in your neck. Roll your head to the right and feel the tension shift; now roll your head to the left.

Straighten your head, bring it forward and press your chin against your chest. Let your head return to a comfortable position and study the relaxation.

Shrug your shoulders and hold the tension. Drop your shoulders and feel the relaxation. Bring your shoulders up, forward and back. Feel the tension in your shoulders and in your upper back. Drop your shoulders once more and relax.

The Pain: An Open and Shut Case

Migraines start when blood vessels in your head constrict for a period of 15 minutes to an hour, then rapidly expand, Dr. Diamond says. The culprit in this process is believed to be serotonin, a hormonelike substance produced by blood platelets.

When you trigger a release of serotonin—by eating certain foods, drinking certain beverages, stressing out or sometimes just oversleeping—the blood vessels in your head narrow. As your kidneys process the serotonin and the level of this hormonelike substance drops, the vessels dilate rapidly, pressing on surrounding nerves and causing pain and inflammation. Dr. Diamond says the ache can last for hours, or days, because the swelling lingers after the blood vessels return to normal.

About one in five migraine sufferers will experience an "aura" minutes before the onset of a headache. Men report seeing flashes of light and zigzag patterns and sometimes experiencing speech impairment, confusion and numbness in their faces and limbs, according to Dr. Diamond.

Heading Off the Ache

Migraine treatments have come a long way over the past 8,500 years or so. (Yes, migraines have really been with us forever.) In ancient Egypt, people with migraines used to nibble on parts of trees—wormwood and juniper were the favorites—to try to relieve the pain. As medical science progressed, doctors began prescribing fun treatments such as placing hot irons on painful spots, cutting a patient's temple and rubbing garlic on the wound and even wrapping an electric eel around a sufferer's head.

Fortunately, such "solutions" are no longer in vogue. If you're looking for ways to stop migraines before they start, experts offer these tips.

Watch what you eat. Many foods can cause the body to boost serotonin levels. Dr. Diamond says these include red wine, aged cheese, processed meats such as hot dogs and sausages, citrus fruits, lentils, snow peas and foods prepared with the flavor enhancer monosodium glutamate, or MSG. For MSG, watch the labels on the foods you buy. Chinese food often has MSG in it, so ask the restaurant to leave it out of your order if you think you're sensitive to it.

Foods affect people in different ways, so it's a good idea to keep a log that lists what you ate in the hours leading up to a migraine attack. Dr. Diamond says you might be able to see patterns emerge and to identify your personal trigger foods.

Try some heavy metal. A study from Henry Ford Hospital in Detroit found that magnesium is in short supply in the brains of most migraine sufferers. So eating foods rich in magnesium, including dark green vegetables, fruits and nuts, might bring some relief.

Kenneth Welch, M.D., chairman of the Department of Neurology at Henry Ford Hospital, stresses that the data on magnesium are preliminary. More work is needed before researchers make a positive link between migraines and this mineral. Still, eating a few more servings of fruits and vegetables won't hurt.

Pop an aspirin. A study of 22,000 American male doctors found that taking one 325-milligram aspirin tablet every other day may help ward off headaches. The doctors in the study who took aspirin reported 20 percent fewer migraines than those who took placebos.

Experts say you should see your own doctor before starting an aspirin routine, since aspirin can cause upset stomach, internal bleeding and other complications that may put you at risk for other health problems.

Sleep on a schedule. Irregular sleep patterns also contribute to migraines, although Dr. Diamond says the exact reason isn't clear. "We see lots of weekend migraines, when people decide to sleep late," he says. "You should try getting the same amount of sleep every night, even on weekends."

Control your caffeine. Too much caffeine—anything more than three cups of coffee within an hour or so—can constrict your blood vessels and trigger a headache, according to Dr. Diamond. But he says slugging a cup of joe just at the start of a headache might keep your vessels from expanding too much and could ward off a migraine.

Chill out—then see your doctor. Once a migraine sets in, Dr. Diamond says, nothing short of prescription drugs can stop it. He suggests riding out the pain by reclining in a quiet, dark room. Never try to exercise during a migraine episode, since a faster pulse only makes the pain worse.

You might want to put your headache on ice, says Lawrence Robbins, M.D., assistant professor of neurology at the University of Illinois at Chicago and at Rush Medical College of Rush University, also in Chicago. You have at least a 50-50 chance of getting some pain relief within two to three minutes of applying a soft cold pack and moderate pressure to your head. Soft cold packs are sold at pharmacies and medical supply stores.

Sometimes, Dr. Robbins admits, a migraine may be so painful that putting something on your head will make it feel even worse. In that case, forget the cold pack.

If you can't control migraines by yourself, see your doctor. A combination of biofeedback, relaxation exercises and medication may solve your problem.

A Drug to Dispel the Agony

A new drug, sumatriptan (Imitrex), shows great promise in fighting migraines. One study showed that 70 percent of patients who took sumatriptan during a migraine episode reported mild or no pain an hour later. The prescription drug is also free of most side effects common to migraine medication, such as sedation, nausea and vomiting.

"It's one of the great discoveries in migraine research," Dr. Diamond says. "It really offers great hope to people who suffer from frequent migraines." Unfortunately, it's not for those who have high blood pressure or heart problems. Ask your doctor if you would make a good candidate.

OSTEOPOROSIS

When Bones Lose Their Strength

If you have guzzled milk since you were a tot and you love to pound around the track, your skeleton is probably full of good, healthy bone. Good thing, too, because as you get older, you're going to need it.

You might know a man who used to stand straight as a flagpole and now has a stoop to his spine. Or maybe you have an older uncle who fell and broke a hip that refuses to mend. These men may have osteoporosis, a gradual thinning of bone that can make aging a perilous journey.

You might think of osteoporosis as a woman's disease, but it does cross gender lines. Everyone loses some bone with age. That's a normal process, and if your bones are in good shape to start with, it shouldn't cause you any harm. But for people with osteoporosis, bones thin at a faster pace, becoming porous and brittle—and breaking with ease. A man's confident stride turns into a tentative shuffle. He's afraid that a fall or slip could lead to a painful fracture.

Not for Women Only

Though osteoporosis strikes four women to every man, don't think you're immune. Approximately 10 percent of all men are affected. In part, this disease is linked to lifestyle factors. The biggest is a diet too low in calcium, a mineral vital to bone building. Although estimates of how many men are short on this crucial nutrient vary from 10 to 25 percent, experts agree that calcium deficiency is extremely common. Another dietary factor is a shortage of vitamin D, which is important to bone health because it helps your body absorb calcium.

Even if your diet is in good shape, if you don't get the right kind of exercise—weight-bearing workouts—your bones may become more porous and more easily broken. A heavy smoking or drinking habit can also contribute to osteoporosis, as can certain prescription medicines, which may erode bone strength particularly if taken for many years or in extremely high doses.

Putting Steel in Your Skeleton

The good news is that the right exercise and diet choices can put a check on osteoporosis. And even if you're getting a late start, you can take steps to halt further bone loss at any age.

Here's how to beef up your bones.

Bear down on exercise. It not only increases bone density but also improves your agility and reflexes, so you're less likely to fall and break a bone, says Susan Allen, M.D., Ph.D., assistant professor of internal medicine at the University of Missouri–Columbia School of Medicine.

But to prevent osteoporosis, you need workouts in which you're truly bearing your weight on your bones. Exercises such as brisk walking or running actually stimulate bone cells to build more bone, particularly in your back and hips, where you most need it, Dr. Allen says.

If you're not sure whether other workouts are weight bearing, just ask yourself whether they involve your feet hitting the ground with at least the impact that brisk walking produces, says Clifford Rosen, M.D., director of the Maine Center for Osteoporosis Research and Education in Bangor. Sports such as tennis and racquetball do, for example, but swimming and biking don't. So vary your routines to include frequent weight-bearing workouts, he says.

Pumping iron is also an ideal way to build bone strength, because it increases the weight of gravity on your bones. It's good sense to make weight lifting part of your weight-bearing exercise. Any lifting done in a standing position is particularly helpful for the spine and hips. If you've never used weights before, be sure to get your doctor's clearance and a trainer's advice on the safest routines.

Pump up your calcium. Calcium is essential to healthy bones. Ninety-nine percent of the calcium in your body is stored in your bones. If you don't get enough calcium, you can't make enough bone—it's as simple as that.

The National Osteoporosis Foundation recommends that men take in 1,000 milligrams of calcium a day, but most men over age 35 fall around 300 milligrams short, says Catherine Niewoehner, M.D., associate professor of medicine at the University of Minnesota in Minneapolis. Ounce for ounce, milk and milk products are the best sources of dietary calcium. One eight-ounce serving of nonfat yogurt provides around 450 milligrams of calcium. A cup of skim milk boasts about 300 milligrams. Many other foods contain calcium, but the nutrient is not as easily absorbed from these foods as it is from dairy products.

Be selective about supplements. "If men are physically active, non-smoking and nondrinking and eat a regular balanced diet that includes dairy products, there's no need for calcium supplements," says Dr. Rosen.

Don't do without D. Bones don't obtain enough calcium for proper mineralization unless the body has an adequate amount of vitamin D, says Michael F. Holick, M.D., Ph.D., director of the Vitamin D, Skin and Bone Research Laboratory at Boston University Medical Center. Without vitamin D, your body ab-

Your Best Calcium Sources

Besides rewarding you with harder, stronger bones, calcium has other vital bonuses. Blood pressure and cholesterol levels tend to rise in men as they age, and calcium battles both.

It's not hard to harvest calcium's powerful anti-aging benefits once you've learned which foods are calcium-rich. Here are the best sources.

Source	Calcium (mg.)
Yogurt, nonfat, 8 oz.	452
Sardines, 7	321
Skim milk, 1 cup	302
Buttermilk, 1 cup	285
Mozzarella, skim, 1 oz.	183
Salmon, pink, with bones, canned, 3 oz.	181
Figs, dried, 5	135
Almonds, unblanched, toasted, 1 oz.	80
Bok choy, cooked, ½ cup	79
Hazelnuts, 1 oz. (16)	55
Mustard greens, cooked, ½ cup	52
Brazil nuts, 1 oz. (16)	50
Kale, cooked, ½ cup	47
Pinto beans, cooked, ½ cup	45

sorbs about 10 percent of the calcium it takes in; with vitamin D, it can absorb 80 to 90 percent. "Vitamin D tells the small intestine 'Here comes the calcium. Open up and let it in,' " explains Dr. Holick. The Recommended Dietary Allowance for vitamin D is five micrograms, or 200 IU—easily found in fortified foods such as milk, breads and cereals.

Besides getting some of your daily vitamin D through food, your body can make it from sunshine, which triggers a vitamin D manufacturing process in your skin. From anywhere in the South to as far north as New York City, 5 to 15 minutes of bright sunshine every day—before you apply sunscreen—will supply your needs, says Dr. Rosen. If you live farther north, however, you can't depend on the sun. In that case, you'll need to be sure you're getting enough vitamin D from dietary sources, he says.

Check out your medicine chest. Certain medications—thyroid medications, anti-inflammatory steroids such as hydrocortisone, cortisone and pred-

(continued on page 220)

Exercises to Bone Up Your Back

Along with weight-bearing exercises such as jogging and weight lifting, exercises that stretch your spine will strengthen the vertebrae most vulnerable to osteoporosis. Try these back extenders suggested by Susan Allen, M.D., Ph.D., assistant professor of internal medicine at the University of Missouri–Columbia School of Medicine.

"To help prevent osteoporosis, do as many of these exercises as you can, once in the morning and once at night," says Dr. Allen.

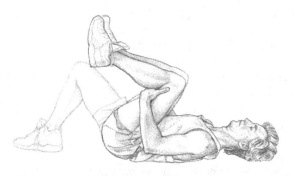

Lie on your back with your knees bent. Bring both knees as close as possible to your chest and hold (with your hands supporting your knees) for five seconds, then lower your legs slowly to the floor. Then bring one knee up to your chest as far as you can, hold for five seconds and lower it slowly to the floor. Alternate right and left legs for ten repetitions each.

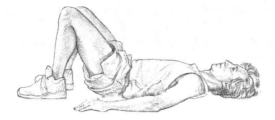

Lie on your back with your knees bent. Press the small of your back against the floor and hold for five seconds. Repeat ten times.

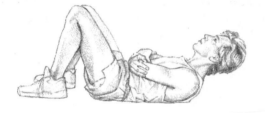

Lie on your back with your knees bent. Place your arms across your middle, cupping the opposite elbow with each hand. Raise your head and shoulders as far as you can without sitting up. Hold for three seconds. Repeat ten times.

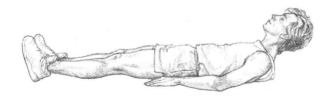

Lie on your back with your legs straight and your arms at your sides. Raise your head and shoulders as far as you can without sitting up. Hold for three seconds. Repeat ten times.

nisone, anticonvulsants such as phenytoin, depressants such as phenobarbital and the diuretic furosemide—can cause osteoporosis, particularly when they're taken regularly in high doses over a number of years. Thyroid medicine in normal doses should pose no problem, however, says Dr. Rosen, and the risk from diuretics can be offset by taking calcium.

The most serious osteoporosis risk is from steroids, Dr. Rosen says. If you need long-term steroid medication, your doctor may advise anti-osteoporosis drugs such as calcitonin (Cibacalcin) in addition to calcium and vitamin D supplements, he says.

Go easy on the booze. "Alcohol actually poisons the cells that build bone," says Dr. Allen. A beer or glass of wine now and then probably won't cause you much harm. But avoid drinking to excess, she says—more than two to three drinks a day.

Quit smoking. Osteoporosis risk doubles in men who smoke cigarettes, says Dr. Niewoehner. Why? Smokers tend to be thinner, and thinner people are at greater risk for osteoporosis, she says. Researchers also theorize that the hormone testosterone may protect men from osteoporosis, just as estrogen protects women, and that male smokers lose more testosterone as they age than non-smokers do. So do your bones a favor and give up the weed. If you need help, talk to your doctor.

OVERWEIGHT

The Keys to Banishing the Bulk

B y the looks of pants sizes in this country, some American men apparently see gaining weight as a constitutional right. It's almost as though smack between the right to free speech and the right to bear arms lies Amendment I-B: the right to eat freely and bear a mighty gut.

That's some dangerous thinking.

Lugging around extra pounds is like wearing a sign that reads "Welcome Age-Related Diseases." That's because conditions that can age your body— high blood pressure, high cholesterol, heart disease, diabetes, arthritis, backaches, sleep apnea and even sexual dysfunction—are firmly linked to the presence of flab.

There is a cancer connection as well. "When you're overweight, you also have increased risk for several cancers, including cancers of the prostate, rectum, liver and bladder," says John Foreyt, Ph.D., director of the Nutrition Research Clinic at Baylor College of Medicine in Houston.

Flab Puts You over the Hill

Of the age-related diseases, high blood pressure has one of the strongest links to overweight. When a heart has to work overtime to carry extra pounds, blood pressure shoots skyward. The Framingham Heart Study, which followed over 5,200 healthy men and women in Framingham, Massachusetts, since 1948, found that overweight men who pared their pounds lowered their blood pressure readings dramatically. A 15 percent decrease in weight resulted in a 10 percent decrease in blood pressure.

Type II diabetes, which often hits men after age 40, is also tied to being overweight. Surplus flesh directly affects the body's ability to balance blood sugar. Many overweight people with diabetes who need regular medication find that once they drop 20 or more pounds, they can also drop their prescriptions.

If arthritis is your main aging concern, there's enormous reason to lighten your load. Researchers at the Boston University Arthritis Center found that overweight people who lost just 11 pounds reduced their risk of developing arthritic knees by almost 50 percent. The connection is obvious: Fewer pounds means less pressure on the joint.

But it's not only for the sake of preventing disease that slimness makes sense. Excess weight can be hard on a man's self-image, too.

What to Do

Unfortunately, it gets harder to control your weight as the years roll by. A man's natural weight increases as his metabolism, the process by which his body burns calories, slows somewhat with age. Reubin Andres, M.D., clinical director of the National Institute on Aging in Bethesda, Maryland, believes it is harmless to gain about five pounds each decade after age 20—but only if you are in good health to start with and remain free of ailments such as diabetes and heart disease. But many experts say any weight gain should be avoided throughout the years.

But it's best to keep the weight off. After following a group of Harvard University alumni for 27 years, researchers found the lowest mortality rate among men who were 20 percent below the average weight for men of similar age and height. This finding held firm even after the researchers accounted for underweight from smoking or illness, which they believe may have distorted the results of previous studies.

The study also showed that men who were only slightly overweight—2 to 6 percent over their desirable weights—still had a significantly greater chance of dying from heart disease and that men who weighed 20 percent more than their desirable weights actually doubled their risk.

But regardless of where you fit on the charts, if you're struggling with more than a few extra pounds, you're probably eating too much—particularly in the fatty foods department—and exercising too little.

What to do about it? Well, you could put yourself on a crash diet. But that probably won't lead to anything but frustration.

"Diets just don't work," says Janet Polivy, Ph.D., professor of psychology at the University of Toronto Faculty of Medicine. "Diets become popular because they work for a week or two and everyone says 'You gotta try it.' Well, speak to those people in a year or two, and you'll find they've failed." When you fall for one of those speedy five-pounds-a-week programs, you lose it, all right—but you lose pounds of fluid, not fat. And as soon as you abandon the diet, the weight comes right back on.

In the long run, what works best to achieve a healthy weight is to modify your eating habits and to get more exercise.

What's a Healthy Weight, Anyway?

You don't need to be a slave to the scale, says John Foreyt, Ph.D., director of the Nutrition Research Clinic at Baylor College of Medicine in Houston. "Your healthy weight is what's produced by healthy eating and healthy exercise," he says. "That's your goal, period."

But maybe you'd feel better with a weight range to aim for. If so, the chart below, from the federal government, will show you approximately where you should stand. Note that it's perfectly all right to add a few pounds as you age. These guidelines were prepared for both men and women; men will generally fall toward the upper end of each range.

Height	Weight (lbs.)	
	Ages 19–34	Ages 35 and up
5'0"	97–128	108–138
5'1"	101–132	111–143
5'2"	104–137	115–148
5'3"	107–141	119–152
5'4"	111–146	122–157
5'5"	114–150	126–162
5'6"	118–155	130–167
5'7"	121–160	134–172
5'8"	125–164	138–178
5'9"	129–169	142–183
5'10"	132–174	146–188
5'11"	136–179	151–194
6'0"	140–184	155–199
6'1"	144–189	159–205
6'2"	148–195	164–210
6'3"	152–200	168–216
6'4"	156–205	173–222
6'5"	160–211	177–228
6'6"	164–216	182–234

Setting the Stage

Most of a man's battle with overweight takes place in his mind, not his mouth, says Thomas A. Wadden, Ph.D., associate professor of psychology and director of the Weight and Eating Disorders Program at the University of Pennsylvania in Philadelphia. "The first step toward feeling more in control is to accept yourself as you are right now." That's right. Say nice things to yourself in the mirror every morning—whatever it takes. Then try these suggestions.

Get ready for the long haul. The key to healthy and successful weight loss at any age is to make the changes very gradually. Losing no more than one-half pound a week is ideal, says George Blackburn, M.D., Ph.D., associate professor of surgery at Harvard Medical School and chief of the Nutrition/Metabolism Laboratory at New England Deaconess Hospital, both in Boston. So aim to attain a healthy weight a year from now, not next week, he says.

Make it a team effort. A good support system makes a huge difference in successful weight loss, says Dr. Foreyt. Ask your family and friends to cheer you on—or to join you in healthy eating. If you feel you have a serious problem with eating compulsively, a support group such as Overeaters Anonymous or professional counseling can be very useful, he says.

Decide to take charge of your cues. Sometimes you can confuse hunger with other feelings or appetites, especially if you're feeling depressed or stressed or just responding to a photo of some feast in a magazine. If it's not your stomach talking, you need to figure out what kind of emotions or discomforts are triggering your urge for food, Dr. Foreyt says. Then develop a problem-solving approach. "How can you answer that need without eating? Walk around the block, call a friend, meditate, take a bath, brush your teeth or gargle with mouthwash," he says. "This breaks the chain and develops an alternate behavior pattern."

Resolve to shut off the fat box. Nothing remote about it. If you watch more than three hours of television a day, you're doubling your chances of a weight problem that won't go away, says Larry A. Tucker, Ph.D., professor and director of health promotion at Brigham Young University in Provo, Utah. Slouched on the couch, you're not burning many calories, and you're likely to be taking in more by chowing down fattening snacks. So turn off the tube (and the junk food habit that usually comes with it) to boost your weight loss campaign.

A Weight Loss Workout Strategy

Activity burns calories, and excess calories are what make you fat. That's one reason why it's crucial to exercise regularly if you're battling overweight. Exercise will also strengthen your heart, improve circulation and boost your self-confidence. In short, it will help counteract many of the harmful effects of overweight. Exercise can even curb your appetite.

If you're not accustomed to exercising, consult your doctor about it before you get started. Here is a strategy to get your program in gear.

Keep it up. "The best predictor of long-term weight management is regular aerobic activity, which boosts your heart rate," says Dr. Foreyt. "Brisk walking is a great choice because it's very easy for most people to do on a reg-

Successful Gut Busters

You're taking your age-beating campaign seriously, and it shows. You have biceps like granite, legs that won't quit and little flab anywhere on your body—with one exception: the gut.

Granted, it's frustrating, but it's normal. An expanding gut is a natural consequence of aging for both men and women, research shows, though with men it tends to be more pronounced. That midriff mound may not be as immovable as you think, however. Here's how to pare it away.

Go easy on the sauce. There really is such a thing as a beer belly, and cutting your alcohol intake may be the key to deflating that keg shape. In a large study, men and women who drank more than two alcholic drinks a day had the largest waist-to-hip ratios, which is how doctors quantify potbellies.

Stop puffing. In the same study, researchers at Stanford University School of Medicine in Stanford, California, and the University of California, San Diego, detected a similar effect for smoking. There were twice as many rotund abdomens among those who lit up as among nonsmokers. See your doctor for help in quitting.

Start huffing. Getting your mountain moving may help it disappear, other research shows. To burn off a belly, exercise must do two things, says Bryant Stamford, Ph.D., director of the Health Promotion Center at the University of Louisville in Louisville, Kentucky. First, it must start out vigorously to trigger a substantial adrenaline release, which frees fat to be used for fuel. You can get this effect from brisk walking, he says. Then the vigorous activity must be followed by prolonged aerobic exercise that will burn up the liberated fat. Walking at a comfortable pace fits the bill. So could a spate of hard digging in the garden followed by some steady raking. "Just step up the pace now and then to boost adrenaline output," he says.

Firm it up. Once the fat is whittled away by low-fat eating and aerobic exercise, daily abdominal exercises can really help improve your shape, Dr. Stamford says. Start with isometric squeezes: Tense your abdominal muscles to the maximum and hold for six to ten seconds. Relax, then repeat several times. Later, he says, you can move to crunches: Lie on your back with your legs apart and knees bent. Cross your arms on your chest. Lift your head up toward the ceiling. Keep going until you can lift your shoulder blades slightly off the ground. Hold for two seconds, then lie back down. Build up gradually to ten repetitions a set.

ular basis. But the effectiveness of any aerobic activity for weight control has been proven repeatedly." Any kind of daily exercise helps. Thirty minutes of aerobic exercise burns flab and tones muscles—as long as you do it regularly.

Burn by building. Aerobic exercise should always be part of the battle plan, but when you bolster it with resistance training such as weight lifting, you stand to win the war. "Muscle tissue needs more calories," says Janet Walberg-Rankin, Ph.D., associate professor in the Exercise Science Program in the Division of Health and Physical Education at Virginia Polytechnic Institute and State University in Blacksburg. "So if you increase muscle mass while you lose fat, you boost your ability to burn fuel." It's later in the day, when you're sitting in a meeting or reading a good courtroom thriller, that your new, ravenous muscle is grinding away calories, she says.

"Resistance training isn't just about lifting barbells, though those are great for the biceps," adds Dr. Foreyt. To really work the different groups of muscles, your best bet is to go to a gym and get the trainer to show you how to circuit-train, he says. You employ a series of different weight machines to lift heavy weights, using muscles in the neck, arms, chest and legs. You can also accomplish the same thing by working with free weights at home, he says. "Pitting your muscles against something that doesn't yield—that's resistance."

And the more you do, the more you'll increase muscle mass. "A typical effective program would be to do your resistance training from 20 to 45 minutes a day, three days a week," says Dr. Foreyt.

Eating to Lose

You may be surprised to learn that the most crucial changes in the way you eat have to do not with eating less but with eating differently.

The latest nutrition research shows that there really is a new way to win at losing weight—without dieting and without hunger. It's based on understanding which kinds of food rev you up and give you real energy and which ones go right into your potbelly. Here's how to eat for health and satisfaction while comfortably controlling your man-size appetite.

Drown it. "Drinking generous amounts of water is overwhelmingly the number one way to reduce appetite," says Dr. Blackburn. Not only does water keep your stomach feeling fuller, but also many people think they're having food cravings when in fact they're thirsty, he says. So aim for 8 cups of fluids daily, sipping ½ cup at a time through the day.

When you're sipping away through the day, keep in mind that caffeine—in cola, coffee or tea—has its drawbacks. Caffeine is a diuretic, which removes water from the body. For that reason, most doctors recommend that people on weight loss programs drink no more than three caffeinated beverages a day.

Phase out fat. Dietary fat makes us gain weight because it's stored in the body far more easily than either carbohydrates or protein. The body burns those for fuel almost immediately, while the more calorie-dense fat burns slower and therefore is more likely to be left over in your spare tire.

Start by cutting fat in the obvious places: Eat fewer fatty meats, fried foods, high-fat dairy products and desserts. Also, beware of salads slathered in oil or other fatty dressings. It's recommended that you keep your total calories from fat to 25 percent or less of your daily diet.

"A high-fat diet has been linked to obesity, which in turn is associated with an increased risk of various cancers. Prudence says that a high-fat diet is a factor in so many illnesses that it only makes sense to eat low-fat foods instead," says Dr. Foreyt.

Don't go hungry. When you replace excess fat calories with carbohydrate calories, you can actually eat more and still lose pounds. In a study at the University of Illinois at Chicago, people on moderately high fat diets were told to maintain their weights for 20 weeks while switching to low-fat, high-carbohydrate diets. They ate to their hearts' content but still lost more than 11 percent of their body fat and 2 percent of their weight. So pile your plate with plenty of carbohydrate-rich pastas (without fatty sauces), low-fat cereals, breads, beans, fresh vegetables and fruits to fill you up while you're dropping down.

Don't be too hard on yourself. If you can't relax and enjoy a treat now and then, you may eventually let slips turn into a downhill slide, says Susan Kayman, R.D., Dr.P.H., a dietitian and consultant with the Kaiser Permanente Medical Group in Oakland, California. There's no use berating yourself for every little bite of cake or steak. If you eat low-fat 80 percent of the time, then when you're out on the town or over at the in-laws, enjoy an occasional higher-fat food without beating yourself up about it, she says.

Keep your eyes on the prize. Here's good news: If you stick with low-fat fare long enough, you'll actually lose your taste for high-fat foods. A four-year study of more than 2,000 people at the Fred Hutchinson Cancer Research Center at the University of Washington in Seattle showed that people who limit their fat intakes lose their taste for fat in six months or less, eventually finding fatty foods unpleasant to eat. So hang in there—it gets easier.

Fire the deadly duo. That's fats and sweets. When the body gets a jolt of sugar, it releases insulin in response. Because insulin is a storage-prone hormone, it opens up fat cells, preparing them for fat storage. So when you eat sugar, keep your fat intake low. Also, fats and sugar taken together can turn up your appetite to unmanageable levels. Eating sweets leads to an increase in the amount of sugar in the blood, which, because of a chain of reactions in the body, pumps up your appetite, says Dr. Wadden. So soothe your sweet tooth with a fresh fruit or bowl of low-fat sugared cereal instead of doughnuts and candy bars.

Eat like you're home on the range. Some researchers support the idea of grazing—eating numerous small meals throughout the day instead of three larger meals—to control appetite and prevent bingeing. "You cannot graze on M&M's, potato chips and Häagen-Dazs," says James Kenney, R.D., Ph.D., a nutrition research specialist at the Pritikin Longevity Center in Santa Monica,

California. "But if you graze on low-fat, high-fiber foods that aren't packed with calories, such as carrots, apples, peaches, oranges and red peppers, you'll keep your appetite down."

Go for the hot stuff. Be lavish with hot spices such as cayenne pepper and horseradish to boost your metabolic rate, which may help your body burn more calories, says Dr. Kenney. "When people eat hot foods, they often sweat, a sure sign of increased metabolic rate. And the faster the metabolic rate, the more heat produced by the body. Remember, whatever warms you up in turn slims you down," he says. But be sure to avoid high-fat dishes, even if they're loaded with spices.

Start with soup. A soup appetizer tends to reduce the amount you eat at a meal, several studies suggest. In one study from Johns Hopkins University in Baltimore, people who had soup before a meal ate 25 percent fewer calories of the entrée than those who started the meal with cheese and crackers. It may be the volume of space that soup takes up in the stomach or the fact that most of soup's calories come from carbohydrates rather than fat, researchers say. Or there may be a psychological factor at work, Dr. Kenney says. "Hot soup is very relaxing if you have a nervous, gnawing appetite."

Surf through the cravings. When the urge strikes for an extra pile of greasy fries, don't confuse the craving with a command, says Linda Crawford, an eating behavior specialist at Green Mountain at Fox Run, a residential weight and health management center in Ludlow, Vermont. Though you might think the craving is going to bear down on you like an 18-wheeler until you have to yield, research shows that food cravings actually start and escalate, then peak and subside. Take your mind off them with a walk or something else that's hard to do at the same time as eating, Crawford says. This will help you ride out the craving. "Just like with surfing," she says, "the more you practice riding a craving wave, the easier it becomes." But if you still have the craving after 20 minutes, go ahead and satisfy it with a small portion—and enjoy it, she advises.

PROSTATE PROBLEMS

Corralling the Male Menace

Lately, your urinary tract is acting like a workaholic. It wakes you up in the middle of the night, interrupts your lunch and yanks you out of important meetings, sending you scurrying to the nearest bathroom. But even though you're in the men's room a lot these days, you never feel that you've finished what you went there to do.

You could blame your bladder, but in all probability, your prostate is the problem.

The prostate, a small gland about the size of a walnut, is wrapped around the urethra, the tube that drains the bladder. The prostate secretes the fluid and enzyme mixture that sperm require for good health and mobility. The prostate usually works so well that most men don't even notice it until they're 40 or 50 years of age, although some guys have trouble in their thirties.

As you get older, the mild-mannered prostate can gradually turn into the gland from hell, becoming vulnerable to infection and disease—including cancer—and often swelling to the point where it interferes with urination.

Virtually every guy will have a prostate problem in his lifetime. Besides being a major nuisance, it's also the clarion call that youth is on the wane.

"Prostate problems go along with gray hair, wrinkles and bifocals. They're one of the first signals that you're getting to the age where you're more likely to be a Boy Scout leader rather than a Boy Scout," says Thomas Stanisic, M.D., a urologist in private practice in Ashland, Kentucky.

No, you don't need an exorcist to rid yourself of these woes, but you should see your doctor, since the symptoms of minor prostate ailments are similar to those of serious disease. Those symptoms include frequent urination, blood in the urine, trouble starting the flow, weak flow and a feeling that even when you're done, you're not quite finished. Let's take a look at the three most common problems.

Chart Your Flow

To see if you have any of the symptoms of prostate trouble, circle the number that most closely describes your experiences. This test, designed by the Male Health Center in Dallas, is not for prostate cancer. Ask your doctor about prostate exams and screening for prostate cancer.

Over the past month, how often have you . . .

1. Had a sensation of not emptying your bladder completely after you finished urinating?
   0   1   2   3   4   5
2. Had to urinate again less than two hours after urinating?
   0   1   2   3   4   5
3. Found that the flow of urine stopped and started several times?
   0   1   2   3   4   5
4. Found it difficult to postpone urination?
   0   1   2   3   4   5
5. Had a weak urine stream?
   0   1   2   3   4   5
6. Had to push or strain to begin urination?
   0   1   2   3   4   5
7. Had to get up to urinate after going to bed on a typical night?
   0   1   2   3   4   5

Add up your score. If you scored ten points or more, visit a urologist for an examination.

BPH: Number One with a Bullet

As a man approaches his mid-forties, his prostate typically begins to swell. In some cases, it can grow to the size of a grapefruit and pinch off urine flow through the urethra, Dr. Stanisic says. The condition is benign prostatic hyperplasia (BPH), and it's the most common prostate problem.

Why does the prostate grow? That's a perplexing question, but some doctors believe the gland's tendency to swell may have something to do with the male hormone testosterone. Eunuchs don't get BPH. For the rest of the male population, however, the condition is common. It affects up to 15 percent of men over age 40 and 60 percent of men over 50.

In advanced cases, an enlarged prostate can completely block the flow of urine. If you wait that long, you're going to need surgery, an operation called transurethral resection of the prostate. It is best described as a Roto-Rooter job in which the doctor inserts a tiny tube into the urethra and shaves away the portion of the prostate that's pressing on the urethra. It's painful and unpleasant and takes a few months to fully recover from.

"Testosterone fuels the prostate," says Kenneth Goldberg, M.D., founder and director of the Male Health Center in Dallas. "We've found that if you can reduce testosterone levels, you slow down the growth of the prostate."

Two medications can help relieve the symptoms of BPH, Dr. Stanisic says. Finasteride (Proscar) reduces the size of the prostate by an average of 20 percent, which is enough to boost urine flow. Another drug, terazosin hydrochloride (Hytrin), relaxes the muscles of the bladder neck and prostate to open up the urethra. So if you have an enlarged prostate, ask your doctor if these drugs can relieve your problem.

Prostatitis: A Disease for All Ages

So what's going on if you are age 35 and have difficult or frequent urination? It could be an infection of the prostate known as bacterial prostatitis.

Bacterial prostatitis can affect men of all ages. It's usually caused by the spread of infection in the bladder or urethra. Although doctors aren't sure how the infection enters the urinary tract, some suspect that an obstruction in the urethra or unprotected anal sex increases the risk. Besides urination problems, the symptoms can include lower abdominal or back pain, discomfort in the testicles and fever.

"It's relatively easy to treat," says Christopher M. Dixon, M.D., assistant professor of urology at the Medical College of Wisconsin in Milwaukee. The ailment is usually treated with antibiotics. In most cases, symptoms improve in about a week, but it may take up to six weeks to evict prostatitis from your body, Dr. Stanisic says.

In some instances, the infection may become chronic, and a man will have recurring bouts of prostatitis for the rest of his life.

Prostate Cancer: The Stealth Killer

Prostate cancer is the most common cancer among men over age 50 and the second leading killer among cancers in men in the United States. More than half of all men over 70 have it, Dr. Stanisic says.

Prostate cancer is rare in men younger than age 45 unless they have family histories of the disease. It is usually curable if detected early, Dr. Stanisic says.

But often this cancer grows silently within the gland without any symptoms until it has spread to the surrounding bone and tissue. That's why it's especially important for men over age 50 to get a digital rectal exam that lets a doctor feel for lumps on the prostate and a prostate-specific antigen blood test that detects a protein that seeps out of the prostate when there is a tumor present.

If cancer is discovered, your treatment will depend on several factors, including the size of the tumor, how fast it is growing and whether the disease has spread beyond the prostate. Treatments include radiation, surgical removal of the prostate and hormonal therapy to reduce testosterone levels.

Taming the Wild Prostate

All right, that's the ugly side of living with a prostate. And like we said earlier, most of us will experience one or more of these problems as we get older. But some doctors believe you can reduce the possibility and impact of these diseases with a few dietary and lifestyle changes. Here's how.

Ejaculate regularly. Tough medicine, we know. But doing so may keep prostatic ducts from getting clogged and backed up. "It can only help," Dr. Goldberg says.

Lower your cholesterol. Cholesterol is converted to testosterone in the body. It has been observed that enlarged prostate tissue is very high in cholesterol. Some doctors claim an improvement in symptoms, if not in prostate size, by getting patients to lower their total blood cholesterol levels to 200 mg/dl (milligrams of cholesterol per deciliter of blood) or less, as recommended by the American Heart Association.

Drop the fat. Avoid foods laden with fat, such as red meats, dairy products and fried foods, Dr. Goldberg says. Limit yourself to one three-ounce serving of meat, fish or poultry a day.

Eat more vegetables. Male hormone levels drop with a vegetarian diet, and that may explain why BPH is rarer in cultures whose diets are largely vegetarian, Dr. Goldberg says.

Get enough zinc. Men with prostate ailments tend to have low concentrations of zinc in their bodies, says Paul M. Block, M.D., a urologist in private practice in Phoenix. The Recommended Dietary Allowance is 15 milligrams a day. Taking zinc supplements or eating foods rich in zinc, including oysters and herring, can help. Oatmeal, wheat bran, milk, peas and nuts also contain the mineral.

Limit spicy foods and alcohol. Both of these may increase bladder irritability, particularly if you have BPH, Dr. Block says. Alcohol can be especially tough, since it's a central nervous system depressant that reduces muscle tone throughout the body, including in the bladder, causing it to retain urine.

Get your exercise. There's no prostate-specific workout, though drinking water, voiding on demand and regular sexual relations help. But you should know that many physicians have observed that men in good shape are less likely to have prostate trouble than their sedentary brothers.

Don't sit for too long. That's your prostate you're sitting on all day, and sitting puts pressure on it, Dr. Goldberg says. Get up and walk around.

Don't hold it in. If you need to urinate frequently, logic may tell you to train your bladder by waiting as long as you can. Logic has been wrong before, and it's wrong here. "You may actually harm yourself by waiting too long," says Patrick C. Walsh, M.D., professor and chairman of urology at Johns Hopkins University in Baltimore. "When urine backs up too far, it can damage the kidneys." Urinate as soon as you feel the need.

Avoid drinking after dark. Forgo liquids after 6:00 P.M. or 7:00 P.M. if your sleep has been interrupted frequently (say, two or more times a night) by the urge to urinate, Dr. Block suggests. Day and night, limit drinks containing caffeine. These make you urinate more and increase irritability of the bladder, causing it to feel full even when it isn't.

Soak it. Sit in a warm bath for 20 minutes at least once a week, Dr. Block suggests. The heat will penetrate the pelvis and increase blood flow, reducing muscle spasms and, possibly, swelling.

RAYNAUD'S DISEASE

Warming Up Those Frigid Digits

*B**rrrrr.* Your hands are so cold they ache, so you rub them together briskly, trying to get the circulation back. Well, that's normal for winter, right? But in fact, it's a muggy summer day, and you've just walked into a meeting in an air-conditioned office. All the other guys are in shirtsleeves, and they're still complaining about the heat.

This has been happening to you a lot in the past few years. Your fingers turn funny colors when they're cold, too. What's going on?

Everyone becomes more sensitive to the cold with age, says Leonard Bielory, M.D., associate professor of medicine, pediatrics and ophthalmology and director of the Division of Allergy and Immunology at the University of Medicine and Dentistry of New Jersey/New Jersey Medical School in Newark. "Even our body temperatures gradually drop from 98.6° to 97°F." And your body's normal response to cold is to divert warm blood away from the extremities and toward vital internal organs. That's why your hands, feet, ears and even the tip of your nose get cold.

But if you have Raynaud's disease, blood vessels in your hands, feet, ears and the tip of your nose go into spasm when you are exposed to cold, and the consequences are more severe than just feeling chilly.

Spasms of Red, White and Blue

Here's the classic profile of a Raynaud's attack, which can last from less than a minute to as long as several hours. First, the small blood vessels constrict, shutting off blood flow. Next, fingers or toes turn an icy shade of pale, then blue, and feel numb. When circulation begins to flow again as the attack subsides, the color turns to red, with tingling and often pulsating pain.

The frustrating thing about Raynaud's is that until you learn the tricks of fending off attacks, ordinary activities are full of hazards. And that can make you feel cautious and fragile. Walking outside on a wintry day, entering an air-conditioned room in summer, opening the refrigerator door or handling a frosty mug of beer or a package of frozen food can trigger an attack. And the symptoms get worse with time.

We Have It Better

This is one condition where men have the health edge over women, though. Researchers aren't certain why, but men develop Raynaud's about half as often as women do, and its onset is later in life. Women usually get Raynaud's sometime between the ages of 15 and 40, whereas it usually shows up in men after 50. One factor may be that our blood usually circulates more efficiently when we're young. A study of 23 men and 26 women at the Mayo Clinic in Rochester, Minnesota, found that under ordinary conditions, the men had greater blood flow in their hands than the women did. Paradoxically, however, the blood flow in women's hands was better under stress.

What Makes It Happen?

Raynaud's can result from infection, repeated exposure to severe cold, a past history of frostbite or smoking, because nicotine constricts blood vessels. Even your workshop, office habits or workouts can contribute. If you often use vibrating power tools or have the painful wrist condition called carpal tunnel syndrome, caused by repetitive motions such as those in typing or racquetball, you may be a candidate. Some heart medications, including beta-blockers such as propranolol, have also been shown to cause Raynaud's, as has ergotamine, a drug used to treat migraine headaches.

Raynaud's disease is usually benign, says John P. Cooke, M.D., Ph.D., director of vascular medicine at Stanford University School of Medicine in Stanford, California. "It's uncomfortable, and nobody likes having blue hands, but it won't hurt you," he says.

But another form of the disease is more serious, and it affects about 25 percent of people with Raynaud's.

Secondary Raynaud's, or Raynaud's phenomenon, usually occurs in people who have or may develop connective tissue disorders such as rheumatoid arthritis, scleroderma (which hardens skin) or a type of lupus that attacks skin, joints and kidneys. Sometimes these conditions run in families. In severe cases of Raynaud's phenomenon, the repeated loss of circulation can result in painful skin ulcers.

Your physician can tell whether you have the primary or secondary form of Raynaud's, says Dr. Cooke. Most conditions related to Raynaud's phenomenon are detectable by blood tests and a physical exam, which includes a technique called nail-fold capillaroscopy. The skin at the base of the fingernail is viewed under a magnifier. Enlarged or deformed capillaries—tiny blood vessels—indicate a disorder such as scleroderma, he says.

Though there's no cure for Raynaud's, there's a great deal you can do to prevent attacks.

Heading Off the Chill

Your main defense is to avoid exposure to cold—both outdoors and in. Here's how to forestall attacks.

Dress for the weather. Don't dash out in your Skivvies to fetch the newspaper when it's cold outside, says Dr. Bielory. Whenever you go out in the cold, be sure to dress warmly and in layers. And don't forget a hat, mittens (they're warmer than gloves) and a muffler over your face and nose. For your feet, choose loose-fitting boots over thick socks.

Keep warm indoors, too. Keep the room you spend the most time in at a comfortable temperature, which may be warmer for you than for other people, Dr. Bielory says. A small space heater may do the trick.

Bundle up in bed. Use flannel sheets and an electric blanket or layers of blankets to keep from getting chilled on winter nights, says Dr. Bielory. Wear socks and a knit cap, too, if you need them. After all, you lose 50 percent of your body heat through your head.

Don't freeze in the fridge. Use oven mitts when you have to reach into the refrigerator or freezer or handle cold or frozen items. Even a cold egg or jar of juice can trigger an attack.

Prep your shower. Run the shower until the water warms up before you get in, says Dr. Bielory. This will prevent you from having to touch cold water.

Think before you drink. In a restaurant, ask for a glass with a stem to keep your cold-sensitive fingers away from the chilled surface. Likewise, on an airplane, ask for your drink to be served in an insulated coffee cup.

Plug yourself in. Try wearing warming appliances such as heated socks or boots or mitten warmers, says Dr. Bielory. You can find these specialty heating products in many outdoor equipment stores, sporting goods stores and catalogs.

No smoking. Whether it's from your own cigarette or someone else's polluting plume, even one puff of tobacco smoke causes spasms that narrow small blood vessels. "Raynaud's patients are sensitive even to other people's smoke," says Frederick A. Reichle, M.D., chief of the Department of Surgery at John F. Kennedy Memorial Hospital and clinical professor of surgery at Temple University Hospital, both in Philadelphia.

Reel in some fish oil. A preliminary study at Albany Medical College in Albany, New York, found that symptoms of Raynaud's stopped completely in 5 of 11 people who took fish oil capsules daily for 12 weeks. The other 6 were able to extend by 50 percent the amount of time they could submerge their hands in cold water before triggering attacks. The researchers caution that these findings have not yet been confirmed, however, and that you should get your doctor's okay and dosage recommendations before taking fish oil supplements.

Use gloves in the workshop and the woods. Another name for Raynaud's is vibration white finger, which refers to Raynaud's disease triggered by the use of handheld vibrating power tools, often among workers in heavy industries such as mining and forestry. If you cut your own wood with a chain saw or have a hobby that involves frequent use of vibrating machinery, you may also be at risk.

In North Carolina State University at Raleigh's Department of Biological and Agricultural Engineering, researchers found that commercial vibration insulating gloves and ordinary work gloves fitted with sponge rubber cushions are equally effective in preventing vibration damage.

Treatment for the Long Run

If simple prevention techniques don't work, you might want to discuss the following options with your doctor before considering the heavy artillery—drugs.

Work on your windup. If an attack sneaks up on you, you can get the jump on it with a simple exercise devised by Donald R. McIntyre, M.D., a dermatologist in private practice in Rutland, Vermont. Swing your arm downward behind your body and then upward in front of you at about 80 twirls per minute, like a souped-up softball pitcher. It's really not as fast as it sounds; give it a try.

The windmill effect forces blood to the fingers through both gravitational and centrifugal force. And it's quick—one man with Raynaud's was able to reverse an attack after just 90 seconds of arm twirling.

Ask about biofeedback. Though research results are mixed, some people with Raynaud's find that they can use biofeedback training to raise the temperature in their fingers, says Jay Coffman, M.D., professor of medicine at Boston University School of Medicine and chief of the peripheral vascular department at Boston University Medical Center/University Hospital. Be aware that biofeedback techniques require considerable time to master at first, he says, and at least a half-hour daily thereafter to maintain. If you'd like to investigate biofeedback, ask your doctor to refer you to a nearby training laboratory.

Consider some medication. In severe cases of Raynaud's, several kinds of prescription medication have proven to help some people, says Dr. Coffman. "The drug of choice for Raynaud's is a class called calcium channel blockers, which relax smooth muscles within the blood vessels, so blood flow increases," he says. The most effective one is nifedipine (such as Adalat), which decreases the frequency, duration and severity of attacks in about two-thirds of those with primary or secondary Raynaud's, he says.

The downside of drug therapy is side effects, which are intolerable for

Do-It-Yourself Raynaud's Therapy

Uncle Sam has found a way to subdue the aching cold spasms of Raynaud's disease—in fingers, at any rate. An Army scientist in Alaska started the Raynaud's conditioning research in 1971, says Murray P. Hamlet, D.V.M., director of research, programs and operations at the U.S. Army Research Institute of Environmental Medicine in Natick, Massachusetts.

Why? "We put a lot of people in cold, bizarre places against their will," he says, "and we'd like them to bring back all their parts." The army has a particular interest in blood flow to the extremities because of injuries in cold climates, Dr. Hamlet says. "And since Raynaud's means abnormal blood flow, it's a good avenue to study."

The procedure involves repeatedly immersing hands in warm water during exposure to warm and cold environments. It was developed at the institute with the help of patients who volunteered for a series of studies. How did it become a home remedy? Accidentally, Dr. Hamlet says. "One day, a lady came back after the lab treatment saying 'If I get a little constriction at home, I just get my pan of hot water and sit out on the porch.'

"The nice thing about this method is that you have control over your disease," he says. "You relieve both symptoms and severity. You have fewer shutdowns, and they aren't as severe. Some people have none at all." Here's how the therapy works.

"You need two cheap styrofoam coolers," Dr. Hamlet says. "Cut holes for your hands in the lids with a paring knife. Fill them both with tap water as hot as you can stand, and put one outside in the cold and

---

about 10 percent of patients, he says. Nifedipine can cause headaches, though in some cases these disappear after a few days. Flushing, anxiety and mild leg swelling may also occur.

Other drugs with similar rates of success block the action of sympathetic nerves, which constrict blood vessels. Side effects from these also affect about 10 percent of patients.

Reserpine (such as Diupres) can cause stuffy nose, slow heart rate or, more worrisome, depression. Guanethidine (such as Ismelin) can cause diarrhea, and prazosin (such as Minizide) can produce palpitations, rapid heartbeat, headache and dizziness.

one in a warm room. Indoors, dress lightly, and put your hands in the hot water for two to five minutes.

"Throw a towel over your hands, run outdoors and stick them in the hot water for ten minutes. Stay lightly dressed, because you want your torso to become chilled outdoors. Throw the towel around your hands, then do the treatment indoors again for two to five minutes while your torso warms up.

"Do 3 to 6 cycles of this a day, every other day for up to 50 cycles, depending on how severe your Raynaud's is," he says.

Whatever is driving your Raynaud's will bring it back in a year or so, he adds, so you will need to repeat the procedure—but only for 10 to 20 cycles.

Why chill your torso? Normally, when your body gets cold, temperature sensors in your skin signal blood vessels to shut down in your hands and feet just temporarily—for up to 15 minutes. This conserves heat in the torso's vital organs. But if you have Raynaud's, the next signal—to restart blood flow in your hands and feet—doesn't work effectively, says Dr. Hamlet. To recondition your response to cold, he says, you want blood vessels in your hands to grow used to staying dilated even when your torso is cold (which is what the hot water signals them to do).

In most people with primary Raynaud's disease, the procedure works quite well, Dr. Hamlet says. If your Raynaud's results from frostbite, it works "to a degree." And the conditioning will help even those with Raynaud's phenomenon, though results don't last as long.

On the brighter side, Dr. Coffman says, "many people with Raynaud's don't need to take their medications during warm weather."

Read up on Raynaud's. You can send for more information on Raynaud's, says Dr. Bielory. Write to Raynaud's Facts, Division of Allergy and Immunology, U.M.D./New Jersey Medical School, 90 Bergen Street, DOC 4700, Newark, NJ 07103-2499. Enclose a self-addressed, stamped envelope.

REACTION TIME

Reversing the Big Slowdown

It's the big company softball game, and all week you've been bragging about your hot hands at the plate and your golden glove at third. But in your first at-bat, you whiff on three pitches, each time swinging long after the ball hits the catcher's mitt. Your luck in the field is no better. By the time you reach down to snag those routine grounders, the ball has already scooted between your legs.

Now you have a new nickname around the office: Molasses.

For a lot of us, a slowdown in reaction time is one of the more harrowing indications that we're getting older. For some guys, the change is too much. They stop playing softball, tennis and other activities that kept them in shape and engaged with other people. They get sluggish and sedentary—and start feeling and looking like age is getting the best of them.

Other guys face the music, make some minor adjustments and stay on top of their games and their lives.

The Secret to Staying Strong and Fast

Let's face it: You're not Brooks Robinson anymore. But then again, even Brooks Robinson isn't Brooks Robinson anymore. "Everyone, including great athletes, reaches his peak fitness level in his mid- to late twenties and then gradually declines," says Ralph Tarter, Ph.D., professor of psychiatry and neurology at the University of Pittsburgh School of Medicine. "As fitness goes, our metabolism slows, and with it, our ability to perform tasks requiring sustained strength and speed."

Fortunately, we have a powerful weapon against this downward decline:

Setting Your Sights

An optometrist or ophthalmologist can put you on a program to improve the clarity and quality of your vision. In the meantime, Arthur Seiderman, O.D., an Elkins Park, Pennsylvania, visual consultant to many professional athletes and author of *20/20 Is Not Enough*, recommends these exercises.

Have a ball. Cut out a variety of letters, small shapes and colored pieces of paper, and tape them to a ball or beanbag. Then play a round of catch or bounce the ball off a wall, spotting and calling out one or more of the letters, shapes or colors before you catch it.

Go for a spin. Cut a piece of cardboard into the shape of a disc, paste different-size letters, numbers, words or figures on it, and put it on a turntable. Set the speed at 33⅓ rpm and call out the information on the disk for one to three minutes. When it gets easier, increase the speed to 45 rpm, then 78 rpm.

Box to the beat. Draw a large box with 16 squares on a chalkboard or piece of paper. Place the numbers 1 through 16 in the squares in random order. Turn on a musical metronome or other rhythm-making device, and point to each of the numbers in numerical order, keeping time with the beat. Try it again in backward order, then repeat.

Flip some flash cards. For this you'll need 50 3- by 5-inch cards. Draw a black dot in the center of each card, below the top edge. Write a different two-digit number on each side of the dot, about ½ inch from the dot. Mark another card with a different pair of two-digit numbers, each placed ¾ inch away from the dot. Continue marking each card, spacing the numbers at ¼-inch intervals until you reach the far corners; then work back toward the center dot.

Hold the stack of cards 14 to 16 inches in front of you. Then flip through the stack while focusing on the center dot and call out the numbers on the card. It should get increasingly difficult to identify the numbers as they are spaced farther from the center. Start slow, then build up your flipping speed.

---

lifelong physical activity. Exercise increases the body's output of growth hormone, a substance that helps maintain muscle mass, bone density and lean body composition. A study by Robert Mazzeo, Ph.D., a kinesiologist (he studies human motion) at the University of Colorado in Boulder, found that regularly active individuals had higher concentrations of growth hormone in their blood

Keep Your Reflexes in Gear

Ever notice how fast David Carradine and Bruce Lee duck and move in those action movies? Their quick reaction times showcase the coordination of mind, body and vision. One of the best techniques you can use to hone and develop all three is practicing one of the martial arts.

What's so special about the marital arts? For one thing, they call for physical fitness. Martial artists spend hours building strength, developing flexibility and performing routines that condition the body for speed. For another, they demand maximum concentration of mind and vision: If you don't pay attention, you or someone else may get hurt. And they're motivational: The belt system of awarding progress encourages you to improve your skills and speed.

According to Charles L. Richman, Ph.D., professor of psychology and director of the Martial Arts Program at Wake Forest University in Winston-Salem, North Carolina, there are more than 100 martial arts styles. All share certain basic postures and rudiments, with some subtle differences. Some, such as tae kwon do and kempo, are more aggressive and emphasize hard contact. Softer styles, such as aikido and judo, emphasize throwing and evading your opponent. And tai chi and kung fu focus on developing fluid, dancelike movements.

For over 15 years, Dr. Richman has studied and taught tae kwon do, a Korean martial art that emphasizes a dazzling array of spins, kicks and punches. Now in his fifties, he knows firsthand just how intertwined aging, fitness and reaction time really are. "Naturally, I have found my reflexes to be slowing when competing against younger, quicker individuals," he says. "However, I have been able to hold my own quite well, speed-wise, against men in my own age group. Overall, I feel my reaction time is still quite good—much better than if I had not made tae kwon do a part of my life."

Whatever form you choose, a martial arts program will help almost anyone develop quicker reaction time, better coordination and greater concentration at any age. It can even help your performance in other activities. "Tae kwon do or any martial art demands physical fitness and mental discipline," says Dr. Richman. "Many principles used in self-defense apply in other sports as well, such as keeping your head still and eyes forward and moving your hips through contact. Since I have been practicing tae kwon do, my golf game has improved considerably."

Consult your phone directory for a martial arts school near you.

than people the same age who didn't exercise and sedentary people who were much younger.

"Even the elderly will see an increase in growth hormone levels from exercise, and with it will come increased strength, balance and speed," Dr. Mazzeo says.

Playing Those Mind Games

Our ability to react to stimuli is controlled by the brain, which processes incoming information and then sends impulses down a pathway to our muscles. "As we age, we see little change in the speed of these impulses. The greatest delays are in the processing of information that is necessary to formulate the messages that tell the muscles what to do," says Lawrence Z. Stern, M.D., director of the Muscular Dystrophy Association's Mucio F. Delgado Clinic for Neuromuscular Disorders at the University of Arizona Health Sciences Center in Tucson.

Why? For one thing, as we age, we lose brain cells that help us process new information. For another, we have lots more information and experiences in our heads than when we were younger. This slows down our ability to make snap judgments. And we get lazy; it becomes easier to rely on old, familiar ways than to deal with new ones.

Your Reaction Time Rx

So how do you keep your mind sharp and your reactions quick?

Use it. "Maintain complex mental activities versus passive ones such as watching television," says Dr. Tarter. "Stay mentally engaged by exposing yourself to demanding tasks and new challenges every single day. When we constantly use the brain and push it to its full capacity, it stays faster, more alert and more efficient."

Check your vision. Before we can mentally or physically react, we must be aware of what is happening in the outside world. For that, we must rely on our senses, particularly vision. "Seventy-five to 80 percent of reaction time is directly related to good visual skills," says Arthur Seiderman, O.D., an Elkins Park, Pennsylvania, visual consultant to many professional athletes and author of *20/20 Is Not Enough*. "That means more than just seeing objects clearly; it also means having the ability to detect, track and recognize fast-moving objects."

Steer clear of alcohol and drugs. Everybody knows that drunk drivers are slow to react behind the wheel, but even one or two drinks can be enough to send your reaction time plummeting, says Dr. Stern. And if you regularly hit the sauce or take any medication that affects the central nervous system, it could put your mind and body in a constant state of slo-mo.

Don't smoke. Tobacco saps speed in more ways than one, says Dr. Tarter.

We all know the effect it has on our cardiovascular system. If our lungs and heart don't work efficiently, neither will our bones and muscles. Smoking also dramatically reduces the amount of oxygen in our bloodstream, and the brain needs a steady supply of fresh oxygen to stay in good working order.

Get some shut-eye. A good night's sleep is nature's built-in mechanism for recharging our mental batteries. "Regular quality sleep every night is essential for the brain to stay alert and perform cognitive tasks at maximal levels," says Dr. Stern.

Zap some aliens. Video and computer games have been shown to dramatically improve mental and motor skills, says Dr. Tarter. "They are often used to help rehab patients develop speed, and even pilots these days practice on video simulators before they climb in the cockpit." If beeps, buzzes and explosions aren't your cup of tea, try some other fast-paced activity, such as Ping-Pong.

RESPIRATORY DISEASES

Keep Them at Bay

You struggle with that last repetition on the leg press. Your breath comes in powerful, lung-expanding grabs of air. But you move the weight inch by inch until finally your legs are fully extended. You've done it. And that last deep breath of success is sweet.

Most of us would like a set of powerful lungs that can withstand any kind of workout. We don't want to suck air on every hill as though we were 100 years old. We don't want to cough every time we take deep breaths. And we don't want to wheeze.

And we don't have to, says Robert Bethel, M.D., a staff physician at the National Jewish Center for Immunology and Respiratory Medicine in Denver.

Our lungs are made to take any workout well into our seventies. Smoking, of course, can change that scenario, clogging up the lungs and making us gasp. Colds, flu, pneumonia and other infectious diseases can do the same, but only temporarily. Other, less common diseases can also affect the lungs.

Strengthening Your Natural Defenses

Every day, your respiratory system draws in approximately 9,500 quarts of air and mixes it with up to 10,600 quarts of blood pumped by the heart into the lungs. Your lungs send oxygen through arterial highways to support the rest of the body and to provide an exhaust system for gaseous metabolic garbage such as carbon dioxide.

Since your lungs are internal organs that draw in the microorganisms of the outside world with every breath, the strength of their natural defense system is particularly important in maintaining oxygen flow to and from the rest of your body. Fortunately for most of us, the lungs' defensive players, including mucus and hairlike filaments called cilia, can sweep pollens, dust, viruses and bacteria out of the airway.

Most of the time they do a great job. But sometimes they're undermined by irritants such as cigarette smoke or overwhelmed by invading microbes.

More than 14 million men and women suffer from chronic obstructive pulmonary disease, which includes both chronic bronchitis and emphysema. And in one year alone, 7 to 8 million men and women had asthma, 129 million had the flu, 4 million had pneumonia, and practically every one of us had some kind of cold virus.

How can you protect your lungs from the diseases and irritants that can slow you down? Here's what experts say.

Keep your cilia sober. Drinking interferes with the cleansing mechanisms that keep your lungs free of disease-causing germs, says Steven R. Mostow, M.D., chairman of the American Thoracic Society's Committee on the Prevention of Pneumonia and Influenza and professor of medicine at the University of Colorado at Denver. "The respiratory system's cilia get drunk right along with the rest of you," he explains. If you're used to having one or two drinks on a daily basis, your cilia will be okay. But if you suddenly decide to drink more than you usually do, your cilia won't be able to do their job.

Add moisture to your environment. To keep your respiratory system in fighting trim, humidify your environment every winter with an ultrasonic humidifier, says Dr. Mostow. The increased moisture will help the cilia sweep out dust, viruses, bacteria and pollens.

Exercise your lungs. Don't just work your biceps. Get into an aerobic exercise program that works your heart and lungs, says Dr. Mostow. It will help keep your lungs functioning at peak efficiency. Walking, running and swimming for 20 minutes at least three times a week will certainly do the job, but check with your doctor before you start, so he can tailor your exercise prescription specifically to your needs.

Banish butts. Smoking a cigarette or even being in a room where others are smoking can damage your lungs, says Dr. Bethel. The smoke may cause your body's natural defense system to release an enzyme that, in trying to attack the smoke's chemicals, literally digests the lung. Not only does this set the stage for future diseases, but breathing can be immediately impaired.

Fighting Sniffles and Sneezes

Colds, upper respiratory infections and bronchitis can be caused by any one of numerous microorganisms that can make you feel as though you lost the ability to breathe.

You get these diseases by inhaling somebody else's germs or touching someone that has a virus, then touching your eyes or nose, allowing the germs to enter your body.

Once the virus has invaded, it sets up shop in your throat and begins churning out baby viruses by the hundreds. These viruses spread throughout your body and trigger those beloved cold symptoms: a stuffy, drippy nose, sore throat, aches and pains and cough.

There's no way to cure a cold as yet, but here's how to deal with its symptoms.

Eat south of the border. Hot peppers and spices such as curry and chili powder cause mucous membrane secretions. The extra fluid can thin out thick phlegm in your nasal passages and lubricate a sore, itchy throat.

Steam your nose. Sip chicken soup or linger in a steamy shower, suggests Thomas A. Gossel, Ph.D., dean of the College of Pharmacy and professor of pharmacology and toxicology at Ohio Northern University in Ada. The fluids you drink or inhale dilute the mucus in your nose and upper throat to help make breathing easier. Use decongestant sprays at bedtime for no more than five days to avoid inflaming tissues.

Look for the big D. The D in many over-the-counter cough suppressants (such as Robitussin DM) is dextromethorphan. Doctors swear by it. Just make sure you follow package directions.

Suck on zinc. Zinc's ability to zap a cold has been suspected for years. And at least one study, at Dartmouth College in Hanover, New Hampshire, indicates that zinc tablets can cut the duration of a cold by 42 percent. But not any zinc tablet will do. You need those marked "zinc gluconate with glycine." They're fairly new on the market, so you may need to ask your druggist for help in tracking them down. If your druggist can't help, write the Quigley Corporation at 10 South Clinton Street, Doylestown, PA 18901.

Nurture your throat. Suck on over-the-counter throat lozenges to soothe your throat, suggests Dr. Gossel. Or aim a medicated spray at the back of your throat, hold your breath and squirt. Follow package directions for both lozenges and sprays.

Relieve the aches. Try aspirin, acetaminophen or ibuprofen to relieve the aches and pains of a cold, says Dr. Gossel.

Fight malaise. The too-tired-to-move feeling that usually accompanies a cold is often caused by dehydration, says Dr. Gossel. Try drinking at least six glasses of water a day to prevent it.

Relax. A study at Carnegie Mellon University in Pittsburgh indicates that the more stress you're under, the more likely you are to get a visit from any cold bug in the vicinity.

The researchers asked 394 men and women between the ages of 18 and 54 about any stress in their lives—recent bereavement, going on a diet, changing jobs, losing money, little sleep and arguing with family members—and then divided them into five groups. Each group received custom-made nose drops containing one of five viruses known to cause colds.

The result? Those who had the most stress in their lives were five times more likely to get colds than those who had the least.

TB Is Back

Tuberculosis (TB), a bacterial lung infection that scientists thought they had virtually eliminated in the United States, is not only alive and well but also thriving.

While the disease had been declining since the late 1940s, the number of cases of TB increased nearly 16 percent in a six-year span between the late 1980s and early 1990s.

Cities have been hit the worst. By the early 1990s, TB had increased to approximately seven times the national average in Atlanta, six times in Newark, New Jersey, and five times in New York City, according to the Centers for Disease Control and Prevention in Atlanta.

The cause? Rampant spread of the bacteria that cause TB among those with AIDS, those who are homeless and those who have newly emigrated to the United States, plus development of drug-resistant strains of the bacteria.

TB is spread by airborne droplets in sneezes, coughs and just plain breathing. The bacteria are inhaled into the lungs. In those with strong immune systems, the bacteria are surrounded by a legion of bacterial fighters that render them harmless. In others, the bacteria settle into the lungs and multiply. With time, they may destroy extensive parts of the lungs and leave cavities. Eventually, the lungs look like Swiss cheese.

Today, ten million Americans carry the disease, many without the typical symptoms of cough, fatigue and weight loss.

"I think the general population is at risk," says Robert Bethel, M.D., a staff physician at the National Jewish Center for Immunology and Respiratory Medicine in Denver. "To a large extent, you can't control whether or not you're exposed to TB. Not that I want to be an alarmist. But if you're on a bus, subway or airline with someone who has active TB and who is coughing, then the people around that person are exposed and vulnerable."

Fortunately, a complicated long-term drug regime can usually fight TB into a dormant stage. But early treatment is important. If you think you've been exposed to TB, check with your doctor. A simple skin test or chest x-ray can usually determine whether you have the disease.

Living with Emphysema and Bronchitis

One disease likely to send your respiratory system into an early retirement is chronic obstructive pulmonary disease. It includes chronic bronchitis, a condition in which the air sacs of the lungs are destroyed, and emphysema, a condition in which lung elasticity is lost and air is unable to flow freely in and out through the airway. It does not include the common bronchitis you might get with a cold—that's simply an irritation of the bronchial tubes that causes a few days of coughing and then goes away.

Both chronic bronchitis—roughly defined as a daily wet cough that lasts for three months or more—and emphysema are usually caused by smoking. Both have early symptoms of shortness of breath, limited ability to exert yourself, hacking up mucus and coughing, and both conditions are on the rise. The number of people who have these diseases has increased 41 percent in the past ten years, and chronic bronchitis and emphysema make up the largest number of respiratory illnesses (other than colds) in people between the ages of 30 and 45. Because more men than women smoke, men are nearly twice as likely as women to get emphysema, but women are rapidly catching up. When it comes to chronic bronchitis, women are more likely to get it. Emphysema and chronic bronchitis together kill approximately 75,000 people a year.

There's no cure for chronic bronchitis or emphysema, but the following strategies can lessen the shortness of breath that eventually comes from an obstructed airway and make life with the diseases a little easier.

Prevent infection. Any type of respiratory infection can make emphysema and chronic bronchitis worse, says Dr. Bethel. As much as possible, avoid being in crowded areas or around people who have infections. And see your doctor if an illness such as a cold or flu is aggravating your breathing problems.

Get shot. Prevent the complications of influenza and bacterial pneumonia by getting immunized against both flu and pneumonia, says Dr. Bethel.

Work with a therapist. If you have emphysema, ask your doctor to recommend an occupational therapist and a physical therapist.

"An occupational therapist can work with people who are short of breath and who are limited in their day-to-day activities," says Dr. Bethel. "The therapist can teach people more energy-efficient ways of doing those activities."

A physical therapist can develop an exercise program that will train your body to use its available oxygen more efficiently. The result will be that the little oxygen you have will go farther.

Medicate your airway. Your doctor will probably prescribe medications that will dilate your airway to its fullest, says Dr. Bethel. Use them according to directions.

Asthma: A Deadly Inflammation

Asthma is different from chronic bronchitis and emphysema in that its obstruction of the airway is both intermittent and reversible.

During an asthma attack, the airway constricts, the airway walls thicken with inflammation, and mucus accumulates within the airway. The result is an obstructed airway that makes you feel as though you were choking to death.

But after an attack, the airway usually returns to normal. Unfortunately, years of these attacks can lead to permanent airway damage.

If you've never had asthma before, breathe easy. Once you're past age 30, you're unlikely to develop it, says Harold S. Nelson, M.D., senior staff physician at the National Jewish Center for Immunology and Respiratory Medicine and a member of the National Asthma Education Expert Panel of the National Heart, Lung and Blood Institute.

"Asthma tends to run in families," says Dr. Bethel. "There may be a predisposition in some people, but we think that asthma is caused by an inflammation of the airway.

"All the mechanisms aren't clear," he adds. "Sometimes the inflammation is caused by allergens that people inhale. Sometimes it's workplace exposures. Exposure to a large number of agents—solder used in the electronics industry or fumes from the making of plastics—may sensitize the airway and make someone asthmatic. And many times people develop asthma, and it's not clear what caused it."

What is clear, doctors agree, is that asthma, which affects about 12 million Americans, is becoming more prevalent and more deadly every year. About 5,000 people die from it each year—and the death rate climbs with age. In a 20-year span, the estimated number of people with asthma rose 71 percent. In a 10-year span, the number of adults who died from asthma increased 56 percent; the number of children ages 10 to 14 increased 100 percent. The deaths of black men rose 68 percent, and of white men, 25 percent. (The deaths of black women rose 65 percent, and of white women, 62 percent.)

What's behind the increase in asthma numbers and deaths is still a mystery, reports the American Lung Association. Any number of things can trigger an asthma attack, including allergies, cigarette smoke and other irritants, a viral infection in your respiratory system and heartburn, which can result in coughing and spasms in your lungs. Even strong emotions and hard exercise—especially in cold weather—can cause troubles, Dr. Nelson says.

New or recurring cases of asthma can start off feeling like regular respiratory tract infections, Dr. Nelson says. If you begin to develop wheezing, tightness in your chest or shortness of breath, see a doctor immediately.

If you're diagnosed with asthma, doctors can prescribe medication to ease the symptoms. Inhalers containing corticosteroids are the most effective way of reducing swelling and helping you breathe easier. Over-the-counter drugs rarely have much effect, Dr. Nelson says.

"This is not something you should treat by yourself," he says. "Asthma is much too serious for that."

Here's what the experts say you can do to handle the disease.

Fight for clean air. "There's evidence that living in polluted environments increases the incidence of lung diseases such as asthma," says Dr. Bethel. That's why you should try to avoid heavily polluted areas such as industrial districts and urban highways.

Air quality is frequently monitored by various agencies to see if it complies with federal and state standards. To find out how badly the area in which you live or work is polluted, call your state's environmental agency. The people there have the information at hand or can refer you to someone who does.

If your area consistently exceeds federal standards, you might want to start lobbying your federal, state and local officials to enforce pollution legislation. They have the authority to fine and even shut down the worst offenders.

Muffle your nose and mouth. Breathing in cold, dry air can constrict the airway and induce wheezing, coughing and shortness of breath. The solution? Wear a scarf that you can draw up over your mouth and nose to breathe through during cold spells. And try to breathe mostly through your nose. Breathing through your nose warms and humidifies the air before it reaches the lungs.

Eat away at it. A review of what 9,000 adults eat every day revealed that higher vitamin C and niacin intakes were associated with fewer cases of wheezing. Good sources of vitamin C include black currants, guava, orange juice and red bell peppers. Good sources of niacin include chicken breast, water-packed tuna and swordfish.

Measure the flow. The home peak-flow meter, a device that measures your breathing capacity, can help identify what's a normal flow and what's not, says Dr. Nelson. Since airflow sometimes drops a couple of hours or days before an impending attack, the peak-flow meter can give you an early warning that allows you to ward off the attack with medication prescribed by your doctor.

Ask your doctor about where to get a peak-flow meter and how to use it.

Open your airway. Prescription medications that treat asthma include anti-inflammatory drugs that suppress airway inflammation, such as steroids, as well as bronchodilators that dilate the airway itself. But noting that some people use only bronchodilators, Dr. Nelson adds, "Anyone with more than the mildest occasional asthma needs to be on anti-inflammatory treatment rather than just bronchodilators. Together, they will decrease symptoms, probably decrease the number of acute episodes that would otherwise need hospital treatment, decrease the need for bronchodilators and, doctors hope, prevent the long-term development of irreversible obstruction."

The Threat of Flu and Pneumonia

Neither flu nor the most common forms of pneumonia are likely to damage your lungs, but they can make you so short of breath that you feel you can't even make it up a flight of stairs.

Flu, which generally causes fever, headache, sore throat, nasal congestion, muscle aches and a feeling of exhaustion, typically strikes between December and March. It's caused by one of two virus strains, A or B, that usually manage to infect anywhere from 33 to 52 percent of Americans each year. Because flu affects older folks so severely, it is the sixth leading cause of death in the United States.

Pneumonia, which is generally characterized by coughing, phlegm, fever, chills and chest pain, can be caused by a variety of infectious agents, including viruses, mycoplasma parasites and bacteria. It occurs in 80 percent of those who have AIDS. Called *Pneumocystis carinii* pneumonia, it is triggered by a parasite and is seen only rarely in people who do not have AIDS.

Fortunately, both flu and the most deadly and common types of pneumonia can frequently be prevented or successfully be treated without leaving permanent damage. Here's how.

Listen to your body. Some types of pneumonia, such as staph or klebsiella, can seriously damage the lung, says Dr. Mostow, and "your lung is never the same afterward." So see your doctor quickly if you have a fever, breathlessness or a nagging cough that won't go away.

Get the pneumonia vaccine. The pneumonia vaccine doesn't prevent pneumonia, says Dr. Mostow, but it can prevent you from dying when pneumonia strikes. The vaccine is effective against 23 different types of bacterial germ—the kinds that are responsible for 90 percent of pneumonia deaths. You need to get the vaccine only once in your life.

Get the flu vaccine. The flu vaccine is highly effective, says Dr. Mostow.

Anyone with chronic lung or heart disease, diabetes, impaired immunity, kidney disease, anemia or another blood problem should get the vaccine every year in the fall, as should anyone over age 65 and anyone who's involved in the care of patients.

Who should not get the shot? Since the vaccine is incubated in eggs, those who are allergic to eggs should avoid it. In general, if you can eat eggs, you can safely receive a flu shot.

See your doctor. If you forget to get your flu shot, there are two prescription antiviral drugs that can stop flu in its tracks, says Dr. Mostow. One is amantadine (Symmetrel), and the other is rimantadine (Flumadine). These two compounds are active against influenza A, the only flu virus that kills. Just one caveat: You must get them from your doctor within 48 hours of when you come down with flu.

If you forget to get the pneumonia vaccine—or if you're unlucky enough to run into one of the pneumonias that's not in the vaccine—your doctor will prescribe an antibiotic that is specifically designed to kill the virus or bacteria that have attacked, says Dr. Mostow. If you have the form of pneumonia that affects those with AIDS, *P. carinii*, then your doctor will prescribe trimethoprim sulfate (Polytrim), a drug that won't cure the disease but will keep it under control.

RESTLESS LEGS SYNDROME

Resisting the Urge
to Get Up and Dance

When you crawl into bed after a long, hard day, you don't expect your legs to want to spring out of bed and start running the 100-yard dash.

But as strange as it may seem, many men will one night park themselves in bed only to find that their legs suddenly have a strong desire to get up and hit the road. To do the lambada. To do anything but lie still. And the only way these guys can suppress this urge is to actually get up and walk about or rub their legs.

It's called restless legs syndrome, and it affects at least 5 percent of all adult Americans at some time in their lives.

Guys who get it say the discomfort is like nothing they've ever known before. Not pain, but bizarre sensations of burning, pulling and crawling . . . like bugs running up the legs.

In most cases, restless legs syndrome poses no health risk; it's merely a nuisance. But that doesn't mean it doesn't have consequences. It can keep you awake for all or a good portion of the night, leaving you sleepy, irritable and non-alert the following day. Long-term sleep deprivation can seriously affect your job performance, mental health and personal safety. And we all know the look of a sleep-deprived man: distant, droopy...like a crotchety old coot.

It's Not in Your Head

These nightly tap-dancing sessions in no way signify any kind of psychiatric disorder, yet the anxiety they create is often enough to make any man think he's losing his marbles. "A severe case of restless legs can virtually incapacitate you any time you lie down," says Mark Mahowald, M.D., director of the Minnesota Regional Sleep Disorders Center at the Hennepin County Medical

Center in Minneapolis. "Facing this problem night after night can literally drive you out of your mind. For many people, it completely interferes with their ability to enjoy happy, productive lives. Some patients have even told us that they would contemplate suicide if the problem wasn't fixed."

Restless legs can hit a man at any age, but as you get older, your chances of experiencing it become much greater. "We see the greatest onset when people reach their forties," says Alexander G. Reeves, M.D., chairman of the Department of Neurology at the Dartmouth Hitchcock Medical Center in Lebanon, New Hampshire. "The discomfort occurs nightly and can last for years or decades, sometimes going into periods of remission or growing more intense."

What makes your haunches so hyperactive? Doctors don't know. Restless legs can sometimes be linked to problems such as neurological disorders, diabetes, anemia, vitamin and mineral deficiencies and sedative withdrawal, but 95 percent of guys with jumpy legs are otherwise as healthy as wild horses.

Don't confuse restless legs syndrome with the occasional bedtime involuntary kick. "We all jerk, twitch or kick several times a night, some more frequently and more intensely than others," says Karl Doghramji, M.D., director of the Sleep Disorders Center at Thomas Jefferson University Hospital in Philadelphia. Unlike restless legs, these quick, sudden movements aren't in tandem with any burning or pulling sensations, nor are they likely to ruin your sleep.

Slamming on the Brakes

Even if restless legs or periodic limb movements aren't making your nights a living hell, have your doc check them out. Remember, there is a slight chance that there could be a more serious underlying medical problem. He can recommend a program to keep your lively limbs under control. In the meantime, give these tips a try.

Shake a leg. Walking, stretching, stomping, massaging—anything you can do to keep your limbs active will provide temporary relief, says Dr. Mahowald. "The only problem is that the discomfort usually returns soon after you stop, and you have to get up and do it all over again."

Get more exercise. Strenuous exercise during the day or a mild nighttime workout, such as an evening walk, can help prevent restless legs, says Dr. Reeves. Or it may make your symptoms worse. "For some, it's a good idea to make your legs tired," he says. "In others, fatigue actually brings on restless legs. So you have to experiment."

Mellow out. "Many guys with restless legs are stressed out," says Lawrence Z. Stern, M.D., director of the Muscular Dystrophy Association's Mucio F. Delgado Clinic for Neuromuscular Disorders at the University of Arizona Health Sciences Center in Tucson. "If you can deal with your worries and eliminate physical tension before going to bed, the time you spend in bed will likely be more relaxing." Try reading, yoga, sex...anything to relax you before hitting the sack.

Alter your nighttime routine. Sometimes you can control restless legs by changing the way you do things before you go to bed or while sleeping, says Dr. Stern. Experiment by sleeping in a new position, changing your bedding and bed clothing or rearranging your pre-bedtime rituals.

Try the E and Q combo. Many men prevent the jitters by taking one or two 400 IU capsules of vitamin E daily, along with one 162.5-milligram tablet of quinine, says Dr. Reeves. Both supplements are available over the counter at any pharmacy. You can also find them in combination capsules. Although quite safe in moderate doses, you shouldn't pop these like candy. Check with your doctor before you make these a nightly habit.

Consider your diet. Restless legs syndrome has been linked to a low intake of the B vitamins, specifically vitamin B_{12} and folic acid, as well as many minerals, including iron, potassium and calcium, says Dr. Stern. So it's important to get enough of them in your diet.

Eat light and early. Do you chow down seven-course meals at 9:00 P.M.? Or make midnight raids on the fridge? If so, your overstuffed stomach may be to blame for your restless legs. "The process of digesting a heavy or spicy meal can trigger restless leg symptoms," says Dr. Stern.

Apply warmth . . . or cold. Here again, you must experiment. Blankets, baths and heating pads help some guys, says Dr. Reeves. Cold-water soaks help others. But do not apply ice directly to your legs; it can cause frostbite or nerve damage.

Quit smoking. You think that taking a long drag on a cigarette is relaxing? It's not in the long run. Cigarette smoking has been linked to restless legs, and many find that the symptoms disappear when they quit, says Dr. Stern.

Cool it on the caffeine. Not just before bed, but during the day, says Dr. Mahowald. The caffeine from a cup of joe can linger in your system for eight to ten hours, so even an afternoon caffeine fix can trigger nighttime jitters— and restless legs. But so can caffeine withdrawal. If you give up your java, do so gradually.

Avoid alcohol and sleeping pills. A nightcap or sleeping pill may knock out some people, but in most cases, it only makes legs more restless, says Dr. Reeves. Besides, steady use of alcohol or sleeping pills puts you at risk of addiction.

Ask about medications. Your doctor can tell you of several drug therapies that have been successful. The most prescribed is Sinemet, a derivative of levodopa, or L-dopa, a medication that is often used for Parkinson's disease. Other classes of drugs are the muscle relaxants known as benzodiazepines (such as clonazepam, or Klonopin); vasodilators, including beta-blockers (such as atenolol, or Tenormin) and calcium channel blockers (such as nifedipine, or Procardia), which are used to treat heart patients; and anticonvulsants, including baclofen (Lioresal) and carbamazepine (Tegretol), which are commonly used to treat muscle disorders.

SEX PROBLEMS AND STDS

Putting Worries to Bed

It was a board game called Life. Everybody in the neighborhood used to play, and you'd all wrestle with challenges and setbacks and eventually wind up with careers, spouses and kids.

But Life's tribulations did not include squares that read "Premature ejaculation—lose your turn" or "You have herpes—go back ten spaces."

Wouldn't it be great if handling such sexual problems were that simple?

In real life, sexual difficulties and sexually transmitted diseases can strain your intimate relationships, damage your self-esteem and, in the case of AIDS, even kill you. At the very least, sexual problems can make you feel as if age is catching up with you, sapping your virility and turning you into an isolated old man.

"Men who have a sexual dysfunction—be it impotence, premature ejaculation or low sexual drive—may be spending up to 80 or 90 percent of their waking hours thinking about it. They lose sleep. They're depressed and anxious. They may be having problems with their relationships and difficulty concentrating on the job. It just ripples into their entire lives," says Roger Crenshaw, M.D., a sex therapist and psychiatrist in private practice in La Jolla, California. "Once a man stops functioning sexually like he thinks he should, he starts to look at himself as aging quickly."

Every year, about six million American men get sexually transmitted diseases. Untreated, these illnesses can lower sexual drive, trigger acute arthritis and some chronic diseases, disrupt the central nervous system and cause dementia. Some diseases, such as hepatitis and syphilis, can lead to death.

But fortunately, there are scores of ways that you can prevent sexual problems and sexually transmitted diseases from developing in the first place, doctors say. Even if you have one, most sexual difficulties and diseases can be remedied, leaving you free to enjoy a lifetime of active and fulfilling sex.

Performance Perplexities

Over 50 percent of American men between ages 40 and 70 have or will have chronic sexual problems sometime during their lives, including premature ejaculation, impotence and inhibited sexual desire, says Irwin Goldstein, M.D., professor of urology at Boston University School of Medicine.

Some sexual difficulties are caused or complicated by ailments such as diabetes or heart disease and require medical attention. But doctors say most of us can head off the heartache of sexual disorders and improve our chances of having vigorous sex lives if we follow these basic guidelines.

Butt out. "Smoking is death to sex," Dr. Crenshaw says. Your penis needs good blood flow to work properly. Smoking constricts blood vessels in the penis and over time will make your erections less firm and sustained. So if you're a stud at age 40 and want to stay that way, quit smoking now.

Stow the booze. Sure, a glass or two of wine or beer can loosen sexual inhibitions, but drink more than that, and you'll hamper your ability to have an orgasm or, worst yet, pull the plug on your ability to get an erection, says Beth Alexander, M.D., sex counselor and associate chairperson in the Department of Family Practice at the Michigan State University College of Human Medicine in East Lansing. Alcohol can also trigger hormonal changes that will decrease sexual desire.

Ask about medications. "A lot of drugs can affect your sexual response," Dr. Alexander says. Medications for high blood pressure, antidepressants such as fluoxetine hydrochloride (Prozac) and lithium, steriods, ulcer drugs and beta-

---

Not Tonight, Dear . . .

Sex may cure some headaches, but more often it triggers them, and that could be a sign of serious illness, says George H. Sands, M.D., assistant professor of neurology at the Mount Sinai School of Medicine of the City University of New York in New York City. Most common is the explosive type of headache that feels like a grenade has gone off in your head as you near orgasm. Any headache that occurs during sex should be checked out by a doctor, since it could be a symptom of a serious condition, such as a cerebral aneurysm.

blockers such as timolol are among the hundreds of drugs that can adversely affect sexual performance. If you suspect a medication is interfering with your sex life, ask your doctor if the drug can be changed or the dosage reduced.

Slow down, you're going too fast. If you're constantly rushing from here to there and working 50-plus hours a week, you may be on the fast track to a sexual problem, Dr. Alexander says. "If you can change things that are stressful to you, do it, because lowering your stress and taking more time for yourself will improve your sexual performance," she says. Find ways to relax regularly—take an evening walk around the neighborhood or take a few minutes to romp with the dog before tumbling into bed.

Sleep on it. Avoid having sex when you're tired; you're less likely to encounter a sexual frustration if you do. "You shouldn't feel like you're expending your last bit of energy to have sex at the end of a long day," says Shirley Zussman, Ed.D., a sex and marriage therapist and co-director of the Association for Male Sexual Dysfunction in New York City. "I recommend that you put time aside for sex. That sounds unspontaneous, but in the long run it adds something to your relationship. Not only can sex happen that way, but you can do it with a certain zest."

Give yourself a break. Every man, no matter how experienced he is in bed, will have an occasional sexual frustration. When it happens, you should avoid dwelling on it. Otherwise, you might be setting yourself up for a chronic sexual disorder, says Marty Klein, Ph.D., a licensed marriage counselor and sex therapist in Palo Alto, California, and author of *Ask Me Anything: A Sex Therapist Answers the Most Important Questions for the '90s*. "Everybody experiences an erection problem or lack of orgasm periodically. So if you believe it's going to happen to you at some point, when it does happen, it's no big deal," he says.

"It's like getting a rash. Everyone gets rashes sometime in their lives. But if you believe that you never will, and then one day you do, you'll totally freak out. This could even set the stage for it happening again and again in the same circumstances."

Ejaculation Problems

Premature ejaculation is a frustrating problem that affects most men at some point in their lives. Fortunately, it is one of the easiest sex problems to fix, according to Dr. Klein.

Then there's the opposite problem: difficulty ejaculating, which affects about as many as 15 in every 100 men. On the surface, that may not seem like such a bad deal, but doctors say it can wound a relationship and cripple a guy's self-image. "At first, the woman may admire the guy's staying power, but eventually, she might begin wondering if she's satisfying him," says Joseph Waxberg, M.D., a psychiatrist and director of the Stamford Center of Human Sexuality in Stamford, Connecticut. If you have this problem, called inhibited ejaculation,

Dr. Sex Will See You Now

Short of meeting his in-laws for the first time, there probably isn't a more terrifying moment for a guy than going to see a sex therapist.

"I've had people come to see me who've carried around newspaper articles about sex therapy for three or four years. It's taken them that long to get in," says Roger Crenshaw, M.D., a sex therapist and psychiatrist in private practice in La Jolla, California.

But sexual therapy is not embarrassing, painful or usually prolonged, doctors say.

"Most sexual therapy doesn't take long," says Joseph Waxberg, M.D., a psychiatrist and director of the Stamford Center of Human Sexuality in Stamford, Connecticut. "If they follow their therapists' instructions, about 90 percent will overcome their sexual dysfunctions."

Try to find a therapist who is a member of either the American Association of Sex Educators, Counselors and Therapists or the American Board of Sexology. That's a sign he has been properly trained.

The therapist should help you feel comfortable. After all, you are going to be discussing some mighty intimate stuff, says Marty Klein, Ph.D., a licensed marriage counselor and sex therapist in Palo Alto, California, and author of *Ask Me Anything: A Sex Therapist Answers the Most Important Questions for the '90s.*

Finally, if the therapist tells you nothing can be done, run, don't walk, to another doctor or therapist, Dr. Crenshaw says.

mention it to your doctor, since diseases such as diabetes and prostate and vascular disorders can cause it.

Also, if you have painful ejaculation, see your doctor. Ejaculation should never hurt and could be a sign of a hernia or prostate infection.

But for men whose ejaculation problems aren't caused by disease, control is something that can easily be learned, says Dr. Goldstein. Here's how.

Use different strokes. Dr. Klein suggests the stop-start technique. Begin by stroking your penis with a dry hand. When you sense you're nearing ejaculation, stop stimulating yourself for a few seconds, so your arousal subsides slightly. Then begin stimulating yourself again. Repeat that three times before allowing yourself to ejaculate, Dr. Klein says. Do that most nights for two weeks; then using the same stop-start method, progressively switch to a lubricated hand, to low-energy intercourse and finally to full thrusting.

Consider drug therapy. If the stop-start method fails, ask your doctor if

Prozac might help. As a side effect, the medication delays orgasm. In studies, Prozac helped men who ejaculated within 30 seconds extend their time to orgasm by more than five minutes, Dr. Crenshaw says.

Prescription drugs such as cyproheptadine (Periactin), an antihistamine, can boost ejaculation in some men, Dr. Crenshaw says.

Involve your partner. If you can masturbate to ejaculation but can't do it with your partner, try this: With your partner straddling your body, mutually masturbate each other. When you feel you're about to ejaculate, insert your penis into your partner's vagina, then thrust once or twice. "If you do that often enough, you'll learn how to ejaculate inside her," Dr. Waxberg says.

If that doesn't work, then unresolved anger, fear of intimacy or other psychological issues within your relationship could be repressing your orgasm, according to Dr. Klein. Talk to your partner or see a sex therapist about it.

Erection Changes

At age 18, your erections were instantaneous, seemed to loom like a redwood tree and were as taut as a drum. Nowadays, they look more like dwarf pines—and slouching ones at that. Should you be concerned? Probably not, doctors say. The angle, size, time between erections and how long you can sustain one all change as you age.

"Those are changes that are normal with aging. They don't mean you're losing it forever," says Saul Rosenthal, M.D., director of the Sexual Therapy Clinic of San Antonio in San Antonio, Texas, and author of *Sex over Forty*. "When a 19-year-old guy has sex, he's ready to go again in a few minutes. At 30, it may take him 20 minutes, and at 45, it could well take an hour before he gets another erection."

Low Sexual Desire

When you and your lover first got together, you counted the hours between your sexual interludes. But gradually, as your passion cooled, hours turned into days, then weeks, and now you actually find yourself trying to avoid having sex.

Up to 48 percent of Americans lose interest in sex at least temporarily at one time or another, researchers estimate. A man's libido naturally diminishes after about age 45, says Helen S. Kaplan, M.D., Ph.D., director of the Human Sexuality Teaching Program at New York Hospital–Cornell Medical Center in New York City. Depression, alcoholism and chronic diseases such as liver disease are some of the physical causes that can accelerate that process, Dr. Alexander says. But physical problems rarely inhibit sexual desire in men younger than 55.

"The problem isn't necessarily that one person is unhappy or uncomfortable with his own desire for sex. The problem is that he usually wants more or less of it than his partner," says Michael Seiler, Ph.D., assistant director of the

Phoenix Institute in Chicago and author of *Inhibited Sexual Desire*. "If you want less sex than your partner, you can feel weird, abnormal and certainly older."

Here are some ideas for rekindling the passion in your relationship.

Talk about it. If your wife wants sex four times a week and you feel like it four times a month, talk about your needs and reach a compromise. Otherwise, the problem will get worse. "A couple needs to talk about their feelings," Dr. Seiler says. "If they can't connect emotionally, the likelihood of them getting together in other ways is remote."

If you feel that your partner is losing interest in sex, avoid saying things such as "This is a major problem" or "You have this bad hang-up," suggests Anthony Pietropinto, M.D., a psychiatrist in New York City and author of *Not Tonight, Dear: How to Reawaken Your Sexual Desire*. Instead, try saying "I've noticed that you haven't seemed too interested in sex lately; is there anything I can do?" The important thing is to keep the pressure off your partner.

Dream on. "Learning to fantasize and playing sexually in your mind can rekindle your sexual desire," Dr. Seiler says. To do it, take five minutes each day to conjure up any sexual image that excites you. It could be a movie star, your spouse or even a former lover. Make a mental note of it. Then when you're in a sexual situation, recall it and see if it arouses you.

Sexual Addiction

We know you're probably thinking "Boy, sex must be a real tough addiction to live with." But in reality, it is. Like people addicted to alcohol, drugs or gambling, men addicted to sex will sacrifice career, family and health for the high that sex provides them.

"We treat people who spend $50,000 or more a year on sex. We had a guy in Texas who had four families in different towns. Can you imagine the energy it would take to keep all those balls in the air? He died of a heart attack in his early fifties," says Patrick Carnes, Ph.D., clinical director of the Sexual Dependency Unit and Sexual Therapy Program at Del Amo Hospital in Torrance, California, and author of *Don't Call It Love*. "The costs of the bingeing, staying out all night and worrying about being discovered take a tremendous toll. Addiction is an incredibly stressful thing, and stress definitely ages you."

Up to 6 percent of American men are addicted to sex, Dr. Carnes estimates. Among the risk factors and signs of addiction are:

- Having been sexually abused as a child.
- Feeling shame about your sexual habits.
- Being unable to stop sexual behavior when you know it's inappropriate.
- Believing your sexual activities are abnormal.
- Engaging in sexual practices, such as prostitution or sex with minors, that are against the law.

If you are an addict, you probably won't have to give up sex. But you can learn to avoid behaviors that trigger your addiction. If you suspect you have a sexual addiction, see a sex therapist, or contact Sex and Love Addicts Anonymous, P.O. Box 119, New Town Branch, Boston, MA 02258.

Sexually Transmitted Diseases

If every American who has a sexually transmitted disease moved to Canada, it would more than double the population of our northern neighbor. About 40 million Americans have sexually transmitted diseases, or STDs. Each year, there are 12 million new cases of STDs—that's 33,000 a day.

"We have a tremendous epidemic on our hands," says Peggy Clarke, president of the American Social Health Association in Research Triangle Park, North Carolina.

Most STDs can be cured, although the longer you go without treatment, the more likely you will have lingering or possibly permanent physical and mental disabilities as a result. You should also be aware that STDs are often symptomless and can hide in a body for years while the person unwittingly infects others.

AIDS: Fighting the Scourge

Many of us know at least one person who has AIDS or has died from it. But behind the grim numbers that tell us more than one million Americans have this fatal viral disease, there is a faint glimmer of hope.

"In the beginning, people were dying within months of their diagnoses. But we've learned so much more about the disease since then, and we now have long-term survivors who are very healthy for good periods of time," says Peggy Clarke, president of the American Social Health Association in Research Triangle Park, North Carolina.

Antiviral drugs such as zidovudine (AZT), didanosine (Videx) and zalcitabine (Hivid) can slow the progress of the disease, which gradually destroys the immune system, allowing life-threatening infections and cancers to invade the body at will.

But there is no cure for this deadly disease. So the best way to fight AIDS is to not get it in the first place. That means using a latex condom or having sex in a monogamous relationship in which both partners have been tested and found to be free of the human immunodeficiency virus (HIV) that causes AIDS. If you use intravenous drugs, don't share needles with others, as the HIV virus may be transmitted through bodily fluids that remain in the needle.

Short of abstinence, latex condoms are your best insurance policy against acquiring an STD or passing it on, Clarke says. If you have or have had a lesion, discharge or rash in the genital area, see your doctor.

The federal Centers for Disease Control and Prevention in Atlanta has identified more than 50 sexually transmitted organisms and syndromes. Here's a quick look at some of the more common ones.

Genital herpes. Nearly 31 million people—one in six Americans—have genital herpes. Herpes, caused by the virus herpes simplex type 2, is a lifelong infection that produces genital sores as often as once a month in some men. Other men never develop symptoms, although they are still infectious. Acyclovir (Zovirox), an oral prescription drug, can ease the symptoms but won't cure the disease. Sores from herpes or any other STD also increase your risk of contracting AIDS, since the virus can easily enter the body through these open blisters.

Syphilis. Known as the Great Imitator because its early symptoms mimic a horde of other diseases, syphilis often begins with a painless sore on the penis or genitals and progresses in three stages that can last more than 30 years. Overall, it can make an aging guy's life miserable, because it can induce heart disease, brain damage and blindness. Untreated, it can also cause death. About 120,000 people get syphilis each year. Antibiotics can cure it but cannot reverse the damage it has caused.

Gonorrhea. Known since ancient times, gonorrhea today strikes about 1.5 million American men and women annually. Often symptomless, this bacterial menace can cause painful urination and penile discharge within two to ten days of infection. Untreated, it can lead to arthritis, skin sores and heart or brain infections. Antibiotics can cure it.

Chlamydia. This condition has symptoms similar to gonorrhea, although it, too, can be symptomless. The most common curable STD in the United States, chlamydia infects about four million people annually. It can cause severe arthritis and infertility in men. Like syphilis and gonorrhea, it is eradicated by antibiotics.

Genital warts. Nearly a million new cases of genital warts occur each year. This STD is caused by the human papillomavirus, some types of which have been linked to cancer of the penis and anus. There is no cure, although the warts can be removed surgically or burned or frozen off. Recurrences are common, however.

Hepatitis B. This disease can lead to cirrhosis of the liver or liver cancer. Up to 200,000 cases are reported annually, despite the fact that it is the only STD that is preventable through vaccination.

For more information about STDs or referrals to self-help groups in your area, phone the Centers for Disease Control National STD Hotline (1-800-227-8922) or write the American Social Health Association, a nonprofit organization that provides educational information on STDs, at P.O. Box 13827, Research Triangle Park, NC 27709.

Skin Cancer

Preventable, Curable but on the Rise

You've got your shaving routine down to a sleepwalking science. You can steer that blade with one eye open. Up neck, over jut of jaw, down cheeks, over weird spot.

Hit the brakes. What weird spot? Where'd that come from? You're awake now—and a little worried. What is it? It's not a zit. It doesn't look like a mole. But no way could this be skin cancer. That only happens to really high-mileage guys, right?

It's hard news to wake up to, but the incidence of melanoma—the malignant and potentially fatal form of skin cancer—is rising faster than that of any cancer in the country. And the incidence of other skin cancers is growing at the rate of 6 percent a year. That's probably because we've been soaking up lots of sun and the earth's ozone layer that used to protect us from the worst of the sun's radiation has taken a beating.

What many people used to think happened only to elderly golfers in the Sun Belt is creeping up on younger men. It's enough to make you think you'll have to hang out in the clubhouse all day and leave the links to those younger fellas. But hang on to your putter. Skin cancer is scary, but it's also nearly 100 percent curable, as long as it's caught in time.

Various Breeds

There are various kinds of skin cancer, but in all cases, the sun's radiation is a major culprit, says Vincent DeLeo, M.D., associate professor of dermatology at Columbia Presbyterian Medical Center in New York City. Every one of us is vulnerable, but if your parents or grandparents have had skin cancer, or if you have fair skin and light eyes, you're at greater risk.

Luckily, the skin cancers that occur most often—the forms known as basal cell and squamous cell—very rarely spread, though if they're stubborn, they can recur, says Dr. DeLeo. They're usually found on sun-exposed areas such as the face. Basal cell cancers look like small bumps, either flesh-toned or brown to gray. They may have tiny ulcers in the center that bleed easily—when you're toweling off, for example. Squamous cell growths are similar, but they may also have a hard spot within the bump.

The great white shark of skin cancers is melanoma. It's less frequent, but it can be fatal—it does spread to other organs of the body. Overall, men are at greater risk for melanoma because they tend to have more sun exposure over the course of a lifetime than do women, says David J. Leffell, M.D., chief of dermatologic surgery at the Yale University School of Medicine in New Haven, Connecticut. But sometimes melanoma develops on an area of the skin that is usually not exposed to the sun. It may start from a mole that has developed unusual changes. It can also develop from a large, flat brown freckle or bleeding spot.

It may sound grim, but let's cut to the chase. Although skin cancer does appear more often as you get older, you have high odds of outrunning it, for two good reasons. One—it's easy to diagnose, and two—in most cases, it's curable.

Who Needs It in the First Place?

If you pass up sun damage, you'll pass up most types of skin cancer automatically, dermatologists say. And though there may be some kinds of skin cancer you can't always prevent—such as melanoma—a little vigilance will go a long way toward saving your hide, says Dr. Leffell. Whether a skin cancer is sun-induced or not, the key to the cure is to catch skin cancer early, he says. Once you know the warning signs, it won't sneak up on you.

Here are your best bets for saving your skin.

Stay out of the sun. If you're like most guys, you don't live in a cave (though your office might feel like one sometimes). If you're exposed to sun, you need to shield your skin.

Wear a full-spectrum sunscreen that blocks both kinds of ultraviolet radiation (UVA and UVB)—and wear it every day, summer and winter, says Perry Robins, M.D., associate professor of dermatology at New York University in New York City, president of the Skin Cancer Foundation and author of *Sun Sense*. Check to be sure that your sunscreen has a sun protection factor (SPF) of at least 15.

Also, try to limit your outdoor activities during the hours when the sun's rays are the strongest—from 10:00 A.M. to 2:00 P.M., says Thomas Griffin, M.D., a dermatologist with Graduate Hospital of Philadelphia and clinical assistant professor of dermatology at the University of Pennsylvania School of Medicine, also in Philadelphia.

Pore over your pores. Twice a year, go over your skin thoroughly (with help from a hand mirror or a significant other). Watch for any spot that changes in color, texture or size (gets bigger) or starts to bleed, says Dr. Robins. If your skin is particularly sun-damaged or you have a family history of skin cancer, you can ask a dermatologist to "map" your body for trouble spots and to keep track of any changes with follow-up visits.

Teach a mole the alphabet. "If you have the ABCDs, get your butt to a doctor," says Dr. DeLeo. *ABCD* can spell melanoma, and although melanoma can be cured, growth of one millimeter's depth can mean the difference between life and death. Early detection is crucial. If you have a mole with the following changes, see your doctor within days, Dr. DeLeo says.

- *A* is for asymmetry (moles tend to be symmetrical; cancers are not).
- *B* is for border (an irregular border).
- *C* is for color change (a dark area arises within a mole, or a mole shows areas of lightening).
- *D* is for diameter (the mole gets larger or is larger than a pencil eraser).

Getting Rid of It

You've seen your doctor, and the unwelcome word is that you have a skin cancer. The next step is to remove it.

For most cancers, local anesthetic is all that you'll need, and the removal won't leave a noticeable scar. Depending on the depth and nature of the growth, your doctor will use one or a combination of procedures. They include burning, scraping or freezing the growth or cutting it out surgically. Some shallow cancers can simply be treated with a topical chemotherapy cream.

For difficult or recurring cancers, a surgeon can remove malignant cells in very thin layers, leaving healthy skin untouched. And even melanoma has a potent new enemy—a melanoma cell vaccine that significantly increases survival rates.

SLEEP APNEA

The Snooze That Can Leave You Breathless

There's nothing restorative about a night's sleep if it involves relentless interrupted breaths and choked gasps. But that's exactly what happens night after night to millions of men who have a disorder known as obstructive sleep apnea.

The scary thing about sleep apnea is that you may have it and not even know it. Unless, of course, you haven't been feeling quite like your youthful, robust, happy-go-lucky self lately. It makes sense: Even though you're getting eight hours of sleep a night, every time you gasp and wheeze you wake yourself up ever so slightly, breaking those eight hours into little pieces.

"These recurrent mini-arousals rob you of the full restorativeness of unfragmented deep sleep," says Stuart F. Quan, M.D., director of the Sleep Disorders Center at the University of Arizona in Tucson. "This chronic sleep deprivation leaves you extremely sleepy and lethargic during your waking hours."

Sleep apnea not only saps your energy but also can leave you feeling irritable, depressed and even a little dopey. It can also take a toll on your physical appearance, producing baggy eyes, poor posture and changes in the way you walk and talk. "Many people come into our offices with obstructive sleep breathing problems who are in their forties, but they look, feel and act ten years older," says Richard Millman, M.D., director of the Sleep Disorders Center of Rhode Island Hospital in Providence.

Even if you're lucky enough to stay cheerful and keep your looks, you're not out of the woods yet. Men with sleep apnea may experience sharp drops in their blood oxygen levels. This can foster serious health problems that we usually associate with aging, including high blood pressure, heart rhythm disturbances, heart attack and stroke. On top of that, as many as one-third of all men

267

with sleep apnea have probably experienced car accidents or dangerous mishaps on the job, says Willard Moran, M.D., clinical professor of otolaryngology at the University of Oklahoma College of Medicine in Oklahoma City.

Sleep apnea can also put severe strain on a man's relationships. The loud gasps and other noises have driven many wives to separate bedrooms. Impotence is also a common problem. "Sleep deprivation inhibits a man's sexual interest and his ability to obtain an erection," says Dr. Quan. "The man is just too tired to keep his mind on the act, and he falls asleep."

When Your Airway Says No Way

Sleep apnea is caused by a closure of the tissues in the upper airway of the nose and throat. As we age, these muscles and tissues—including the tongue, the tonsils, the soft palate and the uvula (the fleshy structure that dangles from the roof of the mouth)—get flabby and lose tone. When we sleep, they relax and close in upon themselves. If this closure is partial, the obstruction will only be partial, so when you breathe, the tissues vibrate against each other, producing the familiar sounds of a snore.

Now suppose that these same tissues over-relax, creating a total airway obstruction. This is sleep apnea. "Sleep apnea can be thought of as the most advanced form of snoring," says David N. F. Fairbanks, M.D., clinical professor of otolaryngology at the George Washington University School of Medicine and Health Sciences in Washington, D.C. "The process in both is the same, only in sleep apnea, no air passes at all."

These pauses can last from ten seconds to a minute. You struggle for air, but nothing happens until your brain jump-starts your breathing by signaling a loud gasping or snorting response. The gasp wakes you slightly, restores tone to the tissues and opens the airway. When normal breathing resumes, you drift back to unconsciousness, only to have the process repeat.

Sleep apnea is usually years in the making. "It's extremely rare for severe apnea to develop out of the blue," says Christian Guilleminault, M.D., professor at the Stanford University School of Medicine Sleep Disorder Center in Palo Alto, California. "Men will usually progress gradually over the years from heavy snoring to mild sleep apnea to more severe."

Sleep apnea can snag you at any age, but it's more likely to get you after you hit your thirties and forties. The age connection is obvious: As we age, we lose muscle tone, and our tissues get flabbier. We become less active and put on weight.

Certain conditions can bring on sleep apnea, too. Among them: bulky throat tissue; large tonsils, adenoids or uvulas; tumors or cysts in the airway; a recessed jaw; or a nasal deformity. All these things can create blockages or cause the airway to collapse while breathing.

Although obstructive sleep apnea affects men of all shapes and sizes, it is much more likely in heavyset men. Neck size seems to be a factor, too. A thick, fat neck promotes collapse of the throat during sleep. A large number of men with sleep apnea have size 17 necks or larger, says Dr. Millman. It's very common among ex-jocks.

An Arsenal of Airway Openers

There is no cure for sleep apnea, but it is treatable. If these tips don't help nip it in the bud, your physician can refer you to a sleep or breathing specialist, who can prescribe a more specific treatment.

Slim down. For can press down on the neck, making the airway more prone to obstruction and decreasing the amount of air you obtain with each breath, says Dr. Guilleminault. A weight loss of just 10 to 25 percent can eliminate sleep apnea or significantly reduce the episodes.

Kick the habit. Cigarette smoke irritates the airway, causing it to swell and narrow, says A. Jay Block, M.D., professor of medicine and anesthesiology and chief of the Pulmonary Division at the University of Florida College of Medicine in Gainesville. It also increases mucus production in your nose.

Clear your nasal passages. Men with nasal obstructions must inhale with greater effort, causing the throat and airway to constrict, says Dr. Millman. Open your nasal passages with an over-the-counter saline solution or ask your doctor about allergy treatments. Nonprescription nasal sprays (such as Afrin) are also good, but be careful—overusing them can make matters worse.

Lock up the liquor. Alcohol causes muscles and tissues to over-relax, says Dr. Millman. If you must drink, do so in moderation, and avoid it within four hours of bedtime.

Dump the downers. Many snorers perceive their excessive sleepiness as a sign of insomnia and turn to sleeping pills. This is the worst thing you can do, says Dr. Quan. Like alcohol, tranquilizers, sedatives and other sleep-inducing medications will exacerbate your apnea by encouraging muscles and tissues to relax.

Don't burn the midnight oil. Sleep deprivation only makes you extra drowsy, which plunges you into a deeper sleep, over-relaxes your muscles and brings on apnea, says Dr. Quan. Try to keep normal bedtimes.

Eat light. Large evening meals and midnight snacks can bring on heavier sleep, which results in increased muscle relaxation and a night full of gasping, says Dr. Fairbanks.

Back off. Apnea is more common when you're on your back, so get in the habit of sleeping on your stomach or side, says Dr. Guilleminault. One thing you can try is a snore ball: Sew a pocket on the back of your pajama top and insert a tennis ball. This will condition you to keep off your back.

Put some slope in your sleep. It's wise to raise your head and shoulders while you sleep. But propping with pillows will only kink your neck and cut off your airway. Get around this by placing bricks or wood blocks under the bedposts to raise the head of your bed several inches, says Dr. Millman.

Try a tongue retaining device. A sleep disorder center or an orthodontist can fit you with a variety of dental appliances to comfortably hold your tongue or pull your jaw forward so that your tongue doesn't fall into the back of your throat while you're sleeping, says Dr. Millman.

Mask your apnea. Perhaps the most effective apnea treatment is a home device called a continuous positive airway pressure machine. This is a mask that fits over your nose and provides air pressure to keep the throat from collapsing. The only drawback to the device, says Dr. Moran, is that many men don't enjoy the idea of going to bed looking like Darth Vader. The device must be fitted by a doctor.

Be wary of medications. According to Dr. Moran, some doctors may prescribe stimulants to maintain tone in the airway while you sleep. But these drugs tend to prevent you from entering deep sleep, which is needed for good health.

Consider corrective surgery. As a last resort, physicians have a variety of surgical procedures at their disposal. Tonsils, adenoids and nasal blockages can be removed. A popular procedure called a uvulopalatopharyngoplasty (UPPP for short) removes, shortens and tightens excess tissue in the airway. Surgery to correct set-back jaws has proven successful in keeping the tongue from falling back into the throat. And extreme, life-threatening sleep apnea often calls for a tracheostomy, a hole in the throat to bypass the obstruction.

SMOKING

Butt Out to Put Time on Your Side

If you're like most guys, you started smoking when you were young and stupid in an effort to look and feel older. If you stayed stupid and continued to smoke—unlike the 24 million or so other guys who have quit over the past 30 years—you got your wish: Nothing ages your appearance, spirit and health more than America's most practiced and most dangerous vice.

Just ask Elizabeth Sherertz, M.D., a dermatologist and researcher at Bowman Gray School of Medicine of Wake Forest University in Winston-Salem, North Carolina. "We found that on average, smokers tend to look between five and ten years older than their actual ages because of the wrinkles caused by smoking," she says. "People who smoke are more likely to develop wrinkles, because smoking damages the elastic tissue that keeps skin tight and probably also enhances the sun's damaging effects to the skin."

Or Richard Jenks, Ph.D., a sociologist at Indiana University Southeast in

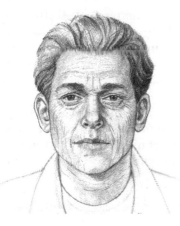

Smoker—behold your future face. Note the wrinkles that radiate from the lips and the corners of the eyes. Note, too, the deeply lined cheeks and the crevices running up and down the lower jaw.

New Albany who studies the effects of smoking on our emotional state, who found that once again, puffers suffer. "Smokers know that their habit is a sure road to health problems, and they're actually even more likely than nonsmokers or ex-smokers to describe it as dirty," he says. "But what my study found was that smokers tend to feel they have less control over their lives, and feel less satisfied with their lives, than nonsmokers."

Or ask any other researcher or doctor who has ever studied the effects that smoking has on our physical and emotional well-being. Study after study—and there have been hundreds of them—backs up what experts already know: If it doesn't kill you—and one in five people worldwide dies from smoking-related diseases each year—it will most certainly take years off your life. Says Margaret A. Chesney, Ph.D., a researcher and professor at the University of California, San Francisco, School of Medicine who has studied smoking issues, "If you want to radically slow down the aging process and live longer, stop smoking."

Why Smoking Kills

The reasons are clear: Cigarette smoke contains about 4,000 chemicals, including minute amounts of poisons such as arsenic, formaldehyde and DDT. With each puff, these poisons are inhaled through the lungs—which retain up to 90 percent of the compounds—and then passed through the bloodstream. Some of these poisons, such as carbon monoxide, are the so-called free radicals that rob red blood cells of oxygen. Free radicals have been linked to a host of problems, ranging from wrinkles to cancer.

Meanwhile, the nicotine in tobacco smoke causes the adrenal glands to se-

Weight Gain Is No Heavy Burden

Wondering what quitting will do to your waistline? Well, fret no more, because it's official: According to the Centers for Disease Control and Prevention in Atlanta, when you quit, the average weight gain is about five pounds. And the weight gain can be prevented through a careful diet and stress management. In fact, some people actually lose weight after they quit.

For many men, quitting smoking is part of an overall get-healthy program that includes regular exercise and improvements in diet, says Douglas E. Jorenby, Ph.D., coordinator of clinical activities for the Center for Tobacco Research and Intervention at the University of Wisconsin Medical School in Madison.

crete hormones that increase blood pressure and heart rate, which makes your heart work harder—the primary reason why smokers are at much higher risk for stroke and heart disease.

Smoking makes you more susceptible to infectious diseases such as colds and flu, since it damages the cilia, tiny hairlike bodies that trap and sweep out foreign bodies from the lungs. Without the cilia to do their work, the tar from cigarettes clogs breathing passages, leading to emphysema and lung cancer. Smoking also hobbles your ability to stay fit, sapping your body and mind of energizing oxygen.

"Even if smoking is not a causal factor in a particular disease, it can certainly exacerbate it," says Douglas E. Jorenby, Ph.D., coordinator of clinical activities for the Center for Tobacco Research and Intervention at the University of Wisconsin Medical School in Madison. "For instance, we know that smoking doesn't cause diabetes, but people with diabetes who smoke have a much worse prognosis than those who don't."

Another case in point: A study by British researchers found that smokers with the human immunodeficiency virus develop full-blown AIDS twice as quickly as nonsmokers, although scientists aren't sure why.

Men Are Better Quitters

The good news is that once guys make up their minds to quit, they're on the road to success, statistically speaking. "Men are much more successful at quitting than women," says Dr. Jorenby.

"When the surgeon general's first report on smoking and health was published in the 1960s, twice as many men as women were smoking," says Dr. Jorenby. "Today, the smoking rate between men and women is almost even, and in the next few years, it will probably cross for the first time—and there will be more women smokers than men." In real numbers, about 28 percent of American men over age 18 smoke. That's a drastic decrease from the 52 percent who smoked when the first surgeon general's report came out in 1964. By comparison, about 24 percent of American women smoke, which is down from 34 percent who smoked in 1964.

Men are better quitters because we apparently don't suffer withdrawal symptoms as severely as women. "There is evidence that equal numbers of men and women attempt to quit, but men succeed at about twice the rate," says Dr. Jorenby. "One reason is that women report more depression when they quit smoking, and we know from various studies that depression makes it more likely that you'll go back to smoking." Men also aren't the primary targets of advertising that presents cigarettes as a way to control weight and appear more glamorous.

Of course, those claims aren't true, since there's little glamour in the way smokers have been treated in society lately. As far as the weight issue, it's apparently a big, fat lie: True, nicotine slightly curbs the appetite, meaning that

Supplements for Smokers

While they're no substitution for quitting, antioxidant vitamins have been shown to offer at least some protection against the harmful effects of smoking. Jeffrey Blumberg, Ph.D., associate director of the U.S. Department of Agriculture Human Nutrition Research Center on Aging at Tufts University in Boston, recommends these vitamins to keep your immune system strong and to offset some of the damage caused by tobacco.

Vitamin C. 250 to 1,000 milligrams daily. The Recommended Dietary Allowance (RDA) is 60 milligrams. Good sources include citrus fruits, broccoli, cantaloupe, red peppers, kiwifruit and strawberries.

Vitamin E. 100 to 400 IU daily. The RDA is ten milligrams alpha-tocopherol equivalents, or 15 IU. Good sources include cooking oils, wheat germ and mangoes.

Beta-carotene. 15 to 30 milligrams daily. There is no established RDA. Best sources are yellow-orange and dark green fruits and vegetables such as carrots, sweet potatoes and squash, as well as spinach and other green leafy vegetables.

smokers consume fewer meals. But when they eat, smokers are more likely than nonsmokers to gravitate toward foods that are higher in calories and fat, says Doris Abood, Ed.D., associate professor of health education at Florida State University in Tallahassee.

In her study, which examined the smoking, eating, drinking and exercise habits of 1,820 Navy men, she also found that smokers exercise less and consume more alcohol, which is notoriously high in calories. And Dr. Abood and other researchers found that the more people smoke, the more bad habits they practice, and to a greater extent.

Still, regardless of these other habits, it's smoking itself that does the most damage, causing nearly 419,000 deaths a year. It also plays a leading role in scores of diseases, from cancer to colds, from heart disease to hip fractures. "The effects of smoking are distributed so much throughout the entire body that it has an impact on virtually any disease you can think of," says Dr. Jorenby.

A Quick Fix

But once you quit, the benefits occur right away. Just one year after you quit smoking, your risk for heart disease is cut in half, and after three years, your risk becomes comparable to that of someone who never touched a cigarette. Your risks for other diseases, such as emphysema, bronchitis and cancer, also diminish. Plus you'll look and feel younger, with more energy and stamina and fewer wrinkles.

Sure, quitting is tough. Fewer than 10 percent of the 20 million smokers who try to quit each year actually succeed, says Rami Bachiman, director of community education for the American Lung Association of New York in New York City. There are various strategies you can use to help you along—keeping

You Gotta Have Heart—And Willpower

Nicotine patches and gum and hypnosis may take some of the sting out of the withdrawal symptoms that come with quitting, but don't expect these aids to replace grit and determination.

Smokers who quit with the assistance of these tools are two to three times more likely to succeed than those doing it cold turkey. Although quitting cold turkey is the most popular method, it is also the least successful, having a success rate of only 5 percent. The smoker using nicotine gum or patches plus enrolling in a comprehensive behavioral smoking cessation program increases his chances of stopping and can anticipate a one year success rate of 23 to 40 percent. Meanwhile, there's a 15 percent success rate using hypnosis.

There are some side effects to nicotine patches and gum, which are prescribed by a doctor usually to heavy smokers who simply can't quit or who have had severe withdrawal symptoms when they've tried.

The patch, an adhesive square that secretes nicotine through the skin and into the bloodstream to help ease the pain of withdrawal, can cause itchiness and minor burning. And smoking even one cigarette while wearing the patch can cause a heart attack.

The effectiveness of the gum, meanwhile, is wiped away if you eat or drink anything—especially diuretics such as coffee and cola—within 15 minutes of chewing it. And although the gum isn't supposed to be used after four months from your last cigarette, 1 in 12 smokers continues using it for over a year after quitting.

The bottom line: If you've tried to quit and failed in the past, ask your doctor about these products. But, says psychologist Mitchell Nides, Ph.D., of the University of California, Los Angeles, you have to "learn" how to be a nonsmoker, and that's something that no pharmaceutical can do by itself.

your hands busy, chewing on carrot sticks, taking deep breaths of fresh air, drinking lots of water or even rewarding yourself with a present. But here's how you can increase your chances of quitting successfully and not relapsing during those crucial first few weeks.

Log your progress. If you're trying to quit by the slow and steady route, the first thing you should do is set a deadline up to three weeks away for when you'll have your last smoke. But in the meantime, log each cigarette you smoke—where you smoke and under what circumstances, advises Don R. Powell, Ph.D., president of the American Institute for Preventive Medicine in Farmington Hills, Michigan, and a former smoker. This will help you identify situations that cause you to smoke and then find alternative behaviors other than cigarettes.

Delay the desire. If you are quitting gradually, each time you get the urge to smoke, hold off lighting up for 5 minutes, suggests Dr. Powell. After a few days, extend the delay to 10 minutes. After another few days, extend it to 15 minutes, and so on. "You'll find that the actual urge to smoke at any given moment fades relatively quickly," he says.

Seek support. Whether you're quitting cold turkey or doing it gradually by slowly decreasing the number of cigarettes you smoke, you'll probably fare better if you have a lot of encouragement. "Having some kind of group support can make a big difference in how you do, whether it's from friends and family or some sort of group therapy," says Dr. Jorenby. There are probably groups in your area offering free counseling and group therapy for people trying to quit. Contact your local chapter of the American Heart Association for more information.

Drink orange juice. The hardest part of quitting cold turkey, which is the most popular method (and the one most men succeed at), is getting through the withdrawal symptoms of nicotine, which last one to two weeks. But you'll get over the irritability, anxiety, confusion and trouble concentrating and sleeping that come with nicotine withdrawal a lot faster if you drink a lot of orange juice during that time.

That's because OJ makes your urine more acidic, which clears nicotine from your body faster, says Thomas Cooper, D.D.S., a nicotine dependency researcher and professor of oral health sciences at the University of Kentucky in Lexington. "Besides," adds Dr. Jorenby, "the citrus taste in your mouth makes the thought of having a cigarette pretty disgusting."

However, if you're quitting with the aid of doctor-prescribed nicotine gum or patches, avoid orange juice and other acidic drinks, because you want to keep nicotine in your system with these products.

Imagine it's the flu. "Before we had nicotine gum and patches, I used to tell people who were quitting smoking to imagine they were having the flu," says Dr. Jorenby. "A lot of withdrawal symptoms are similar to the flu: You fly off the handle easily, you have trouble concentrating, your stamina is down. And as with the flu, there's little you can do other than let it run its course. But you will get over it. As long as you don't relapse and have a cigarette, the withdrawal will be over and done with in a week or two."

Stay out of bars. The greatest chance of relapsing occurs in bars, says Dr. Jorenby. "For many people, having a drink in one hand means having a cigarette in the other. I advise that anyone trying to quit stay out of bars for at least the first two weeks after they stop smoking." Instead, he advises, go to libraries, museums and other public places where smoking is prohibited. "People who quit smoking don't have to swear off going to bars, but we know from many studies that they are at much higher risk of going back to smoking unless they stay away for the first few weeks."

Write a letter to a loved one. When a nicotine fit hits, pick up a pen instead of a butt and write a letter to a loved one explaining why smoking is more important than your life, suggests Robert Van de Castle, Ph.D., professor emeritus of behavioral medicine at the University of Virginia Medical Center in Charlottesville. In the letter, try to explain why you continue a habit that you know will kill you rather than quit and live to see a child graduate from college or get married or to witness other important events.

When Dr. Van de Castle's patients try this letter, he says, they feel so selfish and ashamed that it often gives them the courage to put up with withdrawal symptoms and stay smoke-free.

SNORING

Not as Harmless as You Think

$\mathbf{A}$s a kid, you watched your old man taking a nap and giggled as he sucked in lungful after lungful of air with all the subtlety of a grizzly bear.

Well, you're not a kid anymore, and the sounds that emanate from your own slumber have a striking resemblance to a Harley-Davidson at full throttle. Suddenly, snoring's not so funny. Your spouse can't stand to sleep in the same room with you, and now your kids are the ones standing around giggling. Even more seriously, that snoring may be stealing your health and youthful vitality.

Loud Nights, Foggy Days

Generally, snoring does not pose a health risk for the mild or moderate snorer. But the industrial-strength window rattler does face the possibility of some very serious medical problems—problems that we usually expect to see in an older man.

One such problem is hearing loss. "We've recorded snoring as high as 85 decibels, almost the equivalent of a diesel engine," says Willard Moran, M.D., clinical professor of otolaryngology at the University of Oklahoma College of Medicine in Oklahoma City. "That much loudness at close distances night after night can damage your hearing and your spouse's as well."

The greatest health risk comes from the most advanced form of snoring known as obstructive sleep apnea. Here, unbeknownst to the unconscious man, the airway becomes totally obstructed, and breathing comes to a grinding halt. After a long pause, breathing resumes with a loud snort and a brief partial awakening. These episodes can happen up to several hundred times per night, dropping blood oxygen levels well below normal. This makes your heart pump harder and deprives you of the benefits of deep-stage sleep.

Fortunately, not all snorers have sleep apnea. Still, even the heavy snorer

Spare Your Spouse

The man who snores will never be voted Mr. Popularity by those who must share sleeping quarters with him.

"Snoring has not only driven couples to the point of sleeping in separate bedrooms, it has also caused its fair share of bitter arguments and ugly divorces," says A. Jay Block, M.D., professor of medicine and anesthesiology and chief of the Pulmonary Division at the University of Florida College of Medicine in Gainesville. "Anything that you can do to make your spouse's night more bearable not only will reduce the number of kicks in the shin you receive, it may save your marriage." He recommends the following possible marriage savers.

Buy her earplugs. Heavy-machine operators use them all the time. They are cheap, easy to use and comfortable, and they work well even with real harsh snoring.

Install a white noise machine. Many department stores now sell electronic noise-making devices that produce barely audible sounds that help muffle other more offensive sounds in the room.

Make sure you're the last to go to bed. Let your wife and anybody else in the house get into bed and drift off to sleep for a while before you get into bed. Your snores are less likely to wake them once they're soundly asleep.

may exhibit some aftereffects usually associated with full-blown apnea. He'll wake with a throbbing headache and feel drowsy all day, possibly dozing off on the job or while driving. In other ways, his behavior may start to resemble that of a much older man. He will be moody and sullen, will have difficulty with memory and mental tasks and may lose his sex drive.

"The heavy snorer or apnea sufferer may even appear a bit senile," says Richard Millman, M.D., director of the Sleep Disorders Center of Rhode Island Hospital in Providence. "The real problem is that inadequate sleep and oxygen are robbing him of his alertness, concentration and vigor."

The lack of oxygen in the blood and added strain on the heart can produce cardiovascular problems normally associated with old age, such as high blood pressure, heart failure, stroke, irregular heartbeat and heart attack. "We can't say for certain that snoring necessarily ages you or that you will suffer from one of these problems if you snore," says Dr. Millman. "But a large number of men with long-term sleep breathing problems do look, act and feel older than their true ages. And in general, snorers don't live as long as non-snorers."

The Source of the Racket

Among men ages 30 to 35, 20 percent snore regularly. And by age 60, over 60 percent of men saw lumber in their slumber. There are many potential causes of snoring, ranging from a clogged nose to tonsils to cysts. But a common cause in middle-aged men is flabbiness in the throat membranes.

It's easy to see why snoring becomes more common with time. As we age, some of us start to lose muscle tone and put on fat. One area where fat collects and muscle loses tone is the throat. If the muscles and fleshy tissues in the throat are flabby, they can, in effect, "cave in," partially obstructing the flow of air.

"It's like sucking air through a soggy straw: When you breathe, the airway narrows and partially collapses. The structures in the airway vibrate against each other. The result is the unmistakable sound of a snore," says David N. F. Fairbanks, M.D., clinical professor of otolaryngology at the George Washington University School of Medicine and Health Sciences in Washington, D.C.

This process is years in the making. "Snoring is a progressive condition that gradually develops and increases in intensity as we age," says Christian Guilleminault, M.D., professor at the Stanford University School of Medicine Sleep Disorder Center in Palo Alto, California. "A non-snorer will slowly become a mild or an occasional snorer long before he becomes a heavy snorer."

Snore No More

Snoring does not have to be a life sentence. Today, physicians specializing in sleep and breathing disorders can do wonders for almost all cases of snoring

Am I a Snorer?

If it weren't for kicks from irate bed partners, many guys wouldn't have a clue that they're buzzing like chain saws. But even with black-and-blue shins, some guys still need convincing.

One thing your spouse can do for you (or you can do for yourself if you sleep alone) is tape-record your sleep, suggests David N. F. Fairbanks, M.D., clinical professor of otolaryngology at the George Washington University School of Medicine and Health Sciences in Washington, D.C. For many men, hearing is believing, he says.

If you sleep alone, symptoms that may hint at a snoring problem include morning headaches, frequent awakenings and gaspings at night, daytime sleepiness and dry morning mouth.

and sleep apnea. But even the heaviest of snores may not need a doctor. The following tips may be all you need to quiet the storm once and for all.

Snuff that butt. As if you didn't already have enough reasons to quit smoking. Cigarette smoke greatly irritates the tissues of the nasal passages and upper airway, causing them to swell up and obstruct airflow, says Dr. Fairbanks.

Get lean and mean. Although thin people can be snorers, snoring is three times more prevalent in husky guys, says Dr. Guilleminault.

Eat light. Don't eat a large meal three hours before retiring, and steer clear of midnight snacks, says Dr. Moran. That's because the process of digestion causes muscles everywhere—including those in your throat— to relax.

Unclog your snoot. If your nose feels like it's stuffed to the rim, consider opening things up with an over-the-counter nasal spray (such as Afrin), suggests A. Jay Block, M.D., professor of medicine and anesthesiology and chief of the Pulmonary Division at the University of Florida College of Medicine in Gainesville.

But be careful. Overuse can backfire on you, clogging up your nose even worse. Follow the directions on the package. Constant nasal blockages should be discussed with your doctor.

Bag the booze. Avoid drinking for four hours prior to going to bed, says Dr. Millman. Alcohol causes the muscles in the airway to over-relax. Ditto for sedating medications such as sleeping pills and tranquilizers.

Get off your back. Sleeping on your side may prevent your tongue and the fleshy lobe that hangs from the roof of your mouth from falling back into your airway, says Dr. Moran. One good way to make sure you don't roll over onto your back is to sew a pocket on the back of your pajamas and place a tennis ball inside. The ball will cause such discomfort that you'll either wake up or unconsciously roll off your back.

Raise your head and shoulders. Sleeping on a slight slant can help prevent snoring by keeping the tongue from falling back into the airway. Don't prop your head with pillows, however—this will only kink the airway in your throat, making matters worse. Instead, says Dr. Millman, place a brick under each bedpost at the head of the bed to raise it four to five inches.

Try a whiplash collar. A neck brace may not be your version of an ideal bed partner, but it may keep your chin extended so that your neck won't kink and your throat stays open, says Dr. Fairbanks. To guard against a stiff neck the next morning, Dr. Fairbanks suggests using a foam collar rather than a plastic one. Foam cushions the neck better and is less restraining. But if you do have some morning kinks, gently stretching your neck muscles, giving yourself a gentle massage or taking a warm shower will help, he says.

Hold your tongue. Many sleep disorder centers provide tongue-retaining devices that hold the tongue forward and keep the mouth closed while you sleep, says Dr. Millman. An orthodontist can also create a similar device that achieves the same effect by pulling the jaw forward at night.

Heavy Silencers

When self-help remedies aren't enough, a medical procedure may be in order. Sometimes it may involve having your tonsils or adenoids removed. Other times, when nasal breathing is a problem, it may require an operation to clear the nasal passages.

One of the most frequently performed and successful operations for snoring is called an uvulopalatopharyngoplasty, or UPPP. The surgeon removes excess tissue, shortens the long, limp lobe that hangs from the roof of your mouth and tightens the floppy soft palate, essentially removing the flabbiness that's making all the racket.

A newer and also highly successful technique is called mandibular advancement, in which a set-back jaw is pulled forward to keep the tongue from falling back in the throat.

The most radical snoring treatment is a tracheostomy—an airhole cut in the throat to bypass the obstruction. It is effective, but the big drawback is a permanent hole in your neck.

STEROIDS

Massive Muscles, Major Danger

You'll never take it down from the mantle, no matter how much your wife, roommate, girlfriend or interior decorator begs. It's your trophy, damn it, and you won it fair and square.

Sure, it's dusty, dented and a decade old—but it still has your name on it. It's proof positive that you're an athlete.

Yet lately, you've been feeling less like the bronzed god who won that trophy and more like the stiff little bronzed statue atop it. No matter how long you train, how far you run or how much you lift, it's getting harder to keep up with the young bucks.

And you're thinking that anabolic steroids might give you the extra kick you need to stay on top.

"Forget it. Please forget it," says Thomas Branch, M.D., director of the Emory Clinic's Sports Medicine Center at Emory University in Atlanta. "Of all the things you can do to try to improve as an athlete, taking steroids is the worst."

Men who use steroids to stay young and fit may actually be aging themselves at an accelerated rate. The possible side effects range from heart and liver disease to enlarged breasts, hair loss and sterility.

What price muscles? "You may increase your muscle mass for a brief time, but there's a very high cost to your health," Dr. Branch says. "You risk doing a tremendous amount of damage to yourself, both short term and long term. It's just not worth it."

Watch for the Fallout

Anabolic steroids are synthetic chemicals that mimic the male hormone testosterone. They have limited legitimate medical uses, including treatment

Lyle's Lament: "Steroids Sacked My Life"

Lyle Alzado terrorized NFL quarterbacks for more than 15 years. He was a madman, a wild-eyed giant, an unstoppable 275-pound defensive lineman with a mean streak that was notable even in the brutal world of professional football.

Alzado died in 1992 of a rare form of brain cancer. He blamed more than two decades of steroid abuse for the illness that claimed his life.

He started taking steroids in college to make up for his lack of size. In an interview with *Sports Illustrated*, Alzado told how he mixed, switched and abused steroids and human growth hormone—anything to give him an edge during his career with the Denver Broncos, Cleveland Browns and Los Angeles Raiders. He said he injected so many steroids over the years that doctors had to remove a baseball-size wad of scar tissue from his backside.

He told stories of violent behavior on and off the field. He claimed to routinely chase guys in cars, catch them and beat them up for little or no reason.

Alzado said he was addicted to steroids and couldn't stop using them. "I just didn't feel strong unless I was taking something," he said.

Doctors were reluctant to tie his illness to steroid abuse. But Alzado was certain of it. His dying message was simple: Don't do steroids.

"If I had known that I would be this sick now, I would have tried to make it in football on my own—naturally," he told *Sports Illustrated*. "Whoever is doing this stuff, if you stay on it too long, or maybe if you get on it at all, you're going to get something bad from it.

"If you're on steroids or human growth hormone, stop. I should have."

for some forms of anemia, growth and development problems and osteorporosis. But their ability to increase muscle mass has turned them into the sports world's dirtiest secret.

Although it's a felony to sell steroids or to possess them without a prescription, the drugs remain in wide use. Estimates show that as many as 897,000 American men have used steroids for nonmedical reasons—including 80 percent of weight lifters and bodybuilders.

Once taken, either orally or by injection, steroids flow through your bloodstream, ordering the muscles along the way to produce more protein and heal themselves faster. Dr. Branch says that may help you work out harder, longer and more often.

Scientific studies have shown mixed results about just how effective low doses of steroids are at increasing strength. But Dr. Branch says he has little doubt that steroids can make you bulkier—if you're willing to take them in huge doses, stay on them forever and deal with the inevitable consequences.

"If you take enough steroids and mix them, you'll put on muscle like crazy," he says, "maybe 50 pounds in a few months."

But if you do, be prepared for a lot of hair to fall out. Dr. Branch says steroid use can trigger premature onset of male pattern baldness. Steroids can also make you look like a teenager again—at least when it comes to your complexion. They have been linked with acne on the face, shoulders and back, Dr. Branch says.

And while you may look more manly from the waist up and from the thighs down, you might be doing serious damage to the precious parts in between. "Abusing anabolic steroids is a form of castration," says Lewis Blevins, M.D., an endocrinologist and assistant professor of medicine at Emory University. How do atrophied testicles sound? Impotence? Decreased sperm production, sometimes to the point of temporary sterility? Dr. Blevins says all this could happen with steroid use.

Add in a few other problems—enlarged breasts, insomnia and stretch marks among them—and you get a pretty good indication of some of the effects of steroids.

Then there's liver damage. Your liver has to work overtime to process all the steroids. Dr. Blevins says this can result in any number of problems, from tumor growth to choleostatic jaundice, a dangerous condition in which bile flow in the liver is backed up, causing bile to enter the bloodstream.

Steroids hammer your heart, too, since they make it work harder and harder to keep up with your ever-increasing size. Steroids also raise the levels of low-density lipoprotein, or LDL—the so-called bad cholesterol—in your bloodstream, increasing chances for hardening of the arteries and heart attacks, Dr. Blevins says.

And once you start using them, it may not be a simple matter to stop. Studies show that steroid use can be addictive, just like other controlled substances. Even if you do manage to kick them, Dr. Branch says, you'll quickly lose all the muscle you built when you were using steroids.

There's more bad news. Studies show that even moderate steroid use can affect your mood and behavior. "Anger is common, and so is excessive violence," Dr. Branch says. "And there's more. While some athletes like that angry edge in competition, your personality can change off the field, too. You'll see violent mood swings. I've even seen suicide attempts."

Then there's AIDS. Some forms of steroids are injected. That might mean sharing needles—one of the most common ways to spread the human immunodeficiency virus, which causes AIDS. At least one case of a steroid user getting AIDS has been documented. "It's a very real threat," Dr. Branch says. "As real as any other way to get AIDS."

Steroids also make your tendons harder and more brittle, according to Dr. Branch. "You could grow in size and strength, rupture a tendon and be done athletically for a long time, maybe for good," he says. "It sort of defeats the whole purpose.

"Consider all that, and ask yourself again: Is it worth it?" Dr. Branch says. "It's hard to see where it is."

Stay Off—Or Get Off

It's tough to say what kind of permanent damage steroids can wreak on your body. Most people who use them are reluctant to tell doctors or researchers about their use or the problems the drugs cause.

"I'm not sure everyone knows the full story about steroids when they start taking them," Dr. Branch says. "If they did, I doubt so many people would be using them."

Here's what the experts advise about steroids.

Get off them now. If you're using steroids, stop. Cold turkey. Some of the damage they can do to your body may be reversible if you stop in time, Dr. Blevins says. "Otherwise, you may be a day late and a dollar short."

If you are taking steroids and notice any of the following symptoms, Dr. Blevins advises seeking medical attention immediately: nausea, vomiting, pain under the left side of your rib cage, weight loss or jaundice, which is characterized by a yellow skin tone.

If you have been using steroids for a while and then stop, you may suffer some temporary withdrawal symptoms, such as feelings of depression and anxiety. It may be tough, Dr. Branch says, but stopping is the only way to avoid harm to your body. See your doctor if you think you need help.

Remember: There's no alternative. No matter what the guys at the gym say, there's no safe steroid substitute. Dr. Blevins says "natural" drugs such as human growth hormone—often extracted from cadavers—may be at least as dangerous as steroids.

"None of these drugs is safe," he says. "People are using them for things they're not intended to do."

Compete against yourself. It's always great to win. But Vince Lombardi might have been guilty of overstatement when he said winning is the only thing.

"You should strive to be the best you can be—without steroids," Dr. Branch says. If that means finishing second in a race, so be it. Set your own standards, then go out and try to meet them. It's more satisfying in the long run—and a lot easier on your body.

Do it naturally. You can build impressive muscles without steroids. In fact, Dr. Branch says, they're more likely to stay with you than steroid-created ones. (For tips on how to bulk up naturally, see Resistance Training on page 519.)

STRESS

Virtually No Part
of Your Body Escapes

Most men don't put a high value on relaxation. We score ourselves on measurable things such as achievement and pay, not on emotional tranquillity. "Men tend to look at relaxing as a waste of time," says Paul J. Rosch, M.D., president of the American Institute of Stress in Yonkers, New York. "We feel guilty if we aren't productive."

Okay, we know what you're thinking: "Yeah, I have a little trouble unwinding, but it isn't going to kill me." Well, indirectly, it could. Long-term tension solidly affixes a finger on the fast-forward button of your biological remote. "Stress speeds up your entire system and produces conditions in younger people that are more commonly associated with growing old," says Allen J. Elkin, Ph.D., director of the Stress Management and Counseling Center in New York City. "Virtually no part of your body can escape the ravages of stress."

You Can't Always Run

Despite its bad reputation, stress is one of our bodies' best defense systems. When we sense danger—such as a car coming at us—our bodies release adrenaline and other chemicals that make us more alert, raise our blood pressure and increase our strength, speed and reaction time.

That's great if we're responding to a threat that requires physical action. Unfortunately, says Leah J. Dickstein, M.D., professor of psychiatry at the University of Louisville School of Medicine in Louisville, Kentucky, our bodies don't recognize the difference between physical threats and mental ones. When we get nervous about meeting a deadline, for instance, we may produce the same stress chemicals as when we see that oncoming car. And if we don't burn off these chemicals through physical exertion, they can linger in the blood-stream and start causing problems.

Studies show that stress can reduce the power of our immune systems. A study in Britain exposed 266 people, most of them in their thirties, to a common cold virus and then tracked who became sick. The study showed that 28.6 percent of those with few signs of stress caught the cold. But the figure jumped to 42.4 percent for those who were under high stress.

The reason? Stress may inhibit the disease-fighting cells in our blood-streams. "Everybody gets sick from time to time," Dr. Dickstein says. "But if you're under a lot of stress, a virus may get to you that you would have been able to fight off otherwise."

Considered by experts to be the major health problem facing men today, stress has been linked to heart disease, high blood pressure, stroke, cancer and other illnesses—even impotence. Up to 90 percent of all visits to doctors are for stress-related disorders, according to the American Institute of Stress.

Stress often surfaces as a health problem in men because men wait too long to do something about it. Only 20 percent of the people enrolled in a typical stress management program are males, says Joan Borysenko, Ph.D., president of Mind-Body Health Sciences in Boulder, Colorado. "Men take longer than women to realize that they are in trouble," she says.

Learning to unwind is not easy, particularly if you're the hard-driving, achievement-oriented type. "It takes effort—that's the paradox," says Dr. Elkin. "You have to find what'll do the job for you."

The Road to Calm

There are a number of basic rules for keeping from getting wound too tight. The first is to add balance to your life. Make a special attempt to seek out leisure activities that are different from your work. "Our bodies require variety and change," says Keith Sedlacek, M.D., medical director of the Stress Regulation Institute in New York City. "We have to shift gears, readjust our speeds, or our nervous systems will keep racing right into the next day." An accountant or lawyer who spends his week in analytic, left-brain pursuits might find relaxation in chopping wood, gardening, building a deck or tinkering with a car engine. In fact, almost any white-collar type would benefit from manual labor of some kind.

The second rule is to work up a sweat once in a while. Nothing eases stress more than exercise, according to David S. Holmes, Ph.D., professor of psychology at the University of Kansas in Lawrence. "Regular aerobic workouts reduce stress more effectively than meditation, psychiatric intervention, biofeedback and conventional stress management," he says.

Exercise helps burn off all the stress-related chemicals in your system. During a workout, your body will also release mind-relaxing endorphins, Dr. Holmes says. And exercise strengthens your heart, too, further protecting you against the ravages of stress.

Is Tension Adding Up?

Remember: Stress comes from within. Your attitudes about life have a lot to do with how much stress you feel. This quiz, from the book *Is It Worth Dying For?* by Robert S. Eliot, M.D., and Dennis L. Breo, tests your outlook and overall stress level. Read each statement, then score one point if you almost never feel that way, two points if you occasionally feel that way, three points if you frequently feel that way and four points if you almost always feel that way.

1. Things must be perfect.
2. I must do it myself.
3. I feel more isolated from my family or close friends.
4. I feel that people should listen better.
5. My life is running me.
6. I must not fail.
7. I cannot say no to new demands without feeling guilty.
8. I need to generate excitement constantly to avoid boredom.
9. I feel a lack of intimacy with people around me.
10. I am unable to relax.
11. I am unable to laugh at a joke about myself.
12. I avoid speaking my mind.
13. I feel under pressure to succeed all the time.
14. I automatically express negative attitudes.
15. I seem further behind at the end of the day than when I started.
16. I forget deadlines, appointments and personal possessions.
17. I am irritable and disappointed in the people around me.
18. Sex seems like more trouble than it's worth.
19. I consider myself exploited.
20. I wake up earlier and cannot sleep.
21. I feel unrested.
22. I feel dissatisfied with my personal life.
23. I feel dissatisfied with my work life.
24. I'm not where I want to be in life.
25. I avoid being alone.
26. I have trouble getting to sleep.
27. I have trouble waking up.
28. I can't seem to get out of bed.

Add up your marks. If you scored 29 or less, you show low stress. Totals of 30 to 58 show mild stress. If you scored 59 to 87, you show moderate stress. And if you scored higher than 87, you may be under high stress.

Is Work Wearing You Out?

Everyone feels pressure at work. But sometimes it gets out of hand, leaving you angry, tired and unproductive.

To check your stress level at work, take this quick quiz developed by Paul J. Rosch, M.D., president of the American Institute of Stress in Yonkers, New York. Score one point for each question you disagree with, two points for each one you agree with somewhat and three points for each question you agree with strongly.

1. I can't say what I really think at work.
2. I have a lot of responsibility but not much authority.
3. I could do a much better job if I had more time.
4. I seldom receive acknowledgement or appreciation.
5. I'm not proud of, or satisfied with, my job.
6. I am picked on or discriminated against at work.
7. My workplace is not particularly pleasant or safe.
8. My job interferes with my family obligations and personal needs.
9. I tend to argue more often with superiors, co-workers or customers.
10. I feel I have little control over my life at work.

Here's how to score the quiz: 10 to 16 points means you handle stress well, 17 to 23 points means you're doing moderately well, and 24 to 30 points means you need to resolve problems that are causing excess stress.

Research by Robert Thayer, Ph.D., professor of psychology at California State University, Long Beach, showed that 30 minutes of intense aerobic exercise immediately reduces body tension—and does it more effectively than moderate exercise such as walking. Research at Hofstra University in Hempstead, New York, has also found that weight lifting counters anxiety and depression and boosts self-esteem as well as or better than aerobic exercise.

The third rule is that whatever you choose as a relaxation break, it has to be relaxing to you. "If someone tells you to tie trout flies and you find it boring as hell, you'll actually add to your stress," warns Dr. Rosch.

Finally, you have to carve little breaks into your schedule. "You need to put together a relaxation package, a set of techniques that'll calm you down," says Dr. Elkin.

Here are some ideas to try.

Pad your schedule. "Realize that nearly everything will take longer than you anticipate," says Richard Swenson, M.D., author of *Margin: How to Create the Emotional, Physical, Financial and Time Reserves You Need.* By allotting yourself enough time to accomplish a task, you cut back on anxiety. In general, if meeting deadlines is a problem, always give yourself 20 percent more time than you think you need to do the task.

Don't be listless. So many projects, so little time. To beat stress, you have to learn to prioritize, according to Lee Reinert, Ph.D., director and lecturer for the Brandywine Biobehavioral Center, a counseling center in Downingtown, Pennsylvania. At the start of each day, pick the single most important task to complete, then finish it. If you're a person who makes to-do lists, never write one with more than five items. That way, you're more likely to get all the things done, and you'll feel a greater sense of accomplishment and control, Dr. Reinert says. Then you can go ahead and make a second five-item list. While you're at it, make a list of things that you can delegate to co-workers and family members. "Remember: You don't have to do everything by yourself," Dr. Reinert says. "You can find help and support from people around you."

Just say no. Sometimes you have to draw the line. "Stressed-out people often can't assert themselves," says Joan Lerner, Ph.D., a counseling psychologist at the University of Pennsylvania Counseling Service in Philadelphia. "And so they swallow things. Instead of saying 'I don't want to do this' or 'I need some help,' they do it all themselves. Then they have even more to do."

Give your boss a choice. "Say 'I'd really like to take this on, but I can't do that without giving up something else,' " says Merrill Douglass, D.B.A., president of the Time Management Center in Marietta, Georgia, a company that trains individuals and corporations in the efficient use of time and energy, and co-author of *Manage Your Time, Manage Your Work, Manage Yourself.* " 'Which of these things would you like me to do?' " Most bosses can take the hint, Dr. Douglass says.

Carry a canteen. Keep a plastic bottle of water at your desk and drink often. When you are under stress, you sweat more, and then of course, there's your dry mouth. You'll feel better if you hydrate your high anxiety.

Kill the ump. You can blow off your emotions at a ball game and get some of the tension out of your system, says Roger Thies, Ph.D., associate professor of physiology at the University of Oklahoma Health Sciences Center in Oklahoma City. "By yelling something really nasty, you almost make a joke of it, and you may head off that adrenaline squirt on your heart." (Just make sure the drunken guy in front of you isn't rooting for the other team.) Other places to let off steam: sports bars, pep rallies, political conventions. Places not to let off steam: church services, snow-covered cliffs, your father-in-law's house.

Practice your snorkeling. Want to really relax your muscles? Soak in a hot tub. To get the most relaxation from a hot bath, soak for 15 minutes in water that's just a few degrees warmer than your body temperature, or about 100° to 101°F. But be careful: Longer soaks in warmer water can actually lower your blood pressure too much.

Get a grip. Keep a hand exerciser or a tennis ball in your desk at work and give it a few squeezes during tense times. "When stress shoots adrenaline into the bloodstream, that calls for muscle action," says Roger Cady, M.D., medical director of the Shealy Institute for Comprehensive Health Care in Springfield, Missouri. "Squeezing something provides a release that satisfies our bodies' fight-or-flee response."

Serve soup, live longer. Be a volunteer. Isolation only magnifies your worries. Helping others will give you a sense of accomplishment and self-respect—and remind you that relatively speaking, your own troubles don't amount to a hill of beans in this world.

Here's an added benefit: Self-sacrifice may help you live longer. A ten-year study at University of Michigan in Ann Arbor found that the death rate was twice as high in men who did no volunteer work as in men who volunteered their time at least once a week.

Sit up straight. A good upright posture improves breathing and increases blood flow to the brain. We often slouch when stressed, which restricts breathing and blood flow and can magnify feelings of helplessness.

Pop a bubble. A study found that students were able to reduce their feelings of tension by popping two sheets of those plastic air capsules used in packaging. "Now we know why people hoard those things," says Kathleen Dillon, Ph.D., psychologist and professor at Western New England College in Springfield, Massachusetts, and the author of the study.

Trade in the Jag for a Hyundai. Living beyond your means can actually make you sick. A researcher at the University of Alabama in Tuscaloosa studied British census data on 8,000 households and found that families that tried to maintain lifestyles they couldn't afford were likely to have health problems.

Carry a humor first-aid kit. We could cite you chapter and verse on the value of humor in the workplace. Studies have shown that stress-fighting brain chemicals are released when you laugh. Experts say a good laugh relaxes tense muscles, speeds more oxygen into your system and lowers your blood pressure. Some experts believe all it takes is a smile to ignite a positive mood.

Hold your breath. This technique should help you relax in 30 seconds. Take a deep breath and keep it in. Holding palm to palm, press your fingers together. Wait 5 seconds, then slowly exhale through your lips while letting your hands relax. Do this five or six times until you unwind.

Take a ten-minute holiday. Meditation is a great stress reliever, but sometimes it's hard to find the time or place. Dr. Reinert suggests that you try taking a mini-vacation right at your desk or kitchen table instead. Just close your eyes, breathe deeply (from your stomach) and picture yourself lying on a beach in Mexico. Feel the warmth of the sun. Hear the waves. Smell the salt air. "Just put a little distance between yourself and your stress," Dr. Reinert says. "A few minutes a day can be a great help."

Smell the apples. Keeping a green apple on your desk may calm your nerves. A study found that men doing math problems under time pressure were less stressed if they were exposed to the scent of green apples. There's evidence that the scent of vanilla may also induce relaxation in men, says Alan R. Hirsch, M.D., neurologic director of the Smell and Taste Treatment and Research Foundation in Chicago.

Keep it down. If you work, live or play in a high-noise area, consider wearing earplugs. Make sure the ones you buy reduce sound by at least 20 decibels, says Ernest Peterson, Ph.D., associate professor of otolaryngology at the University of Miami School of Medicine.

You can also use sounds to your advantage. Try listening to gentle music, with flutes or other soft-sounding instruments, says Emmett Miller, M.D., a nationally known stress expert and medical director of the Cancer Support and Education Center in Menlo Park, California. He also suggests taking walks in quiet places and listening to leaves rustle or streams babble. Recordings of ocean waves or gentle rainstorms also help, he says.

Dare to be dull. Join the International Dull Men's Club. "We are regular guys who aren't hyper, self-absorbed or pushy," says president Joe Troise.

A Swift Solution

When you get wound too tight, often the first place you feel it is your neck. Try this four-way neck release recommended by former world-class track and field athlete Greg Herzog in his book *The 15-Minute Executive Stress Relief Program* (repeat each of the following exercises three times).

1. With your right hand, reach over your head and behind your left ear, grasping your neck with your fingers. Pull your head gently toward your right shoulder.
2. Do the same exercise, but this time use your left hand to pull your head toward your left shoulder.
3. Clasp your hands behind your head, with your elbows flared and your head bowed toward your chest. Relax in this position for 30 seconds. Then while pulling down with your hands, slowly push your head back until you are looking at the ceiling.
4. Place the palm of your left hand on your forehead, with the bottom of your palm at the bridge of your nose. Hold your right arm across your body so that you can rest your left elbow on your right wrist. Now push against your left palm with your forehead while keeping your right arm locked. Switch hands and repeat.

"When you can say 'It's okay to be dull,' it takes a lot of life's pressures off." For a $5 membership fee, you get a license that certifies you as a dull person, plus some infrequent newsletters. The address: 300 Napa Street, #10, Sausalito, CA 94965.

Tune out—have a potato. If you want to unwind at the end of the day, eat a meal high in carbohydrates, says Judith Wurtman, Ph.D., a research scientist at the Massachusetts Institute of Technology in Cambridge and author of *Managing Your Mind and Mood with Food*. Carbohydrates trigger release of the brain neurotransmitter serotonin, which soothes you. Good carbohydrate foods include rice, pastas, potatoes, breads, air-popped popcorn and low-calorie cookies. Dr. Wurtman says just 1½ ounces of carbohydrates is enough to relieve the anxiety of a stressful day.

Try some fiber. "Stress often goes right to the gut," says George Blackburn, M.D., Ph.D., associate professor of surgery at Harvard Medical School and chief of the Nutrition/Metabolism Laboratory at New England Deaconess Hospital, both in Boston. That means cramps and constipation. To avoid these problems, Dr. Blackburn suggests eating more fiber to keep your digestive system moving. You should build up gradually to at least 25 grams of fiber per day. That means eating more fruits, vegetables and grains. Try eating whole fruits instead of just juice at breakfast time, and try whole-grain cereals and fiber-fortified muffins.

Tune in—have tuna. It's no help unwinding if you feel sluggish and unalert. Dr. Wurtman suggests a high-protein lunch of lean meat, fish or poultry to prevent the afternoon blahs. Protein is loaded with tyrosine, an amino acid that has been shown to boost mental performance in the face of stress.

Quit the bowling league. Look at your life. Are you doing too much? If you're on the company softball team, coaching Little League, volunteering on a church committee and chauffeuring kids to piano lessons and Girl Scout outings and you don't have a weeknight free, you're choking on more than you can chew. "Prune your activity branches," suggests Dr. Swenson. Decide what gives you the most pleasure, and do only those things.

STROKE

Prevention Starts Now

Come on. Can't we just forget about this one for a couple of decades? We have enough worries already. There's job stress and mortgages and mothers-in-law and prostates. And when are the Cubbies ever going to win another pennant? Can't we get serious about prevention when stroke really becomes an issue?

Sorry. It's already an issue. Despite its reputation as an older man's problem, stroke hits more than 15,000 American men between the ages of 30 and 44 every year. Nearly one in every three strokes is fatal. And the aging effects on those who survive can be brutal. Survivors could suffer brain damage affecting speech, memory, thought patterns and behavior. Sometimes there is temporary—or permanent—paralysis.

But if you start working on it immediately, you can significantly cut your risk of stroke, both now and when you're older. "We're beginning to realize that stroke is not an inevitable process," says Michael Walker, M.D., director for the Division of Stroke and Trauma at the National Institute of Neurological Disorders and Stroke in Bethesda, Maryland. "It's preventable, and it is treatable."

It may mean eating more fruits and veggies, breaking a sweat a few times a week and being vigilant about your blood pressure. But when you weigh the options, it's not a bad trade-off.

A Man's Risk

Stroke is a sudden severe illness that attacks the brain. There are two basic types. Ischemic strokes, which account for about 80 percent of total strokes, happen when blood flow to a part of the brain is cut off, causing brain cells to die from lack of oxygen. This frequently occurs due to hardening and blockages in your carotid arteries, which feed blood from your neck to your head. Ischemic strokes can also be caused by atrial fibrillation, an irregular heartbeat that leads to blood clots that may travel through your body and lodge in the brain's arteries.

Hemorrhagic strokes account for the remaining 20 percent. These strokes are caused by bleeding from either a blood vessel on the surface of the brain or an artery in the brain itself. These strokes can be more deadly than ischemic strokes, with a mortality rate of close to 50 percent.

Men are 19 percent more likely to have strokes than women, according to figures from the American Heart Association. Blacks are at greater risk than whites of dying from strokes. Family history of stroke can play a role, though just how much remains unclear. And the risk of stroke goes up as you age. Statistics show that the incidence of stroke more than doubles each decade for a man once he reaches age 55.

Of course, you have no say over gender, genetics or age. But there are a lot of risks you can definitely control.

High blood pressure, for example. Also known as hypertension, it's the single most important risk factor for stroke. "About half of all strokes are caused by high blood pressure," says Edward S. Cooper, M.D., past president of the American Heart Association.

High blood pressure causes stroke by speeding up atherosclerosis and damaging smaller blood vessels. And in Dr. Cooper's words, it can cause tiny blood vessels in your brain to "blow out like an overinflated tire."

Smoking also puts you at increased risk for stroke by speeding up clogging in the carotid arteries. In fact, smoking and high blood pressure are stronger indicators than even blood cholesterol levels of atherosclerosis of your carotid arteries, according to Jack P. Whisnant, M.D., chief investigator for a study of carotid artery disease at the Mayo Clinic in Rochester, Minnesota.

Men with diabetes are also at greater risk of stroke. And risk factors for heart disease—high cholesterol, obesity, inactivity—can increase athersclerosis and raise the likelihood of stroke.

Saving Yourself from Stroke

Despite hundreds of studies, strokes remain shrouded in mystery. They seem to strike without warning. Sometimes it's hard to tell when you're even in danger.

But early prevention can be the key to improving your chances of avoiding stroke. "The process leading to a stroke begins in your forties, even earlier, so now is the time to intervene," says David G. Sherman, M.D., head of neurology at the University of Texas Health Science Center at San Antonio.

To help lower your risk, try these tips.

Check your pressure. Many people don't even know they have high blood pressure, because it produces few outward signs. That's why the American Heart Association recommends having your blood pressure checked by your doctor or another health care professional at least once a year if it is 130/85 or higher. If your blood pressure is lower, get it checked every two years. Many cases of high blood pressure begin developing between ages 35 and 45.

Research shows that controlling high blood pressure can cut your risk of stroke by as much as 40 percent. Any reading higher than 140/90 is considered high.

Your doctor will be able to prescribe treatments for high blood pressure, from dietary changes to getting more exercise to drug therapy. Follow the advice like your life depends on it. It might.

"Controlling hypertension is absolutely vital in stroke prevention," says Harold P. Adams, Jr., M.D., professor of neurology at the University of Iowa Hospital and Clinic in Iowa City.

Cut the butts. If you really need another reason to quit smoking, here it is. Studies show that kicking the habit can reduce your risk of stroke by 33 percent.

"Don't just cut back on cigarettes," Dr. Adams says. "There's no such thing as moderate smoking. You have to stop altogether, all the way, right now."

Check your neck. Ask your doctor to listen for a bruit, a whooshing sound in the carotid arteries in your neck. This is caused by partial blockage and turbulence in the crucial blood vessels that feed oxygen to the brain.

"This is especially important if you have atherosclerosis causing blocked blood vessels elsewhere in your body," says Patricia Grady, Ph.D., acting director of the National Institute of Neurological Disorders and Stroke.

While you're at it, have the doc check your heart, too. Treating atrial fibrillation can reduce stroke risk by up to 80 percent.

Get some exercise. Physical inactivity may be a risk factor for stroke, but a total exercise time of at least 20 minutes a day, three times a week, could help cut that risk. Walking, tennis, bicycling, stair climbing, aerobics and even gardening and Ping-Pong can be potential stroke busters.

A British study of 125 people showed that the sooner you start exercising, the better. Guys who started regular exercise between ages 15 and 25 had 70 percent less risk of stroke than non-exercisers. And even if you're a little late getting started, you can still benefit from exercise: The study showed that people who began exercising between ages 25 and 40 reduced their risk by 57 percent and that people who started exercising between ages 40 and 55 had a 37 percent better chance of avoiding a stroke.

"Exercise has so many benefits," Dr. Adams says. "If you're not exercising, you could be robbing yourself of years later on."

If it's orange or green, eat it. Continuing research shows just how powerful the nutrient beta-carotene can be in fighting stroke.

As part of the Physicians' Health Study, which tracked the well-being of more than 22,000 doctors over a five-year period, 333 male doctors with signs of heart disease were given either 50-milligram doses of beta-carotene or placebos

Warning Signs You Should Know

Quick action can mean the difference between tragedy and recovery when it comes to stroke. Heed these warning signs from the American Heart Association.

• Sudden weakness or numbness in the face, arm or leg on one side of the body
• Loss of speech, or trouble talking or understanding speech
• Sudden dimness or loss of vision, particularly in only one eye
• Sudden severe headache with no known cause
• Unexplained dizziness, unsteadiness or sudden falls, especially along with any of the previous symptoms

If you notice any of these symptoms, get help immediately by calling 911 or the emergency phone number for your area. A study of response times showed that people with stroke signs who called this emergency number got to the hospital two to three times faster than those who called their doctors or tried to transport themselves to the hospital. And with stroke, minutes matter.

What seems like a stroke may actually turn out to be a transient ischemic attack (TIA). These are sometimes called temporary strokes, since the symptoms quickly disappear. But you shouldn't ignore a TIA, since it is the single most important warning of impending stroke, according to Harold P. Adams, Jr., M.D., professor of neurology at the University of Iowa Hospital and Clinic in Iowa City.

---

every other day. The beta-carotene group suffered nearly half as many strokes, cardiac deaths and other cardiovascular diseases as the doctors who were not given the nutrient.

Dr. Adams says it's too soon to tell if beta-carotene is going to be useful in preventing stroke. But he says that eating a little extra each day certainly won't hurt. Fruits and vegetables are high in beta-carotene, with sweet potatoes, carrots, pumpkin, red peppers, winter squash, apricots and spinach among the best sources.

Pack away some potassium. Researchers at the University of California, San Diego, have found that adding a single daily serving of potassium-rich food to your diet could cut your risk of fatal stroke by as much as 40 percent. The reason for the benefit isn't completely clear. Although potassium is known to help lower blood pressure, the amount of potassium those in the study ate had little direct effect on their blood pressure readings. But studies at the University of Mississippi Medical Center in Jackson showed that potassium may help prevent the formation of blood clots, one of the primary factors in stroke and heart attack.

Potatoes are one of the best sources of potassium you can find. Other good sources include beans, avocados, bananas, oranges, salmon, trout and tomato sauce.

Know the aspirin essentials. Aspirin might help ward off ischemic stroke by thinning potential blood clots, Dr. Adams says. But unless you already have a risk factor, such as atherosclerosis or a prior stroke, it may not do you much good. In fact, research shows that aspirin might be linked to a slightly higher incidence of hemmorhagic stroke.

Even if you're a good candidate for aspirin therapy, just how much you should take remains debatable. Some studies have found benefits with an 81-milligram daily dose (a children's aspirin). Others tout a 325-milligram daily dose (a regular-strength adult aspirin). And now some researchers say that as many as three regular aspirin tablets daily may be necessary. The bottom line: See your doctor before you start an aspirin regimen for stroke prevention.

Go low-fat. What's good for your heart is good for your brain. Keeping your cholesterol in check can slow atherosclerosis and ward off ischemic stroke. So eat a low-fat diet. The current recommendation from most doctors and researchers is to limit fat to no more than 25 percent of your total calories.

"Along with exercise and quitting smoking, what you eat is key to preventing stroke," Dr. Adams says. "What we're talking about is a good diet that will help lessen the risk of hardening of the arteries." This diet does not need to be extreme, he says. It does need to be well balanced and low in fat.

Toast your health—in moderation. Excess drinking means increased stroke risk. Numerous studies show that having more than four drinks a day greatly increases your chances of having a hemmorhagic stroke.

But some studies show a link between moderate alcohol intake and slightly reduced risk of ischemic stroke, at least among whites.

"There may be something about alcohol that helps in small levels. It may prevent both heart attack and stroke. I'm not telling my patients to drink for their health," Dr. Adams says. "If you're not drinking now, I don't recommend starting. If you do have more than a couple of drinks a day, the potential complications of alcohol are probably going to hurt you in the long run. The key to alcohol use is moderation."

Sun Damage

They Call Him Old Sol for a Good Reason

Back when you were knee-high to a newt, romping in the sand, you noticed the older guys all oiled up, roasting under the sun like human shish kebabs. You didn't quite get it, so an adolescent sibling helped you out. Simple, my man. A bronzed torso is a magnet for those bikini-clad girls over yonder. So, you reasoned, it's manly to tan.

Eat those words, tadpole. Tanned skin is damaged skin—skin that's going to get age spots, wrinkles and sags long before they're due. Years of exposure to the sun is also an open invitation to skin cancer and cataracts. In short, if you want to look and feel 80 years old when you're only 50, go work on your tan.

It's the radiation in sunlight that ages you before your time, says Karen Burke, M.D., Ph.D., a dermatologist in private practice in New York City. Two kinds of ultraviolet rays are equal partners in the crime. UVA rays go deep beneath the skin, weakening the fibers that normally keep your skin smooth and taut. UVB rays burn the surface and over the years cause a splotchy, leathery texture—along with skin cancer. Both kinds of rays may contribute to cataracts.

Ready for some good news? If you stop sun damage right now, you can roll back the clock—at least where most skin damage is concerned. "Skin is remarkably resilient," says Doug Darr, Ph.D., assistant research professor of dermatology at Duke University Medical Center in Durham, North Carolina. "It can heal itself over time, and it's never too late to start."

No More Nukes

Here's how to protect yourself from the sun's radiation.

Skip the noontime sun. Whenever possible, avoid the sun when its rays

300

Tanning Parlors: Fountains of Aging

"Tanning parlors and sunlamps are the most worthless things you can pay money for—and very damaging to the skin," says Vincent DeLeo, M.D., associate professor of dermatology at Columbia Presbyterian Medical Center in New York City.

Some tanning lamps generate over five times more ultraviolet radiation (UVA) than you'd get sitting for the same amount of time on a beach at the equator, says a report from the National Institutes of Health.

Ultraviolet rays cause long-term damage to the tissues under the skin. That, says Dr. DeLeo, translates to wrinkles, sags and age spots.

are strongest—between 10:00 A.M. and 2:00 P.M., says Jonathan Weiss, M.D., assistant clinical professor of dermatology at Emory University School of Medicine in Atlanta.

Dress like Dundee. The sun's radiation can blast right through many fabrics. "Wear tight weaves or several layers of clothes in the sun," Dr. Weiss says. Better yet, he says, ask the salesperson at your local clothing or sporting goods store about specially woven clothing that prevents ultraviolet rays from penetrating through to your skin. While you're suiting up, don't forget your broad-brimmed hat.

Get hooked on sunscreen. Applying sunscreen in the morning—every morning—could be your best defense, says Dr. Weiss. He recommends that you make this a morning ritual by slapping on sunscreen along with, or in lieu of, your aftershave. Look for a sunscreen marked SPF 15 or greater. *SPF* stands for sun protection factor. SPF 15, for example, will let you stay out in the sun 15 times longer without damage than you could without any sunscreen. If you're serious about stopping sun damage, don't forget your neck, upper chest, hands and forearms. And save a dab for your bald spot, if you have one.

If sunscreen stings your eyes when you work up a sweat, "take a wax-based sunscreen made for lips, and—after you've used it on your lips—use it around your eyes," says Melvin L. Elson, M.D., medical director of the Dermatology Center in Nashville. "It won't drip."

Protect your eyes. Shades can make you look cool, but the right ones may prevent cataracts by protecting your eyes from harmful ultraviolet rays. Check the manufacturer's label to make sure the sunglasses block at least 99 percent of the sun's ultraviolet rays, advises the American Academy of Ophthalmology. The academy also suggests buying wraparound or close-fitting

A Safe Tan in a Tube

Today's self-tanning lotions won't turn you the awful streaky orange that skin dyes did years ago, thank goodness. The new breeds of tan-in-a-bottle are easy to apply, look natural and won't harm your skin.

You may have tried a bronzing gel for that sun-kissed look. The difference between a bronzer and a self-tanner is that a bronzer is a tinted makeup that washes off the next time you cleanse. A self-tanner, on the other hand, actually interacts with your skin to turn it a natural, golden-looking color, says Yveline Duchesne, international training director for New York City–based Clarins Cosmetics. The tan fades gradually as you shed your dead skin cells, usually within a few days.

The main active ingredient in self-tanning lotions is a chemical called dihydroxyacetone (DHA), which combines with amino acids and keratin on the very superficial cell layers of skin to produce the color.

With the new products, you can be attractively tanned without damage to your skin—if you also continue to wear sunscreen. Most self-tanners have sunscreen with only a low sun protection factor (SPF), so it's best to also use your own sunscreen of SPF 15 or higher. The best timing? Since self-tanners take a few hours to develop, apply them the night before, Duchesne suggests. Then apply your sunscreen the next morning, at least an hour before going out.

Other tips for making the most of your self-tanner:

Always allergy-test. Before you try a self-tanner all over, apply the lotion to a small patch of skin and leave it on overnight to see if your skin is sensitive to DHA. (If it reacts, a bronzing gel or tinted sunscreen is your best bet for color.)

Exfoliate before you apply. DHA can take unevenly in areas where there's a buildup of dead cells. Be sure to include hands, elbows and knees.

Start at the top. Work down from your forehead, covering all exposed areas, but skip the eyebrows, where color can concentrate. Apply evenly, including your ears and under your jaw.

Moisturize the rough spots. Elbows and knees will look more natural if you moisturize first and apply self-tanner lightly.

Wait for results. How often you reapply, not how much, determines the depth of your tan. It takes from three to five hours for color to develop, so don't reapply until you've seen the full results.

Let it dry. Wait a half-hour before dressing or going to bed, since some tanners can stain fabric.

Wash up. Wash your hands after you apply your self-tanner, or you'll end up with tan palms.

frames that stop ultraviolet rays from entering under, over and around the sides of your lens and choosing tints that don't distort your vision. Dark gray and dark green are usually best.

Consider supplements. You might want to try taking extra vitamin E and selenium. Both have been proven to reduce sun damage, says Dr. Burke. Safe daily doses are 400 IU of vitamin E (d-alpha tocopheryl acetate, d-alpha tocopheryl succinate or d-alpha tocopherol—not the "dl" form) and 100 micrograms of the trace mineral selenium, best taken as l-selenomethionine. If you slip up and get sunburned, take four or five extra vitamin E capsules as soon as possible. It will lessen the burn with no side effects, says Dr. Burke.

Ask your doctor why you're sensitive. Certain medications can cause oversensitivity to the sun. These include some antibiotics, diuretics, tranquilizers, antihistamines and drugs for diabetes, says Perry Robins, M.D., associate professor of dermatology at New York University in New York City, president of the Skin Cancer Foundation and author of *Sun Sense*. Some medicated soaps and colognes can also make you more vulnerable to the sun's effects. Consider switching to a different fragrance or hypoallergenic soap if you burn or break out easily. Talk to your doctor if you're concerned about any medications you're taking.

A Quick Read on Repair

If your sun damage is extensive, you might want to check out what a dermatologist or plastic surgeon can do. Here are several popular medical options for reversing the aging effects of the sun.

Retin-A. A dermatological wunderkind in a tube, the cream tretinoin (Retin-A) restores skin tone, smooths texture, removes fine wrinkles and fades age spots. Ask a dermatologist about a prescription, suggests Dr. Elson. Results are gradual but worth the wait, he says.

Chemical peels. Out with the old, in with the new is the philosophy here. With a chemical peel, a dermatologist swabs on an acid, and a few days later your skin strips off, peels down and grows, replacing damaged skin, says Dr. Robins.

Dermabrasion. While you're in the shop, think about how planing works. When a dermatologist uses dermabrasion on your skin, he's essentially planing the sun damage away with a special instrument.

Surgery. Sun-damaged men today are considering surgical repairs ranging from wrinkle filling to eyelid-lifts and even face-lifts, says Geoffrey Tobias, M.D., a plastic surgeon at Mount Sinai School of Medicine of the City University of New York in New York City. If you're curious, contact a board-certified plastic surgeon.

TELEVISION

The Great American Brain Drain

Bob Armstrong is a TV addict and darn proud of it.

"I'm serious about watching television. I watch as much as possible. I have five sets on simultaneously, 10 to 12 hours a day," says Armstrong, a 43-year-old cartoonist in Dixon, California, who is "head spud" of the Couch Potatoes, a tongue-in-cheek support group for TV junkies. "We think that TV viewing is a necessary part of life, like eating and breathing. So what if you gain an extra 20 or 30 pounds doing it? It gives you ballast that will keep you from falling off the couch."

Now before you grab a beer and plop on the couch, consider this unfunny fact: Sitting before the boob tube can make you old in mind and body.

"There's absolutely no question that large amounts of TV viewing can make you feel old and weary before your time," says Kurt V. Gold, M.D., a physical medicine and rehabilitation physician at Immanuel Medical Center in Omaha, Nebraska, who has studied the effects of TV viewing on children. "Just think about what happens when you watch television. You're sitting passively, not using your muscles much. After you've watched a long program, you feel stiff, tired and mentally drained. Over the long run, that can lessen your ability to think and perform physical tasks. As a result, your muscles sag, and your mind stagnates."

Heavy Set

Perhaps the thing television does best, as head spud Bob Armstrong says, is "give you ballast." In one study of more than 6,000 men, a researcher at Brigham Young University in Provo, Utah, discovered that those who spent more than three to four hours a day watching television had twice the risk of middle-age spread as those who watched less than one hour daily.

A study of 800 adults, published in the journal *American Dietetic Association*, found that the risk of obesity may be even greater than that. In this study, those who lounged in front of the tube for 4 or more hours a day were four times as likely to be overweight. How many men have the time to watch that much television every day? A lot of us. In fact, the typical American male watches just more than 3½ hours a day, according to a report from Nielsen Media Research.

Not only are TV addicts more likely to be overweight, they're also less likely to be physically fit, says Larry A. Tucker, Ph.D., professor and director of health promotion at Brigham Young University.

In a study of 9,000 adults at Brigham Young University, light, medium and avid TV viewers were asked to do a three-minute step test. Those who watched television for less than one hour a day were the most likely to sail through the test with hardly a bead of sweat. Those who did regular four-hour-plus marathons of viewing were more likely to struggle—on average, they were 50 percent less fit.

Not only are you less likely to be fit if you consume too many reruns of "Bonanza," your blood is less likely to be fit as well. In one study of 11,947 adults, Dr. Tucker found that people who watched three to four hours of television a day had twice the risk of developing high cholesterol levels as people who watched less than an hour a day. High cholesterol levels spell bad news for a guy's heart.

As Dr. Gold pointed out, TV viewing doesn't just age your body. It can also age your mind.

One Canadian study looked at the effects that television had after being introduced into a village where people had not been able to watch television on a regular basis. The average resident's time in front of a television increased from 0 to 22 hours a week within two years. That increase in viewing slashed participation in community social activities and sports. Researchers also found that those who watched a lot of television were less able to solve puzzle problems. In addition, TV-viewing residents gave up trying to solve these problems much more quickly, says Tannis MacBeth Williams, Ph.D., professor of psychology at the University of British Columbia in Vancouver.

Research has also shown that watching television for long periods leaves people in worse moods than they were in before they started watching. Irritability, difficulty relating to others and boredom may also be linked to excessive TV viewing.

How to Cancel Bad Viewing Habits

"I wouldn't say that television is a total waste of one's leisure time. There are some good programs that inform and entertain us," Dr. Tucker says. "But there is a tendency to overindulge." It's that overindulgence, of course, that we need to avoid. Here are a few ways that you can control your television rather than having it control you.

Be tough on yourself. Set a strict limit on the absolute amount of time

Are You a Victim of Television?

Check each question you answer yes.

1. Do you watch more than two hours a day of television?
2. Do you stop talking with others while you view television?
3. Do you become unhappy or irritated if you have to turn off the television to do something else?
4. Do you occasionally feel extremely tired during a regular day's schedule?
5. Do you frequently eat junk food or unhealthy snack food when you sit down to watch television?
6. Do you frequently experience insomnia and use television as a means of distracting yourself during your sleeplessness?
7. On a pleasant day, are you more likely to stay indoors and watch television than to go do something outside?
8. Is it difficult for you to share or communicate your feelings and experiences with others?
9. Are you actively involved in less than two hobbies, clubs or sports at least four hours a week?
10. Do you frequently turn on the television and search the stations without having a specific program in mind to watch?

Grading Your Quiz

For every odd-numbered question that you answered yes, give yourself two points. These factors were determined by experts to be indicators of too much TV watching.

For every even-numbered question that you answered yes, give yourself one point. These factors, in conjunction with poor viewing habits, signal potential trouble.

Tally your score and use the following scale as a rating guide.

3 or less. No problem.

4 to 6. Potential trouble brewing.

7 to 9. Yes, you're probably watching too much television.

10 or more. Whoa! Your brain is becoming fused to your set.

you will watch each week. "You need to set limits, or your viewing can easily get out of control," Dr. Tucker says. Make a chart and put it on the refrigerator, so you can record the time you spend watching.

Set aside a night. Make the television off-limits one night a week. You may be surprised at the creative things you can find to do, Dr. Tucker says.

Create your own guide. Browse through a programming schedule and mark one or two programs an evening that you want to watch. Then stick to the schedule. Turn on the set when the show begins and turn it off immediately after it ends, Dr. Tucker says. This will discourage you from getting hooked on the next program.

Put a camera on yourself. Before you turn on the television to watch a program, take a moment to visualize yourself walking over to the set and turning it off once the show is over. "That will program it into your brain that the television will actually go off at that time, and you will find something else to do," says Jane M. Healy, Ph.D., an educational psychologist in Vail, Colorado, and author of *Endangered Minds: Why Our Children Don't Think and What We Can Do about It.*

Reward yourself for not watching. For every hour that you don't watch television when you normally would, give yourself a point. After you've accumulated 10 or 20 points, treat yourself with tickets to a baseball game, an evening at a comedy club or a dinner out on the town, says Leonard Jason, Ph.D., professor of clinical and community psychology at DePaul University in Chicago.

Say what? Try turning on the set but turning off the sound, says Dr. Healy. More than likely, you'll quickly find something else to do with your time. "Much of the enticement of television comes from the sound track," says Dr. Healy.

Move it out of sight. Try putting your television in an unusual place, such as a cluttered room with no chairs, so you have to make an effort to watch it. "I've been remodeling my house, and I've put a bunch of furniture in front of my set, so I can't get to it very easily," Dr. Gold says. "You know what's nice? I've been working on my yard and spending time with my family instead of the television."

Get out of the house. Take a stroll, visit a museum or go to the neighborhood basketball courts and get involved in a pickup game of hoops. The bottom line: Get out into the real world. "I'd bet you'd come home feeling energized and ready to do anything but watch television," says C. Noel Bairey Merz, M.D., medical director of the Preventive and Rehabilitative Cardiac Center at Cedars-Sinai Medical Center in Los Angeles.

Call on me. "Arrange to have a friend phone you at the end of your favorite program. That might be all the incentive you need to break your habit, because once you get pulled away from the set, it's going to be easier not to go back to it," Dr. Healy says.

Don't get cable. The fewer viewing options you have, the more likely you'll find something else to do with your time, Dr. Gold says.

THYROID DISORDERS

When Your Body's Thermostat Goes on the Fritz

When your home air conditioner spontaneously comes to life in the dead of winter, or your central heating system starts pumping hot air in the middle of July, you can almost always guess what the problem is: That *&%$# thermostat is acting up again.

Like your home's heating and cooling, your body has its own built-in thermostat: the thyroid. Small and butterfly-shaped, it rests out of sight at the base of the throat, monitoring our body functions and diligently producing the hormones that regulate metabolism, temperature, heart rate and other biological processes.

When all systems are go, your thyroid pumps out just the right amount of hormone to keep your body in fine working order. But just like a real thermostat, an aging thyroid can go out of whack, sending hormone production straight through the roof or bringing it to a virtual standstill.

When the thyroid produces too much hormone, your metabolism takes off like a 45 rpm record played at 78; too little hormone, and your metabolism lags and drags at a snail-like 33⅓.

At the same time, these metabolic changes can produce a wide range of nasty symptoms that can make you look bad and feel worse. Left untreated, a screwy thyroid can eventually trigger heart problems—and can even lead to coma or death.

Ugly scenario? Yes. Inevitable? Not at all. "With early detection and proper treatment, almost all the problems of an abnormal thyroid can be corrected, and the symptoms, reversed," says Brian Tulloch, M.D., clinical associate professor at the University of Texas Medical School at Houston. "And most patients go on to live normal, functional, productive lives."

Hypothyroidism: Life in the Slow Lane

When the thyroid's hormone production trails off to a trickle, a condition called hypothyroidism, your body gradually shows all kinds of signs that it's running on empty: fatigue, chills, dry skin, coarse hair, swelling and puffiness around the face and eyes, to name a few. It can affect your mental functioning, leading to poor concentration, forgetfulness and depression. Even your sex drive can completely sputter and stall.

The difficulty with hypothyroidism is that many of the symptoms associated with it are so vague and common that you might not even suspect the thyroid is to blame. "It's easy to overlook an underactive thyroid, because the symptoms are similar to those associated with other common illnesses and mimic many of the physical changes we associate with normal aging," says Lawrence Wood, M.D., president and medical director of the Thyroid Foundation of America and a thyroidologist at Massachusetts General Hospital in Boston. "Many patients—and even some doctors—just take these symptoms to mean that the body is getting older, so quite often, the problem goes unreported or is undiagnosed."

Generations ago, thyroid enlargement, or goiter, was very common in America due to insufficient iodine in the diet. Today, however, iodine deficiency is not a problem in the typical American diet; the most common cause of hypothyroidism is Hashimoto's disease, a disorder of the body's autoimmune system.

Because hypothyroidism slows down the way the body burns calories, some men would like to think that their increasingly bulging bellies and love handles are really the by-product of a sluggish thyroid. Not the case. "Obesity and major weight gains are rarely related to an underactive thyroid," says Dr. Tulloch. "Most thyroid-related weight gains amount to only a few pounds, and that's due mostly to water retention."

While doctors can't usually make your underactive gland active again, they can make up for its lackluster performance. "All we have to do is restore the right balance of thyroid hormone in the system by replacing what isn't being produced," says Martin I. Surks, M.D., head of the Division of Endocrinology and Metabolism at the Montefiore Medical Center in New York City. Men with hypothyroidism take little tablets containing a synthetic version of the hormone thyroxine. The drawback: They must take them every day for the rest of their lives.

Hyperthyroidism: All Revved Up

Now let's do a 180-degree turn and imagine the thyroid pumping out too much hormone, a condition called (not surprisingly) hyperthyroidism. This time, we have lots of excess hormone pushing the body's metabolism into overdrive, producing a unique combination of hyper-symptoms that include rapid heartbeat, weight loss, weakness, nervousness, irritability and tremors.

The most common cause of hyperthyroidism is Graves' disease, the autoimmune disorder that struck both former President George Bush and Barbara Bush. The former first lady, you may remember, suffered persistent vision problems (including bulging eyeballs) and experienced a period of rapid weight loss—classic Graves' symptoms. And her husband became aware of his Graves' disease after a scare from an irregular heartbeat.

Physicians can treat an overactive thyroid in several ways. The simplest and most prescribed is to use radioactive iodine to reduce the number of overproductive thyroid cells. Doctors can also prescribe drugs that block the production of thyroid hormone or that block the effects of the hormone on the body. And as a last resort, doctors may surgically remove all or part of an overactive thyroid. (Since surgery and radioactive iodine can cause a person to develop hypothyroidism later in life, a lifetime of thyroxine tablets is often necessary.)

Are You at Risk?

We men are lucky: Thyroid problems are much more likely to develop in women. But that doesn't mean we don't get our fair share of cases. Graves' disease is most likely to develop between the ages of 20 and 40. By age 50, at least 1 in every 30 men will have some signs of an underactive thyroid. And 9 percent of those over 60 suffer from some form of hypothyroidism.

Heredity also plays a role. If your family has a history of thyroid disease or autoimmune diseases such as diabetes and rheumatoid arthritis, you're a candidate for thyroid problems as you get older. Another fact to consider: According to a Dutch study, cigarette smoking appears to be a significant factor that produces Graves' disease in genetically predisposed people.

Other risk factors: having had radiation treatments around the head and neck as a child, the use of certain medications such as lithium or going through a particularly stressful time such as losing a loved one.

Thyroid Maintenance

Eating a balanced diet and avoiding cigarettes are about all you can do to prevent thyroid disease. Whether the gland malfunctions is usually beyond your control. But early detection can help you head off thyroid complications.

Have your doctor check out any symptoms or abnormalities that may suggest hypo- or hyperthyroidism. According to Dr. Wood, anyone over age 50, especially if in a risk group, should make a thyroid test part of an annual physical exam. "Regular exams become increasingly important as you get older, because many of the symptoms of thyroid disease become less obvious and harder to detect on your own," he says.

Checking your thyroid usually requires only a simple blood test. If a lump or nodule is present, a doctor may take a sample of thyroid tissue for examination in a relatively painless procedure called a fine needle aspiration biopsy.

TYPE A PERSONALITY

Calming the Hostile Heart

Bumper to bumper—again. Are they ever going to finish this damn construction? Hey, buddy! No way! You're not cutting in front of me, you jerk!"

Does your morning commute often feature this kind of hostile inner monologue? Do you lose your temper every time a traffic light turns yellow? At work, do you constantly interrupt slow-talking friends and colleagues? Even when you're off duty, are you driven to be the best—all the time, at any cost?

If so, you're probably a Type A guy. And you may be putting yourself at risk for a deadly aging problem.

"There seems to be little doubt that Type A behavior is hard on your heart," says C. David Jenkins, Ph.D., professor of preventive medicine and community health at the University of Texas Medical Branch at Galveston. "I can tell you from my own experience. You may be in perfect health otherwise, physically fit and everything—and Type A behavior can still bring on premature problems with your cardiovascular system."

Why Hurrying Hurts

The American Heart Association lists six characteristics of Type A men. They love competition, attempt to achieve many poorly defined goals, have a strong need for recognition and advancement, are always in a hurry, show intense concentration and alertness and are prone to anger. Fewer than half the men in America are Type A, Dr. Jenkins says. But if you're a salesman, taxi driver, newspaper reporter, air traffic controller or other high-pressure worker, the odds are that you fit the profile. Your personality probably drew you to the field. In fact, even if you weren't Type A to start with, Dr. Jenkins says that the demands of these jobs can push you in that direction.

The key problem with Type A behavior is stress. Hard-driving men put themselves under constant pressure, and their bodies react by producing extra amounts of stress-related hormones. These hormones may cause long-term damage. A study at Harvard Medical School in Boston of about 500 men and women showed that Type A's had a 50 percent higher risk of suffering heart attacks than the mellower Type B's.

Dr. Jenkins says the process probably works like this: Every time you lay on the horn at an intersection or argue with the boss, your body produces a stress hormone called noradrenaline. This chemical turbocharges your body, making you more alert and raising your blood pressure temporarily. Dr. Jenkins says it can also cause minor damage to the lining of your blood vessels. Your body repairs the torn lining. Over time, this patchwork of repairs can lead to a buildup of cholesterol in your arteries—setting you up for a heart attack.

Type A men may face other heart-related concerns as well. A ten-year study of 200 young men in rural Kentucky showed that Type A men were more likely than others to increase the number of cigarettes they smoked over the course of the study. They also showed greater increases in blood pressure. Both factors are known risks for heart disease.

Though heart disease is the biggest thing to watch, Type A men may be rushing into other health problems as well. Studies show that Type A men are more likely to grind their teeth, which can lead to jaw pain, headaches and dental troubles. Because of stress, hard-driving men may also suffer from chronic muscle fatigue and soreness in their necks and shoulders—although they're unlikely to report the pain or admit it to themselves.

Scientists are even exploring a possible link between Type A behavior and cancer. There's no concrete evidence on this one. But a continuing study of 3,154 American men shows that Type A guys might be more likely to develop and die of cancer than their Type B counterparts. Scientists speculate that this may be because stress represses the immune system, making the body less able to fight off disease.

A-mazing Advice

You can't really "cure" Type A personality, Dr. Jenkins says. Not that you'd want to; there's nothing wrong with a touch of assertiveness and the desire to do good old-fashioned hard work. But you may want to alter a few daily habits and attitudes to help lower your risk of Type A health trouble. Here are a few suggestions to get started.

Pare your priorities. Sure you want to succeed at everything. But there are only 24 hours in a day—and sometimes something has to give. So be a little more choosy. "I think setting realistic goals is the most important thing a Type A person can do," says Lee Reinert, Ph.D., director and lecturer for the Brandywine Biobehavioral Center, a counseling center in Downingtown, Pennsylvania. "Goals make you focus on what's important, instead of whatever crisis is facing you at the moment."

At the start of each week, make a list of things you feel you absolutely must do. Each time you write something down, ask yourself what would happen if you didn't do it. If you can't come up with a legitimate concern, scratch that item off the list. Now comes the tough part: Cut the final list by five items. You may try delegating a few of the items to co-workers, your spouse or your kids. "What's left is a more achievable set of tasks," Dr. Reinert says. "You'll get a greater sense of accomplishment this way, and you won't be chasing after brush-fires that keep popping up."

Be aerobic. If you're Type A, you may produce excess levels of a blood-clotting chemical called thromboxane. And you'd better do some aerobic exercise to get rid of it—or, researchers warn, it might lead to a heart attack. A Canadian study of 97 college-aged males reported that physically fit Type A's seem to burn off thromboxane while sedentary Type A men don't.

One word of caution: Don't overdo it. Because they tend to exercise like madmen, Type A men lose twice as much training time as the more mellow Type B's to injury. "Get a good workout. Raise your heart rate, but don't try to win at all costs. Don't keep trying to beat your own record," Dr. Jenkins says.

Write your wrongs. Keeping journals helps men discover the roots of their aggressiveness and anger, Dr. Reinert says. "A lot of times, you're not really mad at what's going on right now. You're upset about more of a core issue—maybe an unhappy family relationship," she says. Writing down your thoughts and feelings may help you discover what's really ticking you off. It can also help you detect patterns. Maybe you always get mad when you're waiting in line. Or when Snerdley in accounting won't let you get a word in at the staff meeting. If you anticipate these moments, you can either find ways to avoid them or ask yourself whether they're really important enough to blow your stack over.

Don't take it personally. Is that little old man in the slow-moving Buick really trying to make you mad? Was he awake deep into the night plotting ways to make you late? Or is he just a little old man who needs to use a little extra caution to drive these days? In his book *Anger Kills*, Redford B. Williams, M.D., director of the Behaviorial Medicine Research Center and professor of psychiatry at Duke University Medical Center in Durham, North Carolina, suggests putting yourself in the other person's shoes. When you look at the world from the perspective of the people who anger you, you'll probably be a little less cynical about them—and a little less Type A in the process. Dr. Williams also suggests doing some volunteer work as a way to relieve hostility and gain empathy for other people.

Take ten. Type A men typically schedule their days to the millisecond. That leaves no margin for error—and sets you up for extra stress when things go wrong. So try to give yourself an extra 10 percent pad. If you work a ten-hour day, leave at least one hour free to deal with the unexpected. If that sounds like an awfully big block of time, Dr. Reinert suggests setting aside five or six minutes each hour instead.

These cooldown periods can help you organize your thoughts and create new plans of attack. They can also spark creativity, making the rest of your work time far more productive. "If you don't have a little downtime, you're not giving yourself a chance to absorb all the information that's flying at you," Dr. Reinert says. "You'll be more creative and efficient if you just take time to process."

Scan for stress. Take another 10 or 15 minutes a day to check in with your body. Sit on a comfortable chair in a quiet room, close your eyes and breathe deeply. Tense, then release, the muscles in your feet. Then do your calves. Work up your body, paying special attention to the areas that feel tight or are throbbing (especially your shoulders and neck). "This is a great stress reducer," Dr. Reinert says. "It lets your body relax. And it shows you how needlessly tense you become during the day."

ULCERS

Putting Out the Fire

Ulcers used to be considered sort of a double-edged badge of honor. Sure, they pierced the gut with burning pain, but at the same time, they were thought of as emblems of success. To have one of these raw, craterlike sores eating away at your digestive tract was to say that you were a hard-driving, nose-to-the-grindstone kind of guy—albeit one in a great deal of pain.

But it's not those long hours on the job that cause ulcers, as was once believed. Actually, ulcers are more common among the unemployed. And there's no evidence that spicy food plays any role in their formation, either. In fact, there are numerous causes of this painful problem that afflicts one in ten people at some point in his life.

"It's often not what people think, but there are many causes of ulcers, and age seems to play a role in most of them," says Jorge Herrera, M.D., associate professor of medicine at the University of South Alabama College of Medicine in Mobile.

That seems fitting, since ulcers can make you feel old before your time. That midsection misery can keep you from being as physically active as you'd like—and walking around with a bottle of antacid doesn't exactly scream youth. And while scientists have found no evidence that a bland diet either heals or helps protect against ulcers, more than a few guys still handle ulcers by adopting an old man's diet of bland foods such as applesauce and cottage cheese.

Drugs: A Cause and a Cure

Ulcers form when digestive juices—acids, really—start burning through the delicate pink lining of your digestive organs. This is usually the result of a dete-

rioration in a protective layer that covers the lining of the stomach and duo-
denum, the top part of the small intestine. Many times this deterioration—and
the ulcers it causes—is linked to an infection of the upper gastrointestinal tract
by common bacteria called *Helicobacter pylori,* says William B. Ruderman, M.D.,
chairperson of the Department of Gastroenterology at the Cleveland Clinic
Florida in Fort Lauderdale. The bacteria are spread from person to person, like
other infectious diseases, and can be cured with antibiotics.

Studies show that these bacteria, which also play a role in other gastrointestinal problems, have been found in at least 95 percent of patients with duodenal ulcers, the most common type found in men. In fact, as many as one in
five men with this bacteria will develop duodenal ulcers.

Symptoms of duodenal ulcers, which occur in the uppermost part of the
small intestine, include a burning or "hungry" feeling under the breastbone, a
vague uneasiness of the stomach and even chronic nausea. With duodenal ulcers, the pain is often relieved after eating.

These ulcers typically strike men between ages 20 and 40. But hitting the
midlife mark doesn't put you in the clear. "These bacteria are more common as
you age," says Dr. Ruderman. "For one thing, exposure to these bacteria increases over time. And your body's defenses may get impaired over time." Also,
duodenal ulcers often result from smoking, which causes the production of excessive amounts of digestive acids.

Meanwhile, the other type of ulcer occurs in the stomach itself. Gastric ulcers are usually the result of excessive use of nonsteroidal anti-inflammatory
drugs, which include many over-the-counter pain relievers and even aspirin.
Gastric ulcers typically occur after age 50 and are more common in women than
in men. Eating doesn't ease pain in those with gastric ulcers. Either type of
ulcer, however, can cause stools that are black or maroon and foul smelling, and
you may vomit what appears to be coffee-ground material.

"Again, the age connection comes in because many of the medications that
can lead to gastric ulcers are for conditions that usually occur as you age, such as
arthritis drugs and other painkillers," says Dr. Herrera. "If you take any of these
drugs, including aspirin, for more than three months at a time, you increase your
risk of ulcers significantly."

These drugs do their dirty work by inhibiting the production of mucus and
protective acid-neutralizing agents; aspirin can also weaken the stomach lining
and cause bleeding. "In fact, many patients don't even realize they have ulcers
because of the painkillers in the drugs they take," he adds. "Sometimes they
come into the office for problems with bleeding or their stools, and only then do
they realize they have ulcers."

How to Help Yourself

If you think you have an ulcer, a doctor can prescribe drugs to reduce acid
secretions and ease ulcer pain. In some cases, antibiotics may be prescribed for

the bacterial cause. In the meantime, here's what you can do to prevent ulcers or to lessen their severity.

Choose Tylenol. For headaches and other minor aches and pains, take an acetaminophen product such as Tylenol rather than ibuprofen, most commonly sold as Advil and Nuprin. Ibuprofen is an anti-inflammatory, and products containing it can cause ulcers, says Dr. Herrera. "Sure, they have painkilling ingredients, but so do other medications that won't lead to ulcers. So if you have a headache or other minor problem that requires a painkiller, take Tylenol." And stay away from aspirin, since it can do even more damage than ibuprofen. Aspirin can weaken the stomach lining and cause bleeding.

Stop smoking. Cigarettes do double damage to the ulcer-prone. "Smoking can lead to ulcers because it increases acid production several-fold, especially if you smoke after dinner or before bed," says Dr. Herrera. "That's because acid production is usually worse at night."

Once you have ulcers, the acid created by smoking makes it hard to get rid of them. "It keeps ulcers from healing and makes it more likely that they will come back," adds Mark H. Ebell, M.D., assistant professor in the Department of Family Medicine at Wayne State University in Detroit.

Mellow out. People who view their lives as being too stressful are up to three times more likely to develop ulcers than those who learn to roll with life's punches, says Robert Anda, M.D., of the National Center for Chronic Disease Prevention and Health Promotion in Atlanta. But since we're all under stress, why do some guys get ulcers and others don't?

"It's how you interpret stress," says Dr. Anda. When you feel the weight of the world is on your shoulders and perceive stressful events as negative, you're a prime candidate for ulcers, because this perception results in the production of more stomach acids. On the other hand, men who acknowledge they have stress but view it as a fact of everyday life and don't let it overwhelm them are less likely to get ulcers.

Many men who react negatively to stress find they can change their perceptions by talking about their problems with good friends, doing regular meditation or relaxation exercises or even starting regular exercise programs, says Howard Mertz, M.D., assistant professor of medicine at the University of California, Los Angeles, UCLA School of Medicine.

Reassess your bland diet. While there's no proof that eating a bland diet will help, there is evidence that drinking one may hurt. In fact, the old remedy of drinking milk for an ulcer may actually do more harm than good, says Richard W. McCallum, M.D., professor of medicine and chief of gastroenterology at the University of Virginia School of Medicine in Charlottesville. That's because while milk may initially have a neutralizing effect on these acids, after 30 minutes or so, you get a "rebound effect" in which the calcium and protein from the milk actually stimulate acid production.

UNWANTED HAIR

Neanderthal No More

You're an ace of an uncle. Hysterically popular with the little guy. And why? Because you run him ragged and tell awesome stories. You feel like a kid again when you're with him. Then one evening, when he's exhaling pudding breath into your ear, he says, "You got grandpa ears—all hairy."

Fascinated, he yanks on one. Ow!

You have bristly new hairs cropping up in unusual places—not just in your ears but in your nose, too. And your eyebrows are starting to resemble awnings. What's next, the soles of your feet?

Why are you stuck with all these unwelcome sprouts anyway? "Some guys are just hairy throwbacks who look like they just came out of the branches," says Victor Newcomer, M.D., professor of dermatology at the University of California, Los Angeles, UCLA School of Medicine.

"No one really knows why hairs in the nose bristle, eyebrows bush out and hair sprouts in the ears as you get older," he says. "It's just a fact of life." The extra bristles usually start to appear around your early fifties and can become really apparent in your sixties and seventies, he says. Whether it happens to you is just a question of genetic potluck.

You may also have excessive body hair that started growing around puberty and just never quit. While that's not really related to getting older, you may still be fed up with it. Some men have such heavy growth on their chests, shoulders and backs that they feel uncomfortable about relaxing in just a pair of shorts or swim trunks. But there's no need to stay undercover forever.

Winning the Hair Wars

You're not necessarily stuck with the gorilla look. "Men have been trying to get rid of excess hair for years," Dr. Newcomer says. "And most of them end up shaving, since it's the easiest and simplest way." But if you'd like to try another approach on a problem area, here's a rundown of ways to get rid of unwanted hair.

Scissor strays carefully. Actually, you don't really have a jungle of hair inside the ear canal. Most hair grows on the helix, the inner rim of the ear, and the tragus, the little nubbin on the outside. Unless you have a steady hand, you might want to ask your barber to tidy up your ears, nose and eyebrows with a specially shaped electric trimmer, says Dr. Newcomer. If you want to do these trimming jobs yourself, buy a good pair of small, blunt tipped grooming scissors, he says.

Wax 'em. Have you heard of this one for excess body hair? It works on the chest, shoulders, back, arms, legs and even the face, though few men choose waxing over shaving their beards, Dr. Newcomer says. You can go to a professional for this. Or you can buy a waxing hair removal kit at the drugstore, heat up some wax (not too hot), spread it on your skin with a wooden spatula, let it harden and yank it off. The hair comes away with the wax. (Stop cringing; your wife or girlfriend may do it, too—in some very sensitive places.) For your back, you'll need some help reaching behind.

If you want to go the professional route, check out any full-service hair salon for body waxing services. Many cosmetologists have male clients, and they will perform the same waxing procedure on you that you would do at home, only more quickly.

Is the pain of pulled hair a little too intense? "Go see your dermatologist about an hour before you wax, and have him numb your skin with a local anesthetic," says Seth L. Matarasso, M.D., assistant professor of dermatology at the University of California, San Francisco, School of Medicine. "You'll hardly feel a thing."

If you'd like to try waxing and you happen to use the anti-wrinkling cream tretinoin (Retin-A) or any skin lotion containing glycolic acid, be sure to stop using it a few days before waxing, says Dr. Matarasso. These preparations are exfoliants and actually remove the outer two layers of skin, making the skin much more sensitive, he says. "If you wax on top of denuded skin, you'll give yourself a rip-roaring wound," he says. "You can take off a significant amount of the skin."

After you're waxed, it takes up to six weeks before hair grows back, Dr. Matarasso says. Keep in mind that you have to wait until hair grows back to ¼ inch long before you can have it waxed again.

Melt 'em. Lotion depilatories can be used anywhere on the body except near the eyes and the groin area. The active ingredients in lotion depilatories work by dissolving hair at or just below the skin line, so results last for up to two weeks, says Dr. Matarasso. You'll find them at your pharmacy under brand names such as Neet and Nair. They're simple and painless to use, but some have nasty odors. You apply the thick lotion to the skin, wait for up to 15 minutes and then rinse off with warm water. But be sure to test a small area first, to make sure you're not allergic to any hair-removing product, says Dr. Matarasso.

And Dr. Newcomer cautions, "On the face, don't put on too much, or you'll end up with an irritating rash." If a man has brown hair and oilier skin, he can tolerate more depilatory lotion for a longer time, he says. But thin-skinned blondes have less tolerance. And the hair's texture makes a difference in how long it takes the hair to dissolve. "Big, coarse hair takes longer to dissolve, and fine hair comes off easier," Dr. Newcomer says.

Tweeze bushy brows. Plucking extra hairs above the bridge of the nose with tweezers is a handy way to control the mono-brow look. This method is not strongly recommended for other places, particularly nose hair, says Dr. Newcomer. It's excruciating on sensitive skin, for one thing. And if you're dealing with a large expanse of hair on your shoulders or back, it would take forever—even if you can persuade a friend to help, he says.

Electrocute 'em—maybe. There's one bit of good news about electrolysis, says Dr. Matarasso. If you persist with the treatments, the hair will eventually stop growing back. For a small area of unwanted hair, it might be worth it, he says. Electrolysis is an alternative for any part of the body except eyelashes, nose and ears.

Here's how it works: A licensed electrolysist cleans your skin with alcohol, places a very fine needle into the hair follicle (this part doesn't hurt) and then turns on the electric current that the needle is wired to (this part does hurt). The current will destroy the hair follicle, but sometimes it takes several sessions.

Other problems with electrolysis besides pain? There is some possibility of pigment change in your skin, slight scarring or folliculitis, an inflammation of the hair follicles, says Dr. Matarasso. And though it's highly unlikely with the sterilization techniques used by most electrolysists, there is the potential for the spread of infection, he says.

Your best precautions are to make sure your electrolysist uses a new needle each time and to ask her to wear latex gloves, Dr. Newcomer says. The cost of the procedure varies from about $15 to $100, depending on the length of the session.

If you've wondered whether the home electrolysis units you see in mail-order catalogs work just as well as salon equipment, experts are skeptical.

"Some of these units are supposed to work painlessly with radio waves and destroy the hair follicle at the base," says Carole Walderman, a cosmetologist and esthetician in Baltimore. "But hair is not a conductor of electricity, so how could this method destroy the hair root?"

Even when the galvanic current from regular electrolysis machines cauterizes the follicles directly, Walderman says, you still get up to 90 percent regrowth, which is why repeated treatments are necessary to permanently remove the hair.

VARICOSE VEINS

Put the Squeeze on Pain

You're pulling up your argyles, and all of a sudden, you notice them. Varicose veins, just like your dad's. They look like ropy blue cords snaking up your calves. How long have they been there?

A while, maybe. Men often don't notice when varicose veins first start to show, because they're hidden by the hair on their legs, says David Green, M.D., a dermatologist at the Varicose Vein Center in Bethesda, Maryland. Also, pants cover them up.

Although varicose veins are more common in women, between 10 and 50 percent of adult men have some degree of varicose veins on their lower legs. Most men who get them will first notice the problem before age 50, although it tends to worsen with age.

Cosmetically, varicose veins aren't the eyesore they are to women; it's a lot easier for us to cover them up. But medically, they can be a source of discomfort and pain to anyone who has them. They can throb and feel heavy, making you feel like you're dragging your legs around. At night, they can cause legs to cramp or feel restless, disturbing your much-needed sleep. They can even itch and feel sore. And though it's rare, varicose veins can indicate a clot in a deeper leg vein.

Check Your Genes

Where do they come from? Your genes, for starters. You can inherit the tendency to form varicose veins from either side of the family. If you smoke, they're much more likely to creep up on you, because smoking affects blood flow by interfering with the regulation of fibrin, a blood-clotting protein. And though packing a few extra pounds doesn't cause varicose veins directly, if you are more than 20 percent over your ideal weight, you're only increasing your chances of developing them.

321

Unfortunately, some healthy habits can also aggravate varicose veins. If you pride yourself on your power lifting and work out with heavy weights, your veins may have begun to expand. Likewise, running on hard surfaces such as concrete sidewalks or asphalt can hasten the appearance of varicose veins.

The underlying problem is physiological, too. People with varicose veins have an inherited weakness in the valves inside the leg veins. These valves normally prevent blood from leaking back down as it flows up to the heart. If a valve leaks, gravity can force blood into lower veins when you stand up. Once this process is repeated enough times, vein walls can become permanently stretched.

"Whenever you're standing or sitting with your legs below the heart, gravity's working against you," says Malcolm O. Perry, M.D., professor and chief of vascular surgery at Texas Tech University Health Sciences Center in Lubbock.

Fallout from a Western Lifestyle

There's some evidence that varicose veins are also a product of our own lifestyle. Glenn Geelhoed, M.D., professor of surgery and international medical education at George Washington University Medical Center in Washington, D.C., has found that varicose veins are all but nonexistent in Third World nations, where eating habits include lots of fiber and where people don't sit behind desks all day. But he has found that when these people move West and develop our lifestyle—including a low-fiber diet and hours in front of the television—they also begin to develop varicose veins.

Too little fiber produces constipation and straining on the toilet, and that may be where diet affects vein health most. Western populations on low-fiber diets pass smaller and harder stools than do Third World people, who have few varicose veins, Dr. Geelhoed notes. And when you strain in vain, that ups the pressure in rectal veins, which in turn passes on more pressure to leg veins.

In fact, the famed Framingham Heart Study, in which the health habits of residents of this Massachusetts town were tracked for over 40 years, found that the risk factors for varicose veins are the same as for heart disease—particularly being overweight and sedentary.

You Can Head Them Off

If varicose veins run in the family but haven't yet turned up on you, there's a lot you can do to help forestall them.

Pare some pounds. If you are significantly overweight, a gradual, healthy weight loss plan can be your veins' biggest ally, says Alan Kanter, M.D., medical director of the Vein Center of Orange County in Irvine, California. Extra pounds put unnecessary pressure on your legs.

Power up your diet with fiber. Make sure your diet is high in fiber to keep bowels healthy and stools soft. This will prevent straining due to constipation, Dr. Kanter says. Fiber is found in abundance in fruits, vegetables and whole grains.

Drink up. Another way to soften stools is to be sure you're well hydrated by drinking at least eight glasses of water a day, says Dr. Kanter.

Don't smoke. Or if you do, stop, says Dr. Geelhoed. Smoking increases your risk of developing underlying vein disease, which can contribute to varicose veins, he says.

Leave heavy weights to Hulk. Weight-lifting exercise will help with weight control, but you need to do it right to avoid encouraging a vein problem, says Dr. Kanter. Ask a trainer for guidance on using smaller weights and doing more repetitions rather than straining with heavy weights.

Run on softer surfaces. Plan your running route along soft surfaces such as dirt, grass or cinder track whenever possible, Dr. Kanter suggests. The impact of running on pavement can aggravate vein swelling.

Keep moving on the job. Don't sit for two or three hours straight while you work, says Dr. Perry. Be sure to get up and move around often to keep blood circulating. The Framingham study found that men who spent five or more hours a day in sedentary activities, sitting or standing, had a somewhat higher incidence of varicose veins.

Dealing with the Blues

If you already have varicose veins or detect them developing, here's what you can do to keep them under control.

Sleep on a slope. Put six- by six-inch blocks under the foot of your bed and leave them there, says Dr. Perry. This keeps blood from pooling in your legs when you're sleeping. You can quickly adapt to the tilt.

Wear support socks. For a few small veins, choose high-quality knee-high support socks from a good men's clothing store and wear them regularly, says Dr. Perry. The slight compression will help keep the veins from swelling. For more or larger veins, you may need to use gradient compression stockings, available over the counter in most drugstores.

Get prescription support. If the veins you have are fairly large, even good-quality support socks aren't enough, says Dr. Perry. Ask your doctor to prescribe custom-fitted gradient compression hose instead. "They're hot and heavy, but they help," he says.

Calling In the Big Guns

There are two basic medical treatments available for varicose veins: sclerotherapy (injection) and surgical removal (stripping).

The latest advance in both sclerotherapy and vein surgery is the use of sound wave technology, called duplex ultrasound imaging. The ultrasound

Removing the Webs

Some people call them spider veins—those visible red lines that usually crop up on the legs, especially the thighs, and seem to resemble the fragile patterns of a spider's web.

How do you get rid of them? If they're big enough, usually conventional sclerotherapy is the best bet, says Arthur Bertolino, M.D., associate clinical professor of dermatology at New York University Medical Center in New York City and a dermatologist in Ridgewood, New Jersey.

"The optimal size for treatment is at least as large as the line you'd write on a piece of paper with an ordinary ballpoint pen," he says. "If they're too small, you can't put a needle in."

If you have just a few tiny spiders, consider a cover-up makeup with a greenish base, which conceals red tones, Dr. Bertolino suggests.

But for more than a few on the face or legs, sclerotherapy is usually very successful, he says. A tiny needle is inserted into the vein, and a solution is injected. You can actually see the red network disappear as the clear solution enters the vein, he says.

Side effects? Occasionally, the solution will cause a temporary muscle cramp near the ankle or the back of the lower calf, which your doctor can massage away in a minute or two. Rarely, a skin ulcer may result from fluid that escapes a leaky vessel, or new spider veins called mats may form, he says. There may also be a brownish discoloration of the skin, which almost always fades completely on its own but can often be removed using a copper vapor laser.

The pulsed-dye laser is also used by some physicians to remove dilated facial capillaries, says David Green, M.D., a dermatologist at the Varicose Vein Center in Bethesda, Maryland. The light waves emitted by the laser are absorbed by hemoglobin molecules in the blood. "This vaporizes the hemoglobin, which turns the light energy into heat energy and 'fizzles' the vessel wall," he says.

"Current lasers are not great on veins or capillaries below the waist," Dr. Green says. "But they're great on those above the neck, particularly on the nose and cheeks."

equipment is used to locate deeper problem veins and to guide injections precisely, says Dr. Kanter. And ultrasound is both painless and safe.

Sclerotherapy involves injecting a solution into a vein, causing the vein's walls to be absorbed by the body. No anesthesia is needed, and "you can be up and about your business right afterward," says Dr. Green. A few weeks to months later, the vein shrivels to an invisible thread of scar tissue under the skin. If you have had large varicose veins treated with sclerotherapy, you will need to wear gradient compression socks for up to six weeks afterward, Dr. Green says.

The cost usually ranges from around $100 to several hundred dollars, depending on the number of injections needed. Multiple treatments may be required if you have many affected veins.

Who's a candidate? Virtually anyone, as long as you have no history of blood clotting disorders, Dr. Green says. But although the procedure is simple and effective, there are potential side effects. If the solution escapes the vein, it can cause an ulcer on the skin.

And in up to 20 percent of patients, a brown line appears on the skin, following the course of the vein. In greater than 90 percent of these patients, the discoloration fades completely over months or a year or two, Dr. Green says. If it doesn't, there's still help available.

Lasers can remove the discoloration when wielded by a physician skilled in using the copper vapor laser. One Australian study showed that 11 of 16 patients treated with copper vapor laser therapy for discoloration caused by sclerotherapy had significant improvement after three months.

Surgical stripping is sometimes recommended for severe varicose veins. Although some patients can undergo the surgery with local anesthesia, most surgeons prefer a light general anesthesia, Dr. Perry says. Many patients have the surgery as outpatients, going home late the same day. Compression stockings are worn for several weeks to months afterward.

Even though the affected veins are completely removed, there is no risk to your circulation, because other vessels can easily compensate for the loss of the superficial veins, Dr. Perry says.

While some scarring usually results from surgery, often long lengths of vein can be removed through several tiny incisions.

What are the advantages of surgery? Many vein specialists say that even large varicose veins can be effectively treated with sclerotherapy. But some vascular surgeons point out that there is a high rate of recurrence with the injection treatment, and multiple visits are often required. However, when ultrasound imaging is used to help guide the surgery, preliminary results show a higher success rate in fewer visits.

VISION CHANGES

Set Your Sights High

So you've booked the corner table at Chez Snobbe, and it's time to wow those new clients from overseas. The sommelier hands you the wine list. You sigh nonchalantly, make a crack about bad California Chablis and open the list with a practiced touch of disdain.

Panic time. You can't read it. Your eyes won't focus on the fine print. You can't tell Dom Perignon from Chateau Cheapo, and there's no way to be cool about it. You straighten your arms, hold the list a yard from your face and start to squint.

Just like that, you've gone from high-powered deal maker to good ol' grandpa, sitting there reading the large-print version of Aesop's fables. Geez, what's next—trifocals, a yellow plaid sports coat and a "Honk if you love retirement" bumper sticker?

Calm down. Sooner or later, the eagle eyes of youth are going to fade a bit—for all of us. Nine in ten men between ages 40 and 64 wear glasses or contact lenses to make reading and other close-focus work a little easier.

But don't despair. You may be able to slow the process with regular eye exams, a healthful diet and some do-it-yourself eye exercises. More importantly, you can take steps now to deal with serious vision problems such as glaucoma, cataracts and macular degeneration that could lead to greatly reduced sight or even blindness.

So Long, Bug-Eyes

As a kid, you probably spent half your summers nose-first in the dirt, digging up worms and beetles and slugs and millipedes. Remember how cool they looked? You'd pick one up, hold it right in front of your nose and examine every compound wing, compound eyeball and hairy leg joint.

Just try that now. Odds are you can't begin to focus on it until it's a good seven or eight inches away. That's because the lenses in your eyes begin to stiffen with time. And the less they bend, the harder it is to focus on something close.

The condition is a form of farsightedness called presbyopia, and it's as inevitable as Charlie Brown striking out with the bases loaded. "There's really no way around it," says Richard Bensinger, M.D., a Seattle-area ophthalmologist and spokesman for the American Academy of Ophthalmology. "It's easy to correct, but it means you're probably going to have to wear glasses or contact lenses."

If you do end up needing corrective lenses, the choice between glasses and contact lenses is usually up to you. "In most cases, it's just a matter of preference," Dr. Bensinger says. "Some people like glasses, which they can take off when they don't want them. And some like contact lenses, which allow them to see well without showing people that they need glasses."

Even if you eventually need bifocals, which help correct your vision both near and far, you don't have to advertise it to the world. Doctors have developed blended lenses that eliminate the telltale line across the center of each lens. You could also try bifocal contact lenses, which allow you to change focus as your eyes move up and down. Dr. Bensinger says they can be much more expensive than standard contacts, however, and warns that not everyone can adjust to them.

Your eye doctor might also prescribe so-called monovision contact lenses. You put a distance vision contact in your dominant eye (usually the right) and

Common Eye Myths

Reading in dim light can damage your eyes. Myth. Low light can cause eye fatigue but will not harm your eyes.

Watching television hurts your eyes. Myth. There's no evidence that sitting too close to the television or watching for long periods causes any problems.

Too much reading wears out your eyes. Myth. Again, reading can make your eyes tired, but there's no evidence that it will hurt them in the long run.

Eating lots of carrots improves your vision. Semi-myth. You need vitamin A to see, but just a small amount—less than a carrot's worth a day. A healthful diet, with or without carrots, gives you all the vitamin A you need.

the reading contact in your other eye. "It's not as hard to adjust to as it sounds," Dr. Bensinger says. "You don't have to consciously adjust to it every time you change your focus." Monovision lenses are made like regular contacts and are less expensive than bifocal contacts, he says.

In addition to presbyopia, spots and floaters may appear more often as you get older. These are little specks or dots that pop up occasionally in your field of vision, then disappear after an hour or a day or more. Dr. Bensinger says they're caused when parts of the clear vitreous fluid that fills your eye get a little stringy or lumpy.

"Usually, it's nothing serious," Dr. Bensinger says. "The spots just drift down out of your vision, and that's it. But if you suddenly see lots of spots or flashes of lights in your eyes, that could be a sign that something more serious is wrong, and you should see a doctor immediately."

And if you live in an especially dusty or windy area, you may be at risk of developing pterygiums, fleshy, benign growths around the eyes. These can start growing in your mid-twenties, usually on the sides of your eyes closest to your nose. Dr. Bensinger says they're just a cosmetic problem unless they grow large enough to block your sight. Pterygiums are easily removed with minor surgery.

Taking the Long View

Unless you run into the proverbial sharp stick, your eyes will probably serve you well right through your mid-sixties. You may need a new set of glasses every few years, but you probably won't notice any serious deterioration of vision.

Still, experts warn that you should never take your eyes for granted. Most serious eye diseases are painless and show no symptoms for years. If you don't get your eyes examined on a regular basis, you may not know how bad things have gotten until it's too late to help. Here are some diseases to watch out for.

Glaucoma. This progressive disease causes 12 percent of all blindness in America. It is marked by increased fluid pressure in the eye, which, over the years, can cause irreversible damage to the nerves that send vision impulses to your brain.

Doctors don't know what causes most kinds of glaucoma, and they don't know how to cure it. Vision lost to glaucoma cannot be restored, but when detected early enough, glaucoma can be controlled. Eyedrops or oral tablets can sometimes help lower the pressure in the eye. If that fails, laser surgery may help unclog the eye's natural drains, allowing fluid to escape and lowering pressure. And if that doesn't work, eye surgeons can create an artificial drain to carry away the fluid.

An estimated three million Americans have glaucoma, and half of them don't even know it. Another five to ten million people have the eye pressure buildup that precedes the disease, and far fewer than half of them know it. The best advice for dealing with glaucoma? Find out if you have it—now. "The ear-

Are You at Risk for Glaucoma?

Yes. Everyone is, but some more so than others. To find out where you stand, answer these questions from Prevent Blindness America.

1. Do any immediate family members have glaucoma?
2. Are you over age 40?
3. Are you African American?
4. Do you take steroid medication?
5. Have you had an eye injury or eye surgery?
6. Do you have diabetes?

If you answered yes to any of the questions, schedule an eye exam to discuss glaucoma with your doctor. If you answered yes to two or more, you are at higher risk and probably need to see an eye specialist on a yearly basis.

lier this disease is picked up, the better able we'll be to control it," says Carl Kupfer, M.D., director of the National Eye Institute in Bethesda, Maryland. That means regular eye exams, especially if you're at high risk for glaucoma.

Cataracts. Although they usually don't become a problem until you near retirement age, cataracts often start forming much earlier in life, especially if you have ever had an eye injury or have undergone radiation treatments, chemotherapy or an organ transplant.

Over the years, the once-clear lens in each eye may turn yellow because of protein buildup. In time, the lens may become milky white and translucent, clouding vision to the point where you need an artificial lens implant. This plastic replacement lens does not flex to focus light, as the original lens did. But with corrective glasses, your vision can be restored quite well. "While we can't yet cure cataracts, we can certainly provide patients with good sight," Dr. Bensinger says.

Cataracts, like glaucoma, may have a hereditary link. So if anyone in your family has had cataracts, you may be at higher risk and should have your eyes examined more often than the standard every three years.

Macular degeneration. This insidious eye disease robs you of your fine visual skills. "In more advanced cases, you would be able to tell that someone was standing in front of you, but you couldn't tell who," Dr. Bensinger says. "You could see there was a bus coming down the street, but you couldn't tell which one, because you couldn't read the sign."

The cause remains unknown, but the condition somehow causes deteriora-

Eye-robics: Exercises for Your Eyes

You work out every week to flatten your stomach, build your chest and muscle up your arms. So why not take a few minutes to work out your eyes?

Not all experts think that exercises aid your eyes. But a growing number of vision therapists believe a few daily exercises can help keep your eyes younger.

"The logic behind vision therapy," says Steven Ritter, O.D., of the State University of New York College of Optometry in New York City, "is that if you can harm your visual system with close-up tasks, you should be able to rehabilitate it."

Vision therapists can prescribe as many as 280 different exercises. No single set can cure everybody's vision problems. But you can't go wrong with any of these.

Do the fine-print sprint. If you work at a computer terminal for hours at a time, try this: Tack a page of newsprint to a wall about eight feet from where you ordinarily sit. Interrupt your work every ten minutes or so and look up at the newspaper. Bring the print into focus. Then look back at the computer screen. Do this repeatedly for 30 seconds, about six times an hour. It could help eliminate the blurriness many people experience at the end of the workday.

Hit the wall. If you play handball, racquetball, squash or tennis, this two-person exercise may come in handy. Stand three to five feet from a blank wall. Ask your partner to stand behind you and toss a tennis ball against the wall. When the ball caroms off the wall, try to catch it. This exercise can help improve your hand/eye coordination.

Read your thumb. Hold your thumb at arm's length. Move it in circles, Xs and crosses, closer and farther away. Follow it with your eyes. As you do so, keep as much of the room as possible in your field of vi-

tion of the macula, the central part of the retina responsible for sharp focus. Unfortunately, there's little hope right now for restoring sight lost to macular degeneration, though laser surgery may help stabilize sight for a time. There is some hopeful news, though: Because macular degeneration strikes people over age 60 almost exclusively, you can start now—perhaps with the help of an improved diet—to ward it off before it starts.

Diabetic retinopathy. It primarily strikes people with diabetes and is the leading cause of blindness in people ages 20 to 50. Loss of vision begins to

sion. Continue the exercise with one eye closed. Repeat with the other eye. This can improve your peripheral vision.

Track the flashlight. This amusing exercise can improve your ability to track an object visually. It requires a partner and two flashlights. Stand in a darkened room facing a wall. Have your partner shine a flashlight on the wall and wave the disk of light in sweeping motions. Try to eclipse the circle of light with light from your flashlight while balancing a book on your head. This forces you to track the light with your eyes instead of moving your head.

Call the ball. Write letters or numbers on a softball or styrofoam ball, then screw a hook into the top of it and hang it from the ceiling with string. The smaller the characters, the more difficult the exercise. Give the ball a push. Try to call out the numbers or letters that you see. This exercise helps you keep a moving target in focus.

Bead a string. This exercise trains both eyes to converge on a target. It also trains your brain to not switch off one eye's vision. String three colored beads on a string six feet long. Fasten one end of the string to a wall at eye height, and hold the other end of the string to your nose. Slide one bead close to the wall, place the second bead four feet from your nose, and place the third bead 16 inches from your nose.

Look at the farthest bead. You will see two strings forming a V converging at the bead. Shift both eyes to the middle bead. Notice the X where the two strings seem to converge upon it. Shift both eyes to the nearest bead, and observe a similar X. Shift quickly from one bead to another, always observing the V or the X. If both eyes are working as a team, you should always see two strings crossing when you're focused on a bead. If your eyes aren't working together, you'll see different patterns or just one string.

occur when blood vessels in the back of the eye leak, blurring vision and sometimes denying nutrients to the eye.

"If you have diabetes," Dr. Bensinger says, "I cannot urge you strongly enough to have your eyes checked regularly. It can literally save your sight."

Laser treatments can help slow the damage from leaking vessels. But again, help is available only if you get your eyes examined regularly. "Early detection of diabetic retinopathy is even more of a success story than testing for glau-

(continued on page 334)

Test Your Vision at Home

More than ten million Americans over age 25 suffer some loss of sight. Many don't even know it. These simple tests could help you discover whether your vision needs some attention.

Remember: The tests are not a substitute for a professional eye examination. They can only serve as a warning to see an eye doctor.

These tests were prepared by Prevent Blindness America. For more information, write or call 500 East Remington Road, Schaumburg, IL 60173; 1-800-331-2020.

Vision Test 1: Distance vision (right). If possible, have someone help you with this test. Don't take it if you're tired. And if you have glasses or contacts, be sure you're wearing them. (1) Position the chart ten feet away from you, against a bare wall or door. Make sure the room is well lit, and avoid glare from windows. (2) Lightly cover your left eye with a piece of paper. Keeping both eyes open, tell your assistant (or write down) where the opening is in each C on the chart. Start with the largest C and work down the page. Repeat with your right eye covered. (3) If you don't get all the Cs correct on the next-to-bottom line, repeat the test another day.

Nearly half of all blindness can be prevented. Everyone should have periodic eye examinations.

O Ɔ O U C ꓷ Ɔ C O O

Vision Test 2: Near vision (above). Wear your contacts or glasses only if you use them to read. (1) Sit in a well-lit room away from window glare. (2) Keeping both eyes open, hold the near-vision test about 14 inches from your eyes. (3) Read the test sentence or write it down as it looks to you. (4) Write down where the openings are for each C. If you didn't get them all right, take the test another day.

(continued)

Test Your Vision at Home—Continued

Vision Test 3: Macular degeneration. For this test, wear your glasses or contact lenses only if they're for reading. (1) Have someone hold the grid against a bare wall or door in a well-lit room without glare from windows. Make sure the center dot on the grid is at eye level. (2) Stand 14 inches from the grid. Look at the dot in the center of the grid and cover your left eye with a piece of paper. You should see all four corners of the grid. If the grid looks distorted or you see any blank spots or wavy lines, make a mental note of it. Repeat with your right eye covered.

coma," Dr. Kupfer says. If it's caught early, there's a 95 percent chance you can keep your sight for at least five years, Dr. Kupfer says.

Focusing on Prevention

You can't change your genes, so there's not much you can do about the biggest vision risk factor of all—heredity. Still, here's some advice to give you the best chance of staying 20/20 into the twenty-first century.

Get your eyes checked. Doctors just can't say this enough.

"Regular eye examinations are by far the most important thing you can do to help preserve your vision," Dr. Bensinger says.

If you are between ages 30 and 50 and have no previous eye problems, the American Academy of Ophthalmology suggests seeing an ophthalmologist every three years. If you have a family history of glaucoma or diabetes or are already wearing glasses or contact lenses, your doctor may suggest more frequent visits.

The academy suggests an immediate visit to the doctor for any of the following.

- Sudden vision changes in one or both eyes
- Unexplainable redness
- Seeing a number of spots or floaters or showers of sparks in the corners of your eyes
- Eye pain that won't go away
- Accidental contact with chemicals, especially lye

Hide behind some shades. Sunglasses that block both UVA and UVB rays and visible blue light may help decrease the risk of cataracts, Dr. Bensinger says. Wraparound glasses that cover the sides of your eyes are a good idea, since they shield your eyes completely. And try to wear a hat with a visor to block direct sunlight from your eyes.

"Exposure to sunlight drops the age at which you may develop cataracts," Dr. Bensinger says. "So if you're going to be outside, it makes sense to cut that sunlight as much as possible."

Stop smoking. Cancer. Wrinkles. Stinky clothes. Yellow teeth. Emphysema. If you really need another reason to quit, here it is: Cigarette smoking might cause cataracts. A study of 22,000 physicians at Harvard Medical School in Boston showed that men who smoke 20 or more cigarettes a day have twice the risk of developing cataracts.

The reason isn't known, but researchers speculate that smoking may reduce antioxidant levels in your blood, promoting cataract growth.

Try some see-food. The links between diet and vision are still weak. But there's growing evidence that a substance called glutathione may help control the spread of macular degeneration. It's found in fresh green, red and yellow vegetables. Canned or frozen vegetables lose all their glutathione in processing.

Zinc may help, too. Though there's no hard evidence yet, Dr. Bensinger says taking multivitamin supplements containing zinc "is probably not a bad idea, as long as you're not spending too much money on fancy brands."

Antioxidants—vitamins A, C and E plus beta-carotene—showed promise as cataract fighters in the Harvard Nurses' Health Study. A report in the *American Journal of Clinical Nutrition* claimed that people who eat 3½ servings of fruits and vegetables every day have a lower risk of cataracts, too.

"Eating a healthy diet may delay the usual aging of the lens and so delay cataracts," says Paul F. Jacques, Sc.D., an epidemiologist with the U.S. Department of Agriculture Human Nutrition Research Center on Aging at Tufts University in Boston.

WORRY

Manhood's Secret Burden

It's put-up-or-shut-up time at the Cross Forks Ranch, and Poppa takes young Billy Bob aside to assess the situation.

"Son," he says, "the bankers are taking our farm. And we just invested our last nickel in a phony gold mine. We're finished. But Billy Bob, whatever you do, don't let the womenfolk see you worry."

This is our manly burden. Get out there and handle stuff, damn it. Crush whatever pops up along the way—and keep quiet about it.

Well, it's not always so easy. Maybe you're afraid of being laid off. Maybe you're concerned that you're not being a good father or that you're going to die young, or go broke, or crash your car, or look silly at the next staff meeting.

And maybe these worries have piled up to the point where you feel powerless. You suffer from constant tension headaches, and you feel worn out all the time. Your stomach is in knots. A few years ago, you felt scrappy and young, ready to save the planet from whatever ailed it. But now you're feeling feeble, overwhelmed, unable to deal with even the smallest dilemmas.

"Worries are like a straitjacket," says Mary McClure Goulding, co-author of *Not to Worry! How to Free Yourself from Unnecessary Anxiety and Channel Your Worries into Positive Action*. "You feel like you can't do anything, and so you don't. It's a totally unproductive way to spend the best years of your life. And it's something you need to change—and can change—starting immediately."

The Fretful Facts

Here's the hidden truth: The average guy spends 5 percent of each waking day—about 48 minutes—worrying about one thing or another. That's the same as women, by the way. Surveys show that the most common sources of worry for Americans are family and relationships, jobs and school, health and finances.

For as many as 6 percent of men, worrying gets out of hand. It can even

336

evolve into a clinical condition called generalized anxiety disorder. People with this disorder worry about multiple problems at the same time, including things they have little or no control over, such as the weather or nuclear war. And they worry excessively. Chronic worriers report spending an average of 50 percent of each day worrying, and some report as much as 100 percent, says psychologist Jennifer L. Abel, Ph.D., associate director of the Stress and Anxiety Disorders Clinic at Pennsylvania State University in University Park. Chronic worry typically begins in a man's twenties or thirties.

There's no evidence that worrying directly causes disease, says Timothy Brown, Psy.D., associate director of the Phobia and Anxiety Disorders Clinic at the State University of New York at Albany. Worry can lead to poor sleep, with resulting fatigue, restlessness and irritability. But it's the psychological toll that's usually most devastating. "Worriers can't concentrate, get headaches and may not be able to effectively confront and resolve their problems," he says.

Worriers almost always come from fretting families, Goulding says. You may have learned to worry by watching your mother, father, grandmother or an uncle. Worriers may have low self-esteem, Goulding says, and have often been taught to repress feelings—especially happy ones.

All of which leads to a central problem: a feeling of helplessness. "You don't feel in control of your life," says Susan Jeffers, Ph.D., a psychologist in Tesuque, New Mexico, and author of *Feel the Fear and Do It Anyway*. "You think everything is going to go wrong. That makes it hard to overcome even simple problems without great effort and anxiety."

A study of 24 American college students bears this out. When asked what would happen if they didn't get good grades, the non-worriers typically talked about ending up with bad jobs and earning less money. The chronic worriers talked about those same concerns. But they took their worries much further. Some worried about becoming drug addicts. Others worried they would be in constant physical pain. And others said they would die—or even end up in hell.

"At that point, you have to ask yourself whether worrying is worth the effort," Dr. Jeffers says. "You have to decide whether you're going to spend the rest of your life worrying about things or whether you're going to do something about it. It's a difficult decision, but hopefully, you'll choose the latter."

Worry Whippers

It takes years to build a world of worries. You may need a while to tear it all down. But time is on your side. A study of both young and elderly worriers showed that we tend to worry less as we grow older. The oldest of the 163 people studied by professors at the University of Massachusetts at Amherst were less anxious about social and financial problems and no more worried about health issues. But why wait for things to get better? If you're ready to start banishing worry right now, here's some expert advice.

Let them flow. Go ahead and fret a little. It's better than trying to suppress

Quell the Worrier Within

Call him Wilbur the Worrier. He's the unhappy little doomsayer in your head who won't stop chattering about things that can and will go wrong. It's time to shut him up for good.

"You have to silence that voice of self-harassment," says Mary Mc-Clure Goulding, co-author of *Not to Worry! How to Free Yourself from Unnecessary Anxiety and Channel Your Worries into Positive Action.* "If you listen to it, you'll always keep worrying."

The first step is to become aware of the voice. Sit in a quiet place and listen to your thoughts. When you start hearing negative thoughts, consciously replace them with positive ones. Try some affirmations—simple positive statements that you repeat frequently: "There is nothing to fear." "I'm in control of my life." "I'll handle it." "Everything is working out perfectly."

"Repetition is the key. At first, you don't even need to believe what you're telling yourself," says Susan Jeffers, Ph.D., a psychologist in Tesuque, New Mexico, and author of *Feel the Fear and Do it Anyway.* "Just talking positively changes our energy and helps us move forward."

Goulding says that sometimes it helps to be more direct with your inner critic. Stand up, put your hands on your hips and give ol' Wilbur what-for: "Just shut up! I'm not listening to you anymore!" Curse, swear, do whatever feels good. "Drive that voice away," she says. "And then you can fill your mind with happier thoughts instead."

all the anxiety. "Give up trying to stop those unhappy thoughts," says Daniel Wegner, Ph.D., professor of psychology at the University of Virginia in Charlottesville. "My research shows that the more you try to suppress unwanted thoughts, the more likely you are to become obsessed with them. That's particularly true when you're under a lot of pressure, stress or mental overload. So just when you're trying to avoid unhappy thoughts, you'll actually get sadder than if you'd confront those unhappy thoughts head-on."

Dr. Jeffers likes to point out that 99 percent of what we worry about never happens. "Feel the fear. That's part of being human," she says. "But go out and do things anyway, knowing that most of your fears are unfounded."

Take a worry break. It's one thing to think about your problems. It's another to let them dominate your thoughts. Dr. Wegner says research on chronic worriers shows that if they spend time at night actively worrying about their problems, the degree of worrying in their lives goes down overall. "There's something boring, after all, about thoughts you spend an hour a night thinking about," he says.

Michael Vasey, Ph.D., assistant professor of psychology at Ohio State University in Columbus, suggests setting aside 30 minutes a day, always at the same place and time, to worry. "Focus on your worry for the entire period, and try to think of solutions to the problem," he says. If you're worried that you'll be fired, imagine the scenario—the firing and the consequences—and don't let the image drift away.

You'll probably be more anxious at first, but things will improve. "If you practice focusing on worries and thinking of solutions for 30 minutes each day for several weeks, your anxiety will start to taper off," Dr. Vasey says. "You'll get better at generating solutions or realize it's not worth worrying about."

Edit your anxiety. People who worry can be amazingly creative, Goulding says. They turn any harmless scenario into a disaster by imagining the worst. Try putting that creativity to good use by turning your fears into fantasies. If you worry about a school bus crash, try picturing your little boy grabbing the wheel and steering everyone to safety. Then imagine the parade the town will hold for him. Maybe he'll even get the key to the city.

You're disarming your worries this way, Goulding says. By putting a happy or silly ending on a worry, you're allowing yourself a chance to be positive, she says. And that's a major step toward beating worry.

Tally your troubles. List all your worries. Are you afraid that it's going to rain on your golf outing this weekend? You can't control that, so Goulding suggests that you file it under the heading "Beyond My Skills." Do you worry that other people find you unattractive, even when you really know you're not? That goes on the "Creative Fiction" list. What's the sense of worrying about things in these categories? "There isn't any," Goulding says. "Why worry about the weather? Why worry about things that aren't true?" Once you expose these thoughts as worthless worries, she says, it's easier to dismiss them.

Act now. Some worries are more legitimate. Are you concerned about your health? Well, make a list of what you could do to improve things. Maybe you could start walking every day. Or eat better. Then decide which ones you're going to do. The secret is doing, doing, doing. "When you're actively working on a solution, worry is less likely to be a problem," Dr. Jeffers says. "You'll begin to feel like you're the creator of your life, not a victim of it."

Find a friend. Tell someone special about your fears. "When you talk about your worries, it deflates those worries. They can't be suppressed. That cat's out of the bag. And thank goodness, it is just a cat and not some horrible monster," Dr. Wegner says.

Just be careful that your friend doesn't unintentionally make things worse. Out of kindness, he may tell you it's okay to worry or say "Gee, I understand why you're so worried." Goulding says that might help reinforce your need to worry. If you do share your thoughts, make sure the other person agrees to be honest with you and helps you find positive ways to deal with your worries.

WRINKLES

They're Not beyond Your Control

One day, you throw yourself out of bed, slam through 50 push-ups, bike five fast miles on your exercise bicycle and jump into a cool shower—all before the morning sun hits the sky. You feel great—like you've just downed a wake-up slug from the fountain of youth. You slap a towel around your waist and turn to the sink for a shave.

Yikes! Who the hell is that in your mirror? Some guy with an uncanny resemblance to your father is squinting out of the steam.

Where did all those wrinkles come from? You're too young for wrinkles.

A lot of guys—some younger than you—are walking around with premature furrows and ridges. These lines come from years of roughhousing your face. But with a little care, you can prevent most new wrinkles from forming. And you can repair most of the old ones with a little help from your doctor. You can look on the outside like the young stud you feel inside. Here's the game plan.

Know Thy Enemies

Compare the back of your hand with the skin on the inside of your upper arm. The arm skin is almost as smooth as a baby's bottom, right? It's been in the shade your whole life, that's why. Radiation from the sun causes 80 to 90 percent of the visible signs of aging, including wrinkles, doctors say. If genes are on your side, you may luck out, and your wrinkles won't turn up as early as another guy's. But the bottom line is that if you're sunning, they're coming. No way around it.

Wrinklemeister number two? Smoking. If you smoke, you've upped your skin's aging process by up to ten years. That virile Marlboro man squinting all over the billboards? He's trying to keep the caustic smoke out of his eyes, and he's making crow's-feet in the process. Skin gets a "memory" when it's folded in the same place over and over again, and that memory becomes a wrinkle.

340

In addition to making you scrunch up your eyes (and lips), smoking also diminishes blood flow to the skin. If you don't have good blood flow, oxygen and nutrients can't reach the skin surface as easily to help the skin repair damage. Smoking also sets off enzymes that attack the tissues of your skin the way meat tenderizer weakens the fibers of a steak.

Aside from sunlight and smoking, scowling and smirking can also conspire to give you that distinctive shar-pei look. Raise one eyebrow in that devil-may-care smirk that melts the ladies (you might want to do a reality check on this one), and you're creasing your skin, the same way you do when you're squinting to avoid smoke. Do it too often, and the crease becomes yours for keeps.

The Best Defense

Should you throw in the towel and head straight for Prunesville? Absolutely not. Your first move is to stop new wrinkles in their tracks.

Bathe by the light of the moon. Your number one line of defense is to protect your skin from the sun's harmful rays. You can do this by wearing a hat and wraparound sunglasses and applying a sunscreen every time you will be exposed to the sun.

"Put on a sunscreen after you shave, and it'll become automatic in no time," suggests Melvin L. Elson, M.D., medical director of the Dermatology Center in Nashville. Use a fragrance-free, nongreasy sunscreen lotion, and apply pea-size dabs on your cheeks and forehead, working it into the skin all over your face. Don't forget the backs of your hands, as well as your neck, forearms and bald spot, if you have one.

Make sure your sunscreen is broad spectrum (it stops all kinds of sun radiation) and is labeled SPF 15 or higher, says Albert M. Kligman, M.D., professor of dermatology at the University of Pennsylvania School of Medicine in Philadelphia. *SPF* stands for sun protection factor, and SPF 15, which most dermatologists recommend, means that you can stay out in the sun 15 times longer than you normally could before burning. But remember that although daily use of SPF 15 sunscreen will protect you adequately while you dash in and out of buildings, for long hours in the outdoors you'll need to use higher-SPF products and reapply frequently.

Doctors disagree on how high to go with SPF numbers, however. Some say that numbers over 25 may give a false sense of security. While higher numbers do screen out the burning UVB rays, they may let in more UVA radiation. The UVA rays penetrate deeper into skin and cause most age-related changes such as wrinkles, says Dr. Elson.

Joseph P. Bark, M.D., a dermatologist in Lexington, Kentucky, and author of *Retin-A and Other Youth Miracles*, disagrees. He says research shows that skin will burn somewhat even with SPF 15 sunscreens, and he recommends using the highest SPF you can find, even for everyday use.

And read the sunscreen's contents. "The best of the broad-spectrum sun-

Wrinkle-Free with Retin-A

Retin-A is for acne, right?

Yes, but that's not the only thing.

Many dermatologists are using tretinoin (Retin-A) for the nonsurgical removal of fine wrinkles. The drug encourages your skin to produce collagen, which fills in wrinkles. It also increases blood flow to the skin, giving you a healthy glow.

Retin-A won't eliminate deep lines, and "it's not a face-lift," says Albert M. Kligman, M.D., the professor of dermatology at the University of Pennsylvania School of Medicine in Philadelphia who discovered the prescription drug's smoothing effect on wrinkles. But fine wrinkling, blotching and leathery, sun-damaged skin texture can be dramatically improved, particularly for light-skinned people who have always sunburned easily.

"If you have a lot of wrinkles and you're young, even in your twenties, don't wait until you are 40 or 50 and have deep wrinkles and a lot of blotches," he says.

"If you're a light-skinned person who had a normal childhood in America, you should start Retin-A early and get into a program that will last you the rest of your life."

Retin-A comes in cream and gel forms and is sold in varying strengths. You may find that your skin is red, flaky and irritated at first, but hang in there—it will usually adjust within a month or two.

With your dermatologist's help, you can customize the concentration of Retin-A that best suits your skin. "After you cleanse with a mild soap, let your skin dry completely for 10 to 20 minutes," says Alan Matarasso, M.D., a plastic surgeon at the Manhattan Eye, Ear and Throat Hospital in New York City. "Then apply a pea-size amount of Retin-A everywhere—around your eyes (leaving about a half-inch bare under your eyes), mouth, chest, forearms and backs of hands. If you use Retin-A, you won't need a moisturizer at night unless the Retin-A causes a little redness and flaking. If that happens, use a moisturizer that night and alternate with Retin-A." You can also use petroleum jelly around your eye area.

Is there a downside? Retin-A is a lifelong commitment. Daily applications are required for the first two years. After that, weekend applications are sufficient to maintain the benefits. And because Retin-A increases your skin's sensitivity to the sun, a daily regimen of sunscreen with a high SPF (sun protection factor) is vital.

screens contain titanium dioxide—fine particles that stay in your skin and resist washing or rubbing off," says Dr. Kligman. An example is Sundown.

Wear shades. Years of squinting will make your eyes wrinkle for sure. The best sunglasses for preventing wrinkles are the wraparound kind. Make sure they shield ultraviolet radiation.

Dress for the sun. Innovative clothing manufacturers have come out with basic collections of shirts, swimsuits and casual wear that are specially knit to prevent the sun's radiation from reaching your skin.

Dump that nasty habit. Yeah, yeah, you've been told before that smoking isn't cool anymore. Now you have one more reason to quit.

Learn from your mirror. Stone faces belong on Mount Rushmore, not on you. But you may have a few unconscious face-wrinkling habits that can easily be checked. Set a small mirror near your phone, and watch yourself in conversation. Do you constantly furrow your brow and squint your eyes? Ease up on these contortions, and you'll help prevent future wrinkles.

By the way, forget facial exercises that promise to remove wrinkles. Such exercises are worse than useless. In fact, all that contortion can make wrinkles worse.

Consider supplements. For general skin health, eat a balanced diet full of fruits, whole grains and vegetables. You may also want to try supplements of vitamin E and the trace mineral selenium, which have been proven to decrease overall sun damage to the skin, says Karen Burke, M.D., Ph.D., a dermatologist in private practice in New York City. She recommends 400 IU daily of vitamin E in the form of d-alpha tocopheryl acetate, d-alpha tocopheryl succinate or d-alpha tocopherol, not the "dl tocopherols" form, which is far less active. Take these in combination with 100 micrograms of selenium (best when taken as l-selenomethionine), and you might have an edge on wrinkles.

Sleep on your back. "It's the best position for a younger-looking, unlined face," says Gary Monheit, M.D., assistant professor of dermatology at the University of Alabama School of Medicine/University of Alabama in Birmingham. If you've been burrowing into your pillow face-first for years, lying on your back every night with a pillow under your knees may help you to change the habit, he says.

When You Just Want Them Gone

Now that you've wised up to prevention, chin up. You're holding the line on lines, and if you're religious about the sunscreen habit, some mild repair of wrinkling may take place on its own, doctors say. But if you're declaring total war on wrinkles, here's the lowdown on what a dermatologist or plastic surgeon can offer you.

Retin-A. Tretinoin (Retin-A), derived from vitamin A, has earned its reputation as an excellent wrinkle smoother, particularly for the fine lines caused by years of indulging in the sun. But be warned: Retin-A cream is available only by prescription. The legions of similar-sounding ingredients in many cosmetics and lotions are only that: sound-alikes. See your dermatologist.

Alpha hydroxy acids (AHAs). These acids are a new wrinkle . . . er, development in the treatment of aging skin. They are derived from milk, wine, apples, lemons or sugarcane and available from your doctor in highly concentrated lotions. "Use an AHA moisturizing lotion daily, and it will very gradually peel off the top layers of dead skin, making crow's-feet and fine wrinkles less visible," says Dr. Elson.

So far, AHAs are the only wrinkle fighters to offer any real competition to the big-daddy wrinkle remover—Retin-A. Although results are less dramatic than Retin-A's, AHAs are less likely to irritate your skin. Low-concentration AHAs are also available in several popular cleansers and moisturizers, such as Avon's Anew Alpha Hydrox Skin Treatment System and Eucerin Plus Alphahydroxy Moisturizing Lotion.

Chemical peels. Remember the amazing brush-on, peel-off paint removers advertised in hobby magazines? Same principle here, only you're peeling away a layer or two of skin, not shellac. Chemical peels do what Retin-A does, but all at once. They are effective on deeper wrinkles than Retin-A can reach, says Sorrel S. Resnik, M.D., clinical professor of dermatology and cutaneous surgery at the University of Miami School of Medicine.

For a chemical peel, the dermatologist wipes your face with acetone, a strong cleansing solvent, and then applies acid to your skin with a swab. The skin turns white and stings briefly as the acetone penetrates; then several layers of skin (and fine wrinkles) peel off a day or two later.

Many dermatologists will recommend a series of three to six light peels at intervals of several weeks. This will get nearly the results of a deep peel with less discomfort and a quicker healing time, Dr. Resnik says. (If you have a light peel done on Friday, you'll be pinkly presentable at work on Monday.) Trichloroacetic acid has a good record for safety and effectiveness, and glycolic acid, which is less penetrating, is also popular, he says.

Very deep peels, which can literally remove the top layer of your face, have real risks attached. A deep peel using the chemical phenol must be applied in the operating room because it requires close heart monitoring. And if there's any question of kidney problems, steer clear—your kidneys have to work overtime to process the phenol.

Collagen injections. If you're not peeling off a wrinkle from the top down, you can fill it up from underneath. Wrinkle-filling injections will do the job, though some results may be frustratingly temporary. The injection raises a lump above the skin surface. When the lump fades in as little as six hours—presto! The skin is smooth. Depending on the individual (man and wrinkle), collagen can last from 4 to 15 months, says Dr. Monheit.

Some people may be allergic to the cattle-derived collagen used in this procedure, so the doctor must first perform an allergy test. If you're allergic, ask about a newer method called autogenous tissue implant, says Dr. Elson. A patch of skin harvested from another part of your body is sent out to a company that processes your own collagen from the skin. The processor then returns to your doctor a syringe filled with the collagen for an injection.

Dermabrasion. This procedure is often used for deep acne scars but can be very effective on wrinkles, particularly around the mouth, says Michael Sachs, M.D., a plastic surgeon in private practice in New York City. A special instrument called a dermabrader literally sands away the top layer of the skin. You'll need about ten days to heal. A drawback is that dermabrasion often removes pigment from the skin, adds Dr. Reonilt.

Going All the Way

Think only starlets get their faces lifted? Face-lifts these days are being done on the most macho of men from Hollywood to the Bronx, says Dr. Sachs. Surgery is a serious step, because it's surgery. So weigh your options and choose a surgeon carefully.

If pouchy bags and wrinkles above and below your eyes have given you that hangdog look, ask about a procedure called blepharoplasty. The surgeon removes excess fat and tightens skin, leaving barely visible scars in the brow line or beneath lower lashes.

A fat-melting blepharoplasty can do the same with only a small puncture in the skin, says Dr. Sachs, who invented the procedure. Using a heated probe, a surgeon vaporizes the water content of the fat, which flattens pouches and smooths wrinkles.

Solid silicone implants are another surgical option. These have none of the dangers of the liquid silicone banned for breast implants, says Geoffrey Tobias, M.D., a plastic surgeon at Mount Sinai School of Medicine of the City University of New York in New York City. A surgeon can insert these implants under cheeks and along the jowl line to fill out deep wrinkle folds.

"If two or three wrinkles bother you, take care of them. You'll look and feel better," says Dr. Tobias. "But know that you're never going to be 12 years old again or take 20 years off your face. You have to be realistic."

Part III

Boost Your Youthfulness

ADVENTURE

Take a Plunge into the Wild Side

While many of us spend our summers driving the kids to Disney World, Bart Yasso is going on odysseys less likely to turn his hair prematurely gray. In the past few years, Yasso has run 100 miles through the Himalayas, kayaked 200 miles down the Amazon and ridden his bicycle 3,500 miles from Seattle to Atlantic City. Why?

"I do these things because they're adventurous, and when you do adventurous things, you feel like a kid," says the 37-year-old race services manager in the marketing and circulation departments of *Runner's World* magazine at Rodale Press in Emmaus, Pennsylvania.

Some doctors think Yasso's onto something. If you're looking for a fountain of youth, they say, try tossing more adventure into your life.

"Absolutely, adventure and risk taking can make you feel and think like a person who is years younger. It's believed that when you do thrill-seeking adventures, there's a release of certain chemicals in the brain that are truly uplifting to mood," says Bernard Vittone, M.D., a psychiatrist and director of the National Center for the Treatment of Phobias, Anxiety and Depression in Washington, D.C.

Others say adventure does more than jump-start your emotions. "Adventure creates very positive physiological effects, including increased blood and oxygen flow to many of the tissues in your body. That, along with the emotional lift, can make some people literally look younger," says Mark Weaver, Ph.D., a psychologist with the Experiential Learning Institute in Oklahoma City.

Fear and Fascination

Remember the mixture of anxiety and absolute exhilaration the first time you rode a bicycle, climbed a tree, swam in the deep end of the pool or plunged

(continued on page 352)

What Kind of Gutsy Are You?

What kinds of thrills are most likely to turn you on? What level of adventure is right for you? Take this test to find out.

There are no right or wrong answers. Circle only one number per question. Answer all questions. If no answer feels exactly right to you, pick the one that's closest. To determine your score, total all numbers circled and see the scoring that follows.

1. During the past ten years, how often have you changed residence?
    1. 10 times or more
    2. 5–9 times
    3. 2–4 times
    4. 0–1 time
2. Which adjective best describes your behavior before age 12?
    1. hyperactive
    2. mischievous
    3. basically well behaved
    4. very well behaved
3. In the average week, how many hours of television do you watch?
    1. 0–5 hours
    2. 6–10 hours
    3. 11–20 hours
    4. more than 20 hours
4. How often do you tape shut already-sealed envelopes before mailing them?
    1. almost never
    2. seldom
    3. often
    4. regularly
5. For a sales job, how would you prefer to be paid?
    1. straight commission
    2. mostly commission with a substantial draw
    3. a substantial draw with some commission
    4. straight salary
6. In highway driving, how often do you drive faster than 65 miles per hour?
    1. regularly
    2. often
    3. seldom
    4. almost never

7. If you had lived on the East Coast a century ago, do you think you
   would have joined a wagon train headed west?
   1. definitely
   2. probably
   3. probably not
   4. definitely not
8. Suppose you had equal competence at any one of the following
   activities. Which would appeal to you most?
   1. skydiving
   2. mountain climbing
   3. producing a play
   4. building a house
9. Which opportunity sounds more appealing to you?
   1. starting your own business
   2. purchasing a successful business
10. Which statement describes you better?
    1. I get bored easily.
    2. When necessary, I can tolerate routine.
11. What kinds of risks would you say are the hardest for you to take?
    1. commitment risks (long-term involvement with a person, activity
       or career)
    2. emotional risks (in relationships or showing my feelings)
    3. financial risks (of losing money)
    4. physical risks (of life and limb)

Assume that you are equally capable of all of the activities listed below.
For each set, pick the one that you would most enjoy. (If neither activity
appeals to you, pick the one that's least unappealing.)

12. 1. driving a dune buggy
    2. hiking in the desert
13. 1. skiing down a steep slope
    2. ski touring through woods
14. 1. scuba diving
    2. snorkeling

(continued)

What Kind of Gutsy Are You?—Continued

Circle the number of the word that best describes your reaction to the following activities.

15. Building a cabinet
    1. tedious
    2. satisfying
16. Climbing rocks
    1. exhilarating
    2. scary
17. Attending a rock concert
    1. arousing
    2. jarring
18. Teaching school
    1. boring
    2. challenging
19. With a report due in two weeks, what would you most likely do?
    1. start working on it the day before it's due, then stay up most of the night completing it
    2. work hard on the report for a day or two before it's due
    3. start working on it during the second week
    4. budget time throughout the two weeks to produce the report
20. In general, whose company do you prefer?
    1. people you've recently met
    2. professional colleagues, co-workers or fellow members of a club or church

Scoring

30 or below. Suggests a high need for excitement and a low tolerance for boredom. You're more likely than other men to take physical risk and avoid long-term commitments.

31 or above. Suggests you find it hard to take physical and financial risks but easy to take long-term risks such as deciding to raise a family or committing yourself to a career.

down the tracks of a roller coaster? It's that awe of overcoming your own natural fear of the unknown that makes adventure such a vital part of learning, growing and keeping yourself young, Dr. Weaver says.

"The importance of adventure isn't so much that you climbed a mountain, rafted on an unfamiliar river or even started your own small business. The key point is to achieve something new and to discover how you can reach beyond your comfort zone and stretch yourself as a human being," Dr. Weaver says.

So why do some guys feel the urge to bungee-jump while others spend their evenings nervously reading the fine print in their insurance policies? Some of your adventurousness is learned from your parents. "If you have parents who are always amplifying dangers, you'll learn to view situations as more threatening," Dr. Vittone says. "On the other hand, if you have parents who encourage adventure, you're going to develop a higher threshold of excitement."

But biology plays a role, too. "We all react differently to different types of stimulation," Dr. Vittone says. "There are certain anxiety centers in the brain that are tripped off more easily in some people than in others."

As we age, these anxiety centers in our brains become more sensitive, and we gradually lose our ability to distinguish between the negative sort of anxiety that is associated with work, stress and tension and the more positive types of anxiety that are a natural and exciting part of experiencing something new, Dr. Vittone says. As a result, we may become more fearful and avoid any situations that produce anxiety, including relatively safe recreational adventures such as hiking.

"The problem is people start viewing all those feelings of anxiety in the same negative way instead of realizing that some anxiety can be positive," Dr. Vittone says. "It's that lumping of those positive and negative feelings together that makes people gravitate toward wanting to feel safe and comfortable all the time." So you just settle back in that easy chair with that "I'm not as young as I used to be" attitude and start getting old.

A Prescription for Thrills

Fortunately, you don't have to climb Mount Everest, become a lion tamer or drive a Ferrari at 120 miles per hour to get adventure into your life.

"Since we're all different, there's a range of adventures that people are going to find thrilling," Dr. Vittone says. "For some people, even a minor change in routine can be an adventure. Finding a new way home from work or going to a different health spa could do it. For others, it may take parachuting. Whatever you do, it's that feeling of a thrill that you're looking for."

Here are some ways to safely get more thrills into your day.

Let your mind wander. Why did Columbus sail west across the Atlantic? Because he was curious. "Every adventure starts with curiosity," says Andrea Shrednick, Ph.D., a clinical psychologist in private practice in Los Angeles. "Allow your mind to wander free. Imagine if you had a week all to yourself. Where would you go? What would you do? What would it look like? What would it smell like? What types of foods would you eat? If you allow yourself to daydream like that, it will whet your appetite for the real thing."

Know your limits. Take an honest look at your skills and abilities and see if they realistically match up with an adventure you have in mind. If not, reconsider doing it. "A person who doesn't take a careful inventory of his skills and capabilities is being reckless," says Jasper S. Hunt, Jr., Ph.D., professor of experiential education and leadership studies and director of adventure education programs in the Department of Educational Leadership at Mankato State University in Mankato, Minnesota, and a leader of wilderness survival outings for Outward Bound, an adventure travel club.

Take small steps. Keep your adventures simple at first, then gradually increase the difficulty as your competence and confidence grow. If you want to learn to climb, for example, join your local hiking club and build up your expertise before deciding to tackle Mount McKinley, Dr. Hunt says.

Be prepared. "Every adventure, no matter how small, is a step-by-step process," says Anne Bancroft, a motivational speaker and polar explorer from St. Paul, Minnesota, who was the first woman to travel across the ice and reach both the North and South Poles. "You can't control Mother Nature, but before you start you can test your gear, get yourself in shape and do all the other things that make your chances of a successful trip far greater."

Accept reality. Don't push yourself into a dangerous situation. You're only asking for trouble that way. "If you look at mountaineers, the ones who are still alive to tell about their adventures are not the ones who try to conquer the mountain at all costs. They do their homework and know when it's unsafe and time to back off," Bancroft says.

Have some laughs. "A key to being adventurous is to have fun during your adventures," says Tom Head, a magazine travel writer based in Washington, D.C., who has rafted through the jungles of Central America and swum in the icy lakes of Finland. "The purpose of an adventure is lost if you don't have any fun."

AEROBICS

Move into the Future Youthfully

What do the two months before your high school reunion, the three weeks before softball season and the month of January all have in common?

Chances are it's exercise. You know—you'll actually get out and run a few times a week. Or you'll dust off that old exercise bike in the basement and actually ride it for a change.

But soon enough, that New Year's resolution is out the window, softball season's over, and the reunion is nothing but a pile of snapshots in your dresser drawer.

Then it's back to the grind. From early morning till just about midnight your day is packed—commuting, meetings, deadlines, phone calls, travel, family time, errands, chores. Each day leaves you feeling battered, worn out and…well, older than you used to feel. There's barely time to recover, let alone exercise. Out of all the things to do, that's last on your list.

But consider making it first.

Exercise will help you feel younger, both today and in the years to come. In fact, when it comes to age erasers, aerobic exercise is right at the top of the list. Aerobic exercise helps combat aging by preventing heart disease, maintaining bone and muscle strength and keeping your mind sharp. It may also play a role in fending off diabetes and certain forms of cancer. And it can help take the edge off that daily stress by boosting your mood and energy level.

"The cliché is that if ever there was a fountain of youth, this is it," says William Simpson, M.D., professor of family medicine in the Department of Family Medicine at the Medical University of South Carolina in Charleston. The person who regularly engages in aerobic exercise along with resistance training really has the optimal physical preparation for aging, he says.

A Friend of the Heart

For an exercise to be aerobic, it must rev up your heart rate and use your major muscle groups. Walking, running, biking and swimming can easily fill the bill.

A major benefit of aerobic conditioning is its effect on your heart and cardiovascular system. Evidence shows that aerobic exercise helps decrease the risk of cardiovascular disease, the number one killer of both men and women in the United States, says Alan Mikesky, Ph.D., an exercise physiologist at Indiana University School of Physical Education in Indianapolis. And that's the main reason aerobic exercise should be a priority, he says.

Research shows that aerobic exercise can decrease your risk of a first heart attack. In a study of 16,936 Harvard alumni ages 35 to 74, men who were less active were at 64 percent higher risk for a first heart attack than men who extended themselves more by exercising or engaging in activities such as walking or climbing stairs.

Data also indicate that sedentary men have a 30 to 40 percent greater risk of death from coronary heart disease than men who burn over 1,000 calories a week exercising—the equivalent of walking ten miles (about 40 minutes a day, three to four times a week).

Pump It Up So the Pressure Goes Down

Aerobic exercise can help lower your risk of heart disease by strengthening the heart and making it more efficient. When you exercise, your muscles require more fuel—oxygen, that is. So your heart pumps harder in order to push more blood—the vehicle that transports oxygen—to the outlying muscles. When the heart works harder like this on a regular basis, it grows stronger and more efficient, says Dr. Simpson. "You get a stronger pump working."

Exercise also helps improve the quality of circulation. "Exercise tends to dilate vessels so that the heart can pump more easily to supply blood to the rest of the body," says Dr. Simpson. The result is that resting blood pressure declines. "The heart doesn't have to work as hard against resistance," he says.

Aerobic exercise also helps increase your metabolic rate—the rate at which your body burns calories. At heart-pumping levels, exercise burns enough calories to reduce body fat, thus leading to weight loss.

Keeping trim not only helps you feel better but also can help keep down blood pressure, which is a risk factor for heart disease. Studies indicate that blood pressure can be reduced by exercising at least three times a week.

Clobber That Cholesterol

Exercise may also lower your risk of heart disease by keeping your cholesterol—a major risk factor—under control. Studies show that exercise increases

HDL (high-density lipoprotein) cholesterol, the good kind that helps sweep LDL (low-density lipoprotein) cholesterol, the bad kind, from the arteries. High-intensity exercise has been shown to increase HDL levels 5 to 15 percent.

When men engage in moderate exercise—say, the recommended 30 minutes of exercise three times a week at a minimum of 50 percent of maximum heart rate (220 minus your age)—elevated cholesterol levels tend to decline.

A Good Way to Bone Up

Aerobic exercise is effective in helping to maintain bone strength as well. Weight-bearing exercise places stress on the bone, and that stress helps maintain or increase bone strength.

The decline in bone density that occurs with aging is known as osteoporosis. It is more common in postmenopausal women than in men, because men start off with more dense bones to begin with, says Dr. Simpson. So it takes longer for bone density to decline to the point that men are at risk for fractures.

But that picture may be changing. Because we are living longer, more men are going to run out of calcium—the mineral that feeds the bones—before they die, says Dr. Simpson. So we may end up with a larger number of men with fractures due to brittle bones.

Aerobic exercises that are particularly effective are weight-bearing ones such as walking and running. Even riding a bicycle, either stationary or moving, can be effective. Increase the resistance against which you are pedaling, says Sydney Bonnick, M.D., director of osteoporosis services at Texas Woman's University in Denton. "That strengthens the muscles of the upper hips and thighs so they pull on the bone, which is a good stimulus to bone growth," she says. Swimming is not weight bearing and appears to be less effective.

A Matter of Memory Maintenance

Did you know that exercise can keep you younger by fending off the decline of your mental fitness? Well, it can, according to Joanne Stevenson, R.N., Ph.D., professor of nursing at Ohio State University College of Nursing in Columbus who specializes in how exercise affects memory in the elderly.

Long-term memory—the ability to remember distant events—doesn't generally deteriorate with aging. But short-term memory—the ability to remember recent events—does. Part of the reason for this, says Dr. Stevenson, is that as we get older, brain cells receive fewer nutrients and less oxygen than they used to. Aerobic exercise can decelerate that. It also helps increase the number of brain chemicals called neurotransmitters, so messages can be carried more quickly across brain cells, she says. "Exercise, by maintaining a high nutrient level and high oxygenation level, sort of wards off the process of aging."

Aging can also affect what researchers call fluid intelligence, or your ability to conceptualize. This type of memory requires more oxygen to the brain than any other mental chore. "Real quick thinking and real quick gaining of ideas—getting the whole gestalt—slows down through middle adulthood and into old age," says Dr. Stevenson. "Aerobic exercise would slow down this slowdown," she says, and enable people to maintain mental flexibility and quickness for a longer period of time.

Disease Deterrence

Exercise may play a role in fending off diabetes and cancer as well.

Type II diabetes, a disease in which the body produces less insulin and becomes insulin-resistant, affects 10 to 12 million adults ages 20 and over. Preliminary evidence suggests that exercise helps increase insulin sensitivity and resistance to the disease.

In one study of 5,990 male alumni of the University of Pennsylvania, the incidence of diabetes declined as physical activity went up. For every additional 500 calories burned through activity, the risk of diabetes went down by 6 percent. The study indicates that increasing physical activity may help prevent or delay diabetes and that vigorous activities may have a greater impact than more moderate ones.

Physical activity may play a role in deterring cancer, particularly colon cancer, which is common in men. In a study of 17,148 Harvard alumni, those who were highly active lowered their risk of colon cancer by 15 percent compared with inactive alumni. Researchers suspect that exercise may protect against colon cancer probably by reducing the amount of time that potential cancer-causing agents take to move through the intestinal system.

The Immediate Return

Aerobic exercise can make you feel younger by boosting your self-esteem. Regular exercise produces several rewards—muscle strength, gains in your aerobic fitness level, feelings of control over your environment and positive feedback from friends you exercise with—that can make you feel better about yourself.

Exercise can also improve your mental attitude. One study of 26 college athletes found that a 30-minute session of riding a special exercise cycle reduced anxiety significantly and that the effect continued for as long as an hour after the exercise session.

Aerobic exercise can help fight fatigue. "Despite what people sometimes feel, an exercise program tends to increase energy levels rather than decrease them," says Dr. Simpson. If people stop and pay attention to how exercise affects them, they will realize that they are more alert and more energetic, and that can carry over several hours after the exercise session, he says.

Exercise probably helps reduce anxiety and fatigue by boosting levels of endorphins, the body's natural mood elevators.

Coach's Corner:
Get a Handle on That Heart Rate

One way to assess whether you're working hard enough to reap aerobic benefits is to take your heart rate.

Let's say you haven't been exercising and are just starting out on a program. Begin by aiming for 50 to 65 percent of your maximum heart rate. Take your age and subtract it from 220. That figure is your maximum heart rate. Then take 50 percent and 65 percent of that to get your target heart rate range.

So if you're age 40, here's how to figure your heart rate range: 220 minus 40 is 180; 50 percent of 180 is 90, and 65 percent of 180 is 117. This means you're aiming for between 90 and 117 beats per minute. To assess if you're exercising at that rate, you can take your pulse for 15 seconds and multiply the number of beats by 4.

If the number you come up with is less than your target heart rate, in this case 90, you need to work a little harder. If it's 90, you're working hard enough to improve your fitness level. If your number is over 117, slow down a bit; chances are you're working at a pace that's too fast for your fitness level and you probably won't be able to maintain that intensity for the designated 30 minutes. You can also get your blood pressure too high.

Another method for assessing whether you're working hard enough is the ten-point RPE (rating of perceived exertion) scale. So if you were exercising at an intensity that felt very light for you, you would be a 1 on the scale, whereas if you exercised at a level that was very heavy, you'd give yourself a 10. If you felt your exercise level was moderate, you'd get a rating of 3.

With all these great benefits, it should come as no surprise that exercise may help you live longer. A follow-up to a Harvard study found that by the time they were 80 years old, men who had gotten adequate exercise between the ages of 35 and 79 lived one to two years longer than men who hadn't gotten regular exercise.

What the Doctors Recommend

The general guidelines for aerobic exercise have been to get 30 minutes of continuous aerobic exercise that gets your heart rate up to between 50 and 90 percent of your maximum heart rate at least three times a week. How high you need to raise your heart rate to reap anti-aging benefits depends on your age, sex and current fitness level. Generally speaking, men who have low fitness levels should aim for exercise intensities between 50 and 65 percent of their maximum heart rates. Men of average fitness status should aim for between 70 and 75 percent of their maximum heart rates, and men in excellent shape should aim for between 80 and 90 percent of their maximum heart rates.

Statistics show that only 22 percent of Americans get the recommended 30 minutes three times a week. If that much exercise is out of the question for you, try instead to accumulate 30 minutes of exercise over the course of the day—say, by walking 10 minutes before work, 10 minutes at lunch and 10 minutes after you get home. There is growing evidence to suggest it is the cumulative amount of activity, not the amount done at any one time, that can reap long-term health benefits.

Getting to It

It's one thing to know you should exercise, but it's another to get going and stick with it. Here are some tips to help you out.

Get physical. A physical checkup, that is. If you're just starting an exercise program, see your doctor. He'll check to see if you've ever smoked or whether you have a family history of heart disease, high blood pressure, high cholesterol, premature death or heart attack, says Dr. Simpson. The physical exam will assess your blood pressure and whether you have had any previous injuries to your muscles or bones that could be exacerbated by exercise, he says. If you haven't exercised in the past, are over age 35 and have risk factors for heart disease, your doctor may recommend a stress electrocardiogram (or a treadmill test).

Get some guidance. When you first start out on your exercise program, it's very important to get supervision from someone who knows about exercise, says Janet P. Wallace, Ph.D., associate professor of kinesiology at Indiana University Bloomington. On your own, you'll tend to overdo it, so find a trainer to keep you at the right pace. Ask candidates if they have certification from the American College of Sports Medicine, the American Council on Exercise, the Aerobics and Fitness Association of America or the National Strength and Conditioning Association.

Working with a trainer may also keep you on the exercise bandwagon, says Dr. Stevenson. This is because if you actually make an appointment to work out, you're less likely to forgo exercise for a few hours on the sofa at home.

Make it a priority. Instead of looking at exercise as a leisure activity, look at it as a necessity, says Dr. Mikesky. Make an appointment with yourself to get exercise and don't cancel, postpone or reschedule it. Respect that appointment just like you would any other, says Dr. Mikesky.

Warm up. It's important to warm up and stretch before plunging headlong into your workout session. Warming up increases circulation to the muscles, makes them more pliable and helps prevent injury, says Mark Taranta, a physical therapist and director of the Physical Therapy Practice in Philadelphia. Try walking, jogging slowly or riding an exercise bike at a slow pace for a few minutes until you get a light sweat going. Then stretch for eight to ten minutes.

Make it fun. People are more successful getting into regular exercise programs when they choose activities they enjoy, says Dr. Wallace. If it's boring or too hard, you won't stick with it, so try different things until you find a type of exercise you really like.

Mix it up. "Aerobic activities are not the most exciting activities," says Dr. Wallace, so try combining them with another activity that you like. If you enjoy racquetball or tennis (anaerobic activities), try walking for 15 minutes before or after. Or combine different types of aerobic activities. "If you're at the health club with a lot of aerobic equipment, move from one to the next," she says. Spending ten minutes on each one will be less boring. So try the stair climber, then the bike and then the treadmill.

Couple up. Consider going to the gym with your partner, says Dr. Wallace. A study of 16 married couples at her institution found that the dropout rate for individuals who went to the gym with their spouses was much lower (6 percent) compared with those who went to the gym on their own (42 percent). You don't necessarily have to work out together; just plan on going there together, says Dr. Wallace.

Get in a group. If you really have trouble exercising on your own, aim for a group activity. Join an aerobics class or a running group. Start your own walking club with friends from work. Exercising with others will help you stick with it, says Dr. Stevenson, because you'll have to answer for yourself. If you miss a class one week, the next week someone will be asking where you were, she says.

Give yourself a break. Getting into a regular exercise routine can take some time, so allow yourself to slip up here and there. Take it a week at a time, says Dr. Wallace. "If you blow it one day or one week, you still have next week," she says.

AFFIRMATIONS

Say Yes to Youthfulness

Sometimes it's a real douse-them-in-boiling-oil, stab-them-in-the-back-at-the-staff-meeting kind of world. Deadlines are tight. Pressure is high. And your boss would sooner dance the barefoot cha-cha through a pit of spitting cobras than toss you a compliment.

Hey, if you're not going to say nice things about yourself, who will?

That's where affirmations come in. Affirmations are short, positive phrases about yourself, your life and your world. Experts say that repeating them daily can build your self-esteem, give you a booster shot of vitality and help you see things in a more optimistic light. "There's so much negativity around that it tends to pull you down after a while," says Susan Jeffers, Ph.D., a psychologist in Tesuque, New Mexico, and author of *Feel the Fear and Do It Anyway.* "Affirmations can help you live a happier life and diminish the negative clutter that clouds your sense of purpose. They're extraordinarily powerful little pick-me-ups."

Nixing the Negative

Stop and listen to yourself think for a few minutes. If you're like most guys, the chatter inside your head is overwhelmingly negative. "Any time someone pays you a compliment, you immediately drown it out in a chorus of boos," Dr. Jeffers says. "For some reason, the chatterbox in our minds just doesn't want us to accept the fact that we have something on the ball."

Affirmations can counteract that powerful negative inner voice and eventually reduce it to just a whisper. The more positive things you say—about your successes, your feelings and your ambitions—the less time you have for negative thoughts. And even if you don't believe what you're saying at first, Dr. Jeffers says the optimistic messages will eventually seep into your subconscious and become just as powerful as the negative thoughts once were.

Okay, so it sounds a little hokey. How can chanting a phrase like "I am a successful businessman" really make you a successful businessman?

"The power of suggestion is very strong," says Douglas Bloch, a Portland, Oregon–based counselor and lecturer and author of *Words That Heal: Affirmations and Meditations for Daily Living*. "When you say something out loud and repeat it, it makes that thought concrete. You start to believe it and begin taking action accordingly." In other words, if you say you're a successful businessman, you'll probably start acting like one. And success is likely to follow.

Lest you doubt optimism's strength, consider this study. Researchers at the University of Pennsylvania in Philadelphia reviewed campaign speeches from all major candidates for president of the United States from 1948 to 1984. The result? The politicians who consistently delivered the most positive, action-based speeches on the campaign trail won nine of the ten elections. Candidates who wrung their hands and ruminated about issues—are you listening, Jimmy Carter?—were swamped.

Words for Winners

Want to be strong, assertive and successful? Start talking like it! "So much of what we say to other people is full of pain words—phrases like 'I can't' or 'I should,' " says Susan Jeffers, Ph.D., a psychologist in Tesuque, New Mexico, and author of *Feel the Fear and Do It Anyway*. "If we replace these pain words with power words, it really changes our attitude and outlook. Power words are like affirmations you can build into everyday speech and use all the time."

Pay attention to what you say for a few days, suggests Dr. Jeffers. If you hear yourself repeating pain phrases like the ones in the left column, try replacing them with the power phrases on the right.

Pain Phrases	Power Phrases
I can't.	I won't.
I should.	I could.
I hope.	I know.
If only.	Next time.
It's not my fault.	I'm responsible.
It's a problem.	It's an opportunity.
What will I do?	I can handle it.
Life's a struggle.	Life's an adventure.

"It's attitude," Dr. Jeffers says. "When we tell ourselves that we'll fail, that it's going to be a struggle, we set ourselves up for failure. But when we tell ourselves we'll handle whatever happens in our lives, we gain inner strength. And we set ourselves up for success."

Affirmations also are surefire stress busters. "You should have a list of affirmations ready that you can start repeating when you feel stressed," says Emmett Miller, M.D., a nationally known stress expert and medical director of the Cancer Support and Education Center in Menlo Park, California. "They don't have to be complicated. Just thinking to yourself 'I can handle this' or 'I know more about this than anyone here' will work. It pulls you away from the animal reflex to stress—the quick breathing, the cold hands—and toward the reasoned response—the intellect, the part of you that can really handle it."

The Two Ingredients for Success

Before you start using affirmations, you must have two things. The first is patience. "It may take a while to overcome all the negativity you've built up," Dr. Jeffers says. "Some of the effects of affirmations are immediate—you'll start feeling a little more optimistic right away. But only with repetition can you build a positive framework of inner thoughts that will last your whole life."

The second thing you need, of course, is affirmations. Here are some hints about how to create and use them.

Get personal. Affirmations are for you and you alone. So examine your life for areas that could use improvement. Do you want to be more confident? Would you like to be less angry? Do you want to get along better with your mother-in-law? Pick one or two goals to start with, Dr. Jeffers says, and write down the rest to address later.

Keep it short and sweet. Maybe you've decided that one of your goals is to stop worrying so much. Put your thoughts in positive form, state your affirmation in one sentence and always form it in the present tense to make it more immediate. "I let go and trust" or "It's all working out perfectly" may work for you. Try saying it a few times to see if it clicks. "You can feel the tension releasing immediately if it's working," Dr. Jeffers says.

Pick affirmations that state the positive, says Dr. Jeffers. These are better than phrases that negate a negative. For example, say "I am creating a successful career" instead of "I am not going to ruin my career."

Be realistic. Affirmations are tools to help you achieve goals. They are not magic incantations, so don't ask for too much too fast. "There's a fine line between positive thinking and wishful thinking," Bloch says. You'll probably have the most success if you choose affirmations that deal with emotions, confidence and self-esteem. Try to avoid affirmations that deal solely with material wealth. "It's probably not going to work if you keep repeating 'I am now driving a beautiful red sports car. I am now driving a beautiful red sports car,'" says Bloch.

That doesn't mean you won't eventually get your dream car. If you use af-

Affirmations: A Starter Set of Sayings

Affirmations usually work best if you tailor them for your needs. But if you've never created one before, experts suggest you try a few of these phrases first.

I am alive with possibility.
I'll handle it.
I feel myself growing stronger.
It is all happening perfectly.
There is nothing to fear.
I am confident and self-assured.
I deserve to be happy.
I forgive myself and others.
I accept myself as I am.
My prayers are always answered.

firmations correctly, Bloch says they can help. An affirmation such as "I am confident and successful" could lead to another one like "I am now ready to find a high-powered job" and maybe even to a real-life conversation along the lines of "I'll take that sports car now, Mr. Salesman, and make it red."

Repeat, repeat, repeat. Say your affirmations daily. Dr. Jeffers suggests at least 20 or 30 repetitions per day. And make sure you say them out loud. "There's something about hearing them that makes them more powerful," Dr. Jeffers says. It's a good idea to set aside a regular time to say them, then add more whenever necessary.

If you feel the need to say affirmations in a public setting, it's okay to say them to yourself, according to Dr. Jeffers.

Play back the positive. In addition to your daily oral repetitions, try putting your affirmations on tape. Dr. Jeffers suggests playing them as you drift off to sleep and right after you wake up. "Those are times when you're particularly likely to absorb the message," she says. Other good times: during a workout, when you're walking the dog and while you're cooking dinner. If you don't like the sound of your unaccompanied voice, play some soothing background music while you record your affirmations.

Surprise yourself. Hide reminders in unexpected places. Write your affirmations on random dates in your date book. Put them on a book marker in a home repair manual. Tape them to the inside cover of your tool chest. "Seeing your affirmations in odd places at odd times is a great way to reinforce the message," Dr. Jeffers says. "It's a jolt of positive energy."

Explore the spiritual. Affirmations work best when you tap into a higher power, Bloch says. "We derive strength from the feeling that we are not alone. It's comforting and freeing to ask for spiritual guidance," he says.

Try an affirmation like "I am truly blessed" or "Wherever I am, God is." You could even use Bible verses as affirmations: "The Lord is my shepherd; I shall not want." If religious references make you uncomfortable, try looking inward toward what Dr. Jeffers calls your higher self. She suggests affirmations like "I trust in myself" or "I am one with the universe." She explains, "You don't have to believe there's a god. You just have to believe that you can reach a higher plane in your life through reflection and trust."

Don't stop. Affirmations are a long-term commitment, Dr. Jeffers says. Keep using them even when things are going well. "Otherwise, you may find yourself falling back into habits that pull you down," she says. "There can be a lot of negativity in the world, but the proper use of affirmations helps us see the opportunity for growth in all things."

ALCOHOLIC BEVERAGES

A Few Nips
Can Give You an Edge

You sliced the fat, salt and cholesterol in your diet. You exercise enough to exhaust a Marine drill sergeant. You live right, but you do one thing that makes you feel a little guilty. At day's end, you swig a cold one.

Well, drink up—in moderation, doctors say—because a glass or two of alcohol a day may relieve stress, help you think more clearly, fend off heart disease and promote longevity. "If you take a look at mortality studies, the people who live the longest drink a glass or two of alcohol a day. So if someone can control his alcohol consumption, then a glass of wine, a can of beer or a mixed drink a day can extend his life," says Eric Rimm, Sc.D., a nutritional epidemiologist at the Harvard University School of Public Health in Boston.

In fact, death rates for men who savor one or two drinks a day are 16 percent lower than for guys who drink more or nothing at all, Dr. Rimm says.

To Your Health

In moderate amounts, alcohol helps inhibitions melt and tensions float away, says Frederic C. Blow, Ph.D., research director of the Alcohol Research Center at the University of Michigan in Ann Arbor. By decreasing sexual inhibitions, alcohol can help people relax, therefore making sex more enjoyable.

A standard drink is a 12-ounce beer, a 5-ounce glass of wine or a cocktail made with 1½ ounces (or one shot) of liquor. Having one or two a day can help keep your mind sharp, says Joe Christian, M.D., Ph.D., chairman of the Department of Medical and Molecular Genetics at the Indiana University School of Medicine in Indianapolis.

In a 20-year study of 4,000 male twins, Dr. Christian found that men who drank one or two alcoholic beverages a day had better learning and reasoning skills in their sixties and seventies than those who drank less or more. He suspects that moderate amounts of alcohol improve blood circulation to the brain.

Most of us have heard about French studies that concluded that drinking moderate amounts of red wine lowers heart disease risk. But other studies have shown that beer, liquor and white wine are about equally protective of the heart.

In Oakland, California, researchers at Kaiser Permanente Medical Center followed 56,926 men for seven years. While they concluded that white and red wines were most protective—reducing heart disease by 30 percent—researchers also found that beer and liquor were only slightly less protective.

"It doesn't matter what you drink. If you look at the studies, they show it could be hard liquor, wine or beer," says William P. Castelli, M.D., director of the Framingham Heart Study, which has followed the more than 5,200 people of Framingham, Massachusetts, since 1948.

The Benefits of Moderation

Overall, worldwide studies have consistently found a 20 to 40 percent drop in heart disease risk among moderate drinkers. That's about the same reduction in risk as lowering cholesterol or blood pressure or doing regular aerobic exercise, says Michael Criqui, M.D., professor of epidemiology at the University of California, San Diego, School of Medicine.

At Harvard, for example, Dr. Rimm and his colleagues studied 44,000 male health care professionals, including dentists, pharmacists, veterinarians and optometrists, for two years. The researchers concluded that men who reported drinking up to two drinks a day had a 30 percent lower risk of developing heart disease than men who reported drinking less than one-half drink a day.

Another study by the American Cancer Society followed 276,802 men ages 40 to 59 for over 12 years. Men who reported drinking one or two drinks a day were 20 percent less likely to die of heart disease than men who never drank.

In small amounts, alcohol increases the amount of HDL (high-density lipoprotein) cholesterol in your bloodstream. HDL, the good cholesterol, helps sweep LDL (low-density lipoprotein) cholesterol, the bad kind that can clog and damage arteries to the heart, from the bloodstream. Dr. Criqui also suspects that alcohol prevents blood clots that can lead to heart attacks and stroke.

In a British study comparing 137 men who had strokes with 137 men who hadn't, researchers found that the men who abstained from alcohol were nearly 2½ times more likely to have strokes than moderate drinkers.

But if one drink is good, why isn't three or even four drinks a day better? "Alcohol is clearly the most mixed of mixed blessings," Dr. Criqui says. "At one to two drinks a day, we don't see most of the complications of alcohol. However, the medical problems as well as the personal and social problems of heavy drinking are well known. There are terrible family problems, broken homes and spousal and child abuse. All that is associated with heavy alcohol use."

In addition, the risks of stroke, heart disease, liver disease and alcoholism all rise with more than a couple of drinks a day. "Some people may be predisposed to alcoholism, and because we can't tell who those people are before they start drinking, it would be unwise to tell non-drinkers to start drinking," Dr. Criqui says. "On the other hand, if you drink three or more drinks a day, cut back, because you're probably doing yourself more harm than good."

If you do drink, here are some ways to moderate your alcohol use.

Don't binge. One or two drinks a day means exactly that. "The best evidence is the drinking has to be done in small amounts spread over several days," Dr. Criqui says. "Drinking seven drinks on Friday night and seven more on Saturday can dramatically increase your blood pressure and actually increase your potential for blood clots."

Set a limit. If you know how much you're going to drink before you take your first sip, it will be easier to stick to that limit, says William R. Miller, Ph.D., research director at the University of New Mexico Center on Alcoholism, Substance Abuse and Addiction in Albuquerque.

Make it last. If you drink slowly, you'll give your liver a chance to metabolize the alcohol, so it won't build up in your body. Try to drink no more than one alcoholic drink an hour, says Sheila Blume, M.D., medical director of alcoholism, chemical dependency and compulsive gambling programs at South Oaks Hospital in Amityville, New York.

Chow down. Eating will slow the rate at which alcohol is absorbed into your bloodstream. But avoid salty foods, such as peanuts and pretzels, that will make you thirsty and tempt you to drink more, Dr. Miller says.

Be merry. Dance, play billiards or video games or talk to someone, Dr. Miller suggests. You'll probably drink less if you do.

Dilute your drink. Start out with a regular drink, but when it's half gone, add water or club soda to it. Every time your glass is half empty, add more water or club soda, Dr. Blume says.

Drink water. "If you're thirsty, your body wants water, not alcohol," Dr. Miller says. "All this nonsense about alcohol being a thirst quencher isn't true. It actually makes you thirstier. So if you drink a big glass of water first, you're more likely to drink alcohol in moderation."

Try grape juice. Grape juice, like red wines, contains resveratrol, a chemical produced in the grape's skin to fight off fungus. Researchers suspect that the chemical lowers the risk of atherosclerosis. So instead of sipping on wine, try drinking an eight-ounce glass of grape juice every day, Dr. Castelli suggests.

Call a cab. Alcohol is involved in nearly half of the fatal automotive accidents in the United States. If you weigh 150 pounds and have four drinks before you get behind the wheel, you're four times more likely to get into an accident than if you were sober, says Steve Creel, a California Highway Patrol public affairs officer. If you have ten drinks, your risk is 65 times greater. Even if you don't drink enough to be legally intoxicated, you can be arrested for drunk driving if the police believe you are endangering yourself or other motorists, Creel says. So if you drink at all, have a designated driver or get a taxi ride home.

ALTRUISM

Helping Others to Help Yourself

You know Frank, the guy who always comes in whistling on Monday mornings? You always thought he must have an incredible wife, a trust fund or some other secret weapon against the Monday blues. And this time, you're determined to find out what it is.

"So, Frank, what were you up to this weekend?"

"Oh, not too much. Shot a few hoops with Robert and worked with William a while."

Robert? William? You thought Frank's kids were named Joe and Mike, or something like that. You ask a few questions, and a different picture of Frank's weekend starts to emerge. Seems Robert is a kid whose father disappeared before he was born, and William is a parks worker who has spent his life struggling to read the signs on the subway.

Frank spent time with his family, sure, but he also worked in a few hours just being company for Robert and then helping William learn to read—like he does several times a month. It makes him feel good about himself, like a kid again, he says.

Back at your desk, you wonder if Frank's onto something.

What's in It for You?

According to experts on altruism, Frank knows what he's doing. Helping other people produces a health-promoting euphoria that can keep you feeling young and alive at any age. But there's a particular kind of helping that returns your energy tenfold, says Allan Luks, an attorney who heads New York City's Big Brother/Big Sister organization and the author of *The Healing Power of Doing Good*.

When you connect one-on-one with a stranger in need, you tap into altruism's most powerful age-erasing benefits. Writing a check for charity or helping your own family and friends is fulfilling, too, but giving to a stranger has the most direct effects on your physical and emotional health, says Luks. Why? Because helping a stranger in need begins to break down the sense of "them versus us"—and that empathy is the key to experiencing the lasting gratification that altruism brings, he says.

Luks led a national survey of volunteers, which he chronicles in his book. More than 20 volunteer organizations across the country participated in the survey, and more than 3,000 volunteers responded to detailed questionnaires. They described the type and frequency of helping activities they were involved in, the state of their health and their perceptions of the physical and emotional benefits of helping.

The results? More than 95 percent of the volunteers reported a warm burst of happiness and pleasure when they first started to volunteer. When they kept it up, they found that a lasting sense of calm and relaxation entered their lives. And over time, their self-esteem rose solidly—and stayed there.

It's common for men in their forties to have times when they feel as though the juice has gone out of life, Luks says. And altruism may be just what the doctor ordered. Helping other people is a prescription for a new lease on life. But Luks wonders why only one-third of volunteers nationally are male. "When men measure themselves only by jobs and pay, they're missing out on some of the greatest feelings going," he says.

Problems and pain don't vanish completely when you volunteer, Luks says, but they can be alleviated when you focus outside yourself. Helping someone else helps you leave your worries behind.

An Exercise in Youthfulness

Getting into altruism can make your older years not only happier but healthier, according to Howard F. Andrews, Ph.D., an epidemiologist and senior staff associate in neurology at the Columbia University College of Physicians and Surgeons in New York City.

Dr. Andrews's analysis of the data from Luks's research concluded that helping others can significantly improve your overall health and relieve depression. It also reduces pain to the point that people who regularly help others make fewer visits to doctors.

One man's altruism is helping to fight the war on poverty. Millard Fuller is president and founder of Habitat for Humanity International in Americus, Georgia, the organization of volunteers that builds houses for people in need. And here's what motivates him. "A miserly spirit is a dying spirit," Fuller says. "My advice is to give. It's the only way of life that makes sense."

You, too, can build that kind of ageless spirit, whether you're helping a new homeowner climb out of the cracks with sweat equity or giving in some other way. Here's how.

Search for a cause. If you're at a loss where to begin, think of what you care about and head for the phone book, says Luks. "If you're concerned about a certain health problem or social cause, you'll often find a local nonprofit group in the telephone book," he says. "And many communities have volunteer action centers of some sort listed under 'Volunteer.' "

Rehearse it first. Everybody needs a push to get started, and you can give yourself one by mentally visualizing yourself in a helping situation, Luks says. Just try it on for size: "Here's me helping to paint a house" or "Here I am volunteering in a hospital." Adds Luks, "Then when you call an organization in the area you've chosen, say 'Do you use volunteers? I'm thinking about volunteering. Can you send me some literature?' They'll be glad to hear from you."

Work one-on-one. Meeting and spending time with the person you're helping will have a much greater impact on you than if you limit your helping to less personal tasks, such as collecting clothes or canned goods for the poor, says Luks. Of the volunteers he surveyed, only 5 percent of those who had one-to-one contact with the people they were helping did not report a blast of good feelings. But people who never encountered those they helped were three times less likely to experience that buoyant, youthful feeling.

Join a team. It's even more effective to help strangers in company, such as through your involvement with a supportive organization of volunteers. Dr. Andrews's analysis of Luks's data suggests that people who helped strangers through a group rather than on their own made significantly fewer visits to the doctor and reported more positive effects and lasting good feelings from helping.

Stay with the program. Those warm holiday feelings can make every guy feel like putting on a Santa suit. But people who help frequently year-round will continue to experience the good feelings altruism brings the giver, Luks's national survey showed. So make your volunteer activity a regular routine to reap its fullest benefits, Luks says.

Use your know-how. When you use your own particular skills and knowledge to help others, the experience is even more satisfying, Luks says. He cites surveys that asked people who were already volunteering why they continued, and one of the frequent reasons given was that they were able to use their skills to do something useful. Using your own talents to help or support someone else gives you a particularly strong sense of usefulness, which in turn reduces stress, he says. If you're a lawyer, volunteer at a law clinic. If you can teach, you can tutor. If you can grow a vegetable, you can feed the hungry. The opportunities are limitless, Luks says.

Take a volunteer vacation. You can use your hard-earned time off to loll in a hammock with a six-pack. Or take a volunteer vacation and find satisfying adventure along with your altruism. For example, Habitat for Humanity International will connect you with a nearby group working on housing for the poor, Fuller says. Write them at 121 Habitat Street, Americus, GA 31709-3498, for more information.

Or combine travel and volunteering as a member of the EarthCorps. Earth-Corps volunteers join Earthwatch expeditions and assist scientists on ecological research projects and "digs" all over the globe. "You can help conserve endangered species, environments or cultures on 1 of 165 projects in 58 countries and 25 states," says Mary Blue Magruder, Earthwatch's director of public affairs. You can write to Earthwatch at P.O. Box 403 R.P., Watertown, MA 02272, for details.

Beating Burnout

No man can save the world by himself (though you might like to try). To keep your spirits up and fight the good fight, you have to take care of yourself, too. Here are Luks's tips for beating "volunteer burnout."

Set your own timetable. Start gradually and volunteer at a pace that's right for you, Luks says. If it starts to feel like a weary obligation, you're doing too much, or you're in the wrong volunteer activity.

Don't aim too high. If you try to fix everything all at once, you'll set yourself up for disappointment, Luks says. Don't take on total responsibility for even one person or blame yourself for circumstances you can't control.

Make it contagious. A good way to deal with "beginner's nerves" and take the first step toward getting involved is to pursue a volunteer activity as a family or with a buddy, Luks says. You will strengthen your own relationships as you get healthier from helping, he says.

Change course when you need to. If one challenge isn't bringing you satisfaction and well-being, it's perfectly okay to look for another, Luks says. Nobody is indispensable, and you need to find the helping activity that's right for you. You'll know it's the right fit when you feel more energetic after a volunteering session than you did when you started.

ANTIOXIDANTS

Rustproofing Your Body

Don't take this personally, but you might be getting a little rusty around the edges.

Not that you're actually forming little orange and brown flakes around your ears, but the same process that transforms the shiny new chrome on your car into a corroded piece of scrap metal could be, at this very minute, turning you into the biological equivalent of a bucket of rusty bolts.

Ironically (no pun intended), the culprit is something you'd least suspect: oxygen. The very stuff that keeps us alive and kicking. Go without it for a minute, and your face turns blue. But take in lungful after lungful over a lifetime, and bit by bit, you do your body harm.

Just as oxygen in the air can rust metal, the oxygen your body uses in every one of its activities, from digestion to exercise, may attack your body's molecules, cells and tissues, weakening them and changing their structure. Scientists now speculate that this "oxidation" process explains why our bodies deteriorate with age and how certain chronic diseases, like cancer or heart disease, develop.

If you were a car, you could get a nice coat of wax to keep out the rust. But how do you rustproof your body? You certainly can't stop breathing. A man needs a special line of defense, and that's where diet and nutrition come in. A handful of nutrients—vitamin C, vitamin E and beta-carotene—have been identified as having the power to protect cells from the damage of oxidation. Not surprisingly, they are known as antioxidants.

Free Radicals: The Bad Guys

While oxygen serves as the catalyst that triggers this "rusting" process, there are actually other substances responsible for the dirty work. Scientists call these marauding thugs free radicals. No, they aren't a bunch of long-haired, renegade hippies on the loose; they're oxygen by-products. Here's what happens.

To get the energy they need, your body's cells use oxygen to burn fuels such as glucose (blood sugar). In the process, some of the oxygen molecules lose electrons. Those molecules are now free radicals, and they try to replace the electrons they lost by raiding other molecules in the cell. The problem is, the molecules that they vandalize also become free radicals.

"Soon a chain reaction of electron theft begins that can produce widespread damage to the chemistry and function of the cell," says Denham Harman, M.D., Ph.D., professor emeritus of medicine and biochemistry at the University of Nebraska College of Medicine in Omaha.

Wrinkled skin, shrinking muscles, weak bones—these and other physical woes of growing old may be due in part to this destructive oxidation process, the sum of millions of continuous free radical reactions. But of even greater concern to researchers is the notion that these free radicals are causing some of aging's most insidious diseases.

For example, atherosclerosis (hardening of the arteries), the leading cause of heart disease and stroke, is due to the buildup of LDL (low-density lipoprotein) cholesterol, the so-called bad cholesterol. But it probably isn't until free radicals oxidize the LDL cholesterol that it assumes its potentially deadly form, according to Balz Frei, Ph.D., associate professor of medicine and biochemistry at the Boston University Medical Center.

If we could stop or slow down the free radical chain reaction before it starts, then LDL cholesterol may never go "bad" in the first place, says Dr. Frei. Or DNA molecules, the genetic material within our cells, may never mutate to lead to the formation of cancer. Or tissues in the eye may be more resistant to cataracts. In other words, it would be possible to slow the aging process, extend life expectancy and improve the quality of life.

The Good Guys

You don't expect the body to just sit there and take it while these free radicals run rampant, do you? No, sir. From the get-go, your body starts producing certain enzymes to combat the invading free radicals. The problem is that it doesn't produce enough of them to stop all the invaders. It needs outside help—fast.

Enter dietary antioxidants—nutritional "scavengers" that roam the body in search of free radicals, squelching the offending particles before they can even launch their first attack. "Because of their unique molecular structures, antioxidants can give up one or more of their electrons to free radicals without becoming harmful themselves," says Dr. Frei. "They actually render the free radical harmless and head off the destructive chain reaction before damage can occur or spread out."

Most researchers have focused their attention on three of the antioxidant nutrients: vitamin C, vitamin E and beta-carotene, a substance that the body converts to vitamin A. Numerous studies have shown that high dosages of each

A Word about Vitamin A

Besides being an antioxidant protector, beta-carotene is a great source of another important nutrient, vitamin A. The body converts beta-carotene into vitamin A on an as-needed basis.

But be aware that vitamin A and beta-carotene are not the same thing. Vitamin A will not give you the same antioxidant protection as beta-carotene, and too much vitamin A can be highly toxic.

For this reason, nutritionists recommend that you don't go beyond the daily Recommended Dietary Allowance (RDA) for vitamin A (1,000 micrograms retinol equivalents or 5,000 IU) and that you avoid all vitamin A supplements or supplements containing more than 100 percent of the RDA for vitamin A unless prescribed by a doctor. "We get all the vitamin A we need from meats and vegetables or from foods containing beta-carotene," says Jeffrey Blumberg, Ph.D., associate director of the U.S. Department of Agriculture Human Nutrition Research Center on Aging at Tufts University in Boston.

Excessive doses of beta-carotene are not nearly as dangerous as those of vitamin A, says Dr. Blumberg. He says it is almost impossible to consume toxic levels of beta-carotene, but too much can produce an unusual side effect: It can make your skin turn orange.

---

of these nutrients result in low instances of many chronic diseases.

In his research, Dr. Frei has found that vitamins E and C can protect LDLs from oxidative damage. "These studies suggest that antioxidant nutrients, vitamin C in particular, are capable of preventing heart disease or at least slowing down its progression," he says.

Scientists have also noticed a relationship between antioxidants and the incidence of cataracts. A study by Canadian researchers suggests that dietary supplementation of vitamins C and E can reduce your risk of cataracts by at least 50 percent.

Paul F. Jacques, Sc.D., an epidemiologist at the U.S. Department of Agriculture (USDA) Human Nutrition Research Center on Aging at Tufts University in Boston, has found another link between lower antioxidant levels and cataracts. In one study, he observed that the risk of developing cataracts was five times higher in people with "lower levels of all types of carotene, including beta-carotene," in their blood.

Dr. Jacques has also studied the role of the antioxidant vitamin C in fighting high blood pressure, or hypertension. According to his research, rates of high blood pressure are approximately two times higher in subjects with low intakes of vitamin C in their diets (less than the Recommended Dietary Allowance, or RDA, of 60 milligrams).

There is also a growing body of evidence that antioxidants may be our best source of cancer protection as well. Researchers at the Harvard School of Dental Medicine in Boston have shown in experiments on hamsters that a mixture of beta-carotene, vitamin E and vitamin C produces significant protection against oral cancer.

And the research doesn't stop there. Gladys Block, Ph.D., professor of public health nutrition at the University of California, Berkeley, School of Public Health, has reviewed 180 studies comparing the effect of fruits and vegetables and their antioxidant nutrients on various cancers. "One hundred fifty-six of these studies have shown a statistically significant reduced risk of cancer at virtually all cancer sites," she says.

Among Dr. Block's findings is that a low intake of vitamin C doubles your risk of developing oral, esophageal and stomach cancer. And vitamin E and beta-carotene may be protective against lung and stomach cancer.

How Much Does a Man Need?

The National Research Council's Food and Nutrition Board has established the RDAs as guidelines for how much of each nutrient we need to consume each day to meet our basic health needs and prevent deficiency diseases. For men ages 25 to 50, the daily numbers are 60 milligrams of vitamin C, 10 milligrams alpha-tocopherol equivalents (or 15 IU) of vitamin E and 1,000 micrograms retinol equivalents (or 5,000 IU) of vitamin A or 6 milligrams of beta-carotene.

Nutritionists agree that the best way to meet these antioxidant requirements is to eat a balanced diet consisting of a wide variety of fruits and vegetables. "Four to five servings of fruits and vegetables per day should easily provide you with most, if not all, of the RDAs for the antioxidants as well as other important vitamins and minerals," says Diane Grabowski, R.D., nutrition educator at the Pritikin Longevity Center in Santa Monica, California.

That's fine for basic health, but to get the same disease-fighting results seen in scientific studies, you need to surpass the RDAs. Even the most healthful diets fall short in equaling the same amount of antioxidants used in research.

That's where vitamin supplements can play a role. A supplement is an excellent means of ensuring your maximum antioxidant protection as well as correcting any deficiencies in your diet. But popping a vitamin tablet alone isn't the answer. "These nutrients are not 'magic bullets' and work best in conjunction with other healthy nutritional practices such as eating low-fat, high-fiber meals," says Jeffrey Blumberg, Ph.D., associate director of the USDA Human Nutrition Research Center on Aging at Tufts.

Your Antioxidant Arsenal

Much of your antioxidant protection can come from the foods you already love to eat. "A good rule of thumb is to eat from a rainbow of colorful fruits and vegetables," says Diane Grabowski, R.D., nutrition educator at the Pritikin Longevity Center in Santa Monica, California. "In general, the darker green or more vibrantly colorful fruits and vegetables have the richest antioxidant content."

Here are some of the very best sources available.

Sources of Vitamin C

Food	Portion	Vitamin C (mg.)
Orange juice, fresh	1 cup	124.0
Broccoli, fresh, boiled	1 cup	116.0
Brussels sprouts, fresh, cooked	1 cup	97.0
Red bell peppers, raw	½ cup	95.0
Cranberry juice cocktail	1 cup	90.0
Cantaloupe, cubed	1 cup	68.0

Sources of Vitamin E

Food	Portion	Vitamin E (IU)
Sunflower seeds, dried	¼ cup	26.8
Sweet potatoes, boiled	1 cup	22.3
Kale, fresh, boiled	1 cup	14.9
Yams, boiled or baked	1 cup	8.9
Spinach, boiled	1 cup	5.9

Sources of Beta-Carotene

Food	Portion	Beta-Carotene (mg.)
Sweet potato, baked	1	14.9
Carrot, raw	1	12.2
Spinach, boiled	½ cup	4.4
Butternut squash, baked	½ cup	4.3
Fresh tuna, cooked, dry heat	3 oz.	3.9
Cantaloupe, cubed	1 cup	3.1
Beet greens, boiled	½ cup	2.2

Research is under way to determine the exact amount of antioxidants we need for optimal disease protection. Until then, most researchers believe we can best protect ourselves with a combination of diet and supplements. Dr. Blumberg suggests that you try to get all or as much as possible of the RDA of each antioxidant from the food you eat. He suggests that for added protection, you take daily supplements containing 100 to 400 IU of vitamin E, between 500 and 1,000 milligrams of vitamin C and between 6 and 30 milligrams of beta-carotene.

Boosting Your Defenses

Here are some tips on how you can help antioxidant nutrients work more effectively.

Don't pig out. Digestion requires oxygen—lots of it. The more calories we consume, the more oxygen is required, and the greater our chances for free radical formation. Cutting back on the amount we eat can trim our risk of oxidative damage, says Dr. Harman. That doesn't mean you should starve yourself or do anything to reduce your intake of the essential nutrients, he warns. Instead, focus on trimming those nonessential calories from your diet, like desserts, candy and soda.

Get some fresh air. Free radicals are also generated in the environment by some industrial chemicals, heavy metals, fumes, car exhaust, air-conditioning and other airborne pollutants. While we can't escape all these man-made contaminants, anything that limits our exposure to them is beneficial, says Dr. Harman. For example, if you work in a factory or an office, you can take a walk at lunchtime to briefly get away from impurities that may be circulating around your workplace. Open windows. Or use a commercial air-purifying device.

Snuff out the cigarettes. Cigarette smoke contributes huge amounts of free radicals with every puff. Antioxidants can prevent much of the oxidative damage caused by smoking, says Dr. Frei. But if you avoid the habit in the first place, those antioxidants will be available to fight free radicals elsewhere in the body.

Go easy on the hard stuff. The occasional beer with the boys won't cause any harm and may actually lower your risk of heart disease, but frequent alcohol consumption can increase the number of free radicals in the body, says Dr. Frei. Not only that, but people with alcoholism show reduced levels of antioxidants in their systems. According to a study done at the King's College School of Medicine and Dentistry in London, alcoholic patients showed significantly lower levels of vitamin E and beta-carotene, which coincided respectively with higher incidences of liver damage.

Work out in moderation. When it comes to exercise, remember the adage "Train, don't strain." As beneficial as exercise is to our health, the extra oxygen we take in whenever we work out subjects muscles and other tissues to additional oxidative damage. Pushing the body beyond its limits can lead to an overproduction of free radicals, and that can have a devastating effect on the way you look and feel. "This may be why athletes who overtrain find that their performances suffer or they become sick," says Robert R. Jenkins, Ph.D., professor of biology at Ithaca College in Ithaca, New York.

Does this mean you shouldn't exercise? No! Most doctors and scientists believe that any oxidative damage is minimal with normal exercise and offset by the added benefits that exercise provides. According to a British study of endurance runners, regular, non-exhaustive exercise enhances the levels of some antioxidant enzymes in the blood. And a study conducted at the Washington University School of Medicine in St. Louis found that high doses of vitamin C, vitamin E and beta-carotene, while not preventing the body from undergoing any exercise-induced oxidative stress, do seem to reduce oxidative damage in the body.

Regular, moderate exercise seems to strike the perfect balance, says Dr. Harman. And no matter what, keep up your intake of antioxidant vitamins.

ASPIRIN

The Handy Heavyweight of Health

Sometimes life leaves you feeling like Rocky Balboa's personal punching bag. Your back's aching from too much tennis. Your ankle's swollen from slipping on a patch of ice. Your head's pounding from a little too much "friendly advice" from the boss.

So you reach into the medicine cabinet and pull out aspirin, the heavyweight champion of nonprescription drugs. A couple of little white pills can whip common headaches and minor pain, knock out swelling, bring fever to its knees and leave arthritis begging for mercy.

But now research shows that aspirin may pack an even more powerful anti-aging punch—by lowering your risk of heart attack, stopping migraines before they start, reducing your chance of developing gallstones and maybe even helping to prevent digestive tract cancers.

The Heart of the Matter

Doctors have been backing aspirin for nearly 2,000 years. Hippocrates himself told his Greek friends to chew on willow bark whenever they had pain or fever. Turns out that the bark contained salicylic acid, an unrefined form of aspirin.

Aspirin works by inhibiting the body's production of prostaglandins, chemicals that help deliver pain messages from the site of an injury to the brain. But there's an important side effect, too. Prostaglandins aid in blood clotting, so aspirin use reduces clotting. And while that can be a problem in some instances, evidence is growing that this may help prevent heart attacks by halting clots in the coronary arteries that feed the heart.

The landmark Physicians' Health Study looked at 22,000 healthy male doctors ages 40 to 84, half of whom took a standard 325-milligram aspirin tablet every other day. The results showed that men who took aspirin instead of a placebo (a fake pill) had a 44 percent lower risk of suffering a first heart attack.

"We didn't expect to see such a dramatic difference between these two groups," says Charles H. Hennekens, M.D., professor of medicine, ambulatory care and prevention at Harvard Medical School in Boston who headed the study. "Despite the fact that the participants were all middle-aged and older men—which in and of itself puts them at risk for heart disease—this was one of the lowest-risk groups ever studied."

Doctors now prescribe aspirin therapy for men who fall into high-risk groups for heart disease. William P. Castelli, M.D., director of the famous Framingham Heart Study in Framingham, Massachusetts, says those groups include all men in America 50 years of age or older; men 40 or older with strong family histories of heart disease or uncontrolled risk factors like high blood pressure, high cholesterol and cigarette smoking; and men over 30 with excessively high cholesterol levels or diabetes.

Aspirin's anti-aging powers may reach even farther than your heart. Aspirin could help you ward off some forms of stroke by reducing blood clots. Experts warn, however, that aspirin therapy could put you at slightly higher risk for hemorrhagic strokes, which are caused by ruptured blood vessels. See your doctor before you start taking aspirin for stroke prevention. The Physicians' Health Study also showed that men who took aspirin every other day had a significantly reduced need for surgery to repair other blocked blood vessels in the body.

And aspirin might boost your chances of avoiding colon cancer. In one study of more than 600,000 people, those who took aspirin 16 or more times a month had a 50 percent lower risk of developing such cancer. Clark W. Heath, Jr., M.D., vice president for epidemiology and statistics at the American Cancer Society, says that's because aspirin appears to slow down the development of adenomas, polyps that are probably precursors to colon cancer.

On the headache front: The Physician's Health Study also found that those who took aspirin every other day developed 20 percent fewer migraine headaches. Aspirin, however, does little to stop migraines that are already under way, according to Seymour Diamond, M.D., director of the Diamond Headache Clinic in Chicago and executive director of the National Headache Foundation.

People at risk of developing gallstones may benefit from aspirin, too. A British study of 75 patients predisposed to stone formation found that the 12 regular aspirin users in the group got no stones, while 20 of the 63 non-users did.

Helpful—But Not Harmless

So where's the catch? Well, aspirin is a drug, and like most drugs, it has side effects that may outweigh its benefits for some men.

For starters, aspirin can irritate the lining of your stomach. If that happens, you may feel a burning sensation, though usually the damage is not serious. In rare cases, aspirin use can trigger intense abdominal pain, ulcers or even gastrointestinal bleeding.

Aspirin can also cause tinnitus, or ringing in the ears. The condition is usually temporary, and aspirin will cause no permanent damage to your ears. If aspirin makes your ears ring, doctors suggest trying a product containing acetaminophen.

Tablet Tips

Intrigued by aspirin's possibilities? Before you give it a tryout, just remember.

Don't play doctor. Aspirin therapy carries risks. Talk to your physician about whether it's right for you. "You should consult your doctor before taking aspirin for a sustained period of time," says James E. Muller, M.D., co-director of the Insti-

Painkillers: Choose Your Weapon

Long before aspirin won fame for fighting everything from heart disease to gallstones, it was just a humble old headache pill. But aspirin may not be the best choice for minor aches and pains anymore. Other over-the-counter drugs can handle many of aspirin's smaller chores without causing side effects like upset stomach or ringing ears.

Every nonprescription painkiller relies on one or more of three drugs: aspirin; ibuprofen, which is found in brands like Advil, Nuprin and Motrin; and acetaminophen, found in Tylenol, Panadol and some Anacin products. The choice among them isn't that difficult when you know what each one does best.

Minor aches and fever. All three take care of this, but you might want to consider acetaminophen here, because it's easier on your stomach lining than the others.

Headaches. For everyday tension headaches, each of the three pain relievers can do the job, says Frederick Freitag, D.O., a member of the board of the National Headache Foundation.

Toothaches. Ibuprofen is your best bet here. It out-performed aspirin and acetaminophen in a study reported in *American Pharmacy*.

Sore muscles. Ibuprofen and aspirin get the edge here because they are anti-inflammatory agents that help reduce swelling of sore or bruised muscles. Ibuprofen is less irritating than aspirin to most people's stomachs.

Sprains and tendinitis. Again, aspirin and ibuprofen get the nod because they help cut swelling.

tute for Prevention of Cardiovascular Disease at New England Deaconess Hospital in Boston.

Easy dose it. If a little aspirin works wonders, why not take a lot? Simple: Test results show that taking large doses of aspirin does no more good than taking smaller doses.

Most research has focused on those who take a 325-milligram tablet—the size of a regular-strength aspirin—every other day. The Physicians' Health Study found that an aspirin every other day helped cut heart attack risk.

A Dutch study showed that smaller doses—perhaps one-tenth the size of a regular tablet—may provide essentially the same results. "This study adds more weight to the view that doses of aspirin currently used for prevention may be higher than need be," says Dr. Muller.

Your doctor should be able to set a proper dosage for you, Dr. Muller says. He also warns not to cut down on your dosage if a doctor has already prescribed aspirin.

Avoid a gut reaction. Try to take aspirin with a meal, because you'll be less likely to feel stomach pain or nausea. If you're between meals, try swallowing aspirin with a full eight-ounce glass of water.

Bypass your belly. Some regular-dose and low-dose aspirins have special coatings that let them pass through your stomach and digest in your small intestine, which is a little easier on your digestive system. Look for brands that are buffered or "enteric-coated."

Focus on healthy living. No matter how powerful aspirin proves to be, it won't solve all your problems. It may help prevent a heart attack, but so do a healthy diet and regular exercise.

"First of all, you should do everything you can to reduce the risk factors such as high cholesterol, smoking, overweight and lack of exercise," says Alexander Leaf, M.D., founder of the Cardiovascular Health Center at Massachusetts General Hospital in Boston.

BREAKFAST

Make a Big Deal of Your Morning Meal

Wake up and smell the coffee.

A good breakfast can kick your body and brain into high gear, giving you sufficient energy for the rest of the day—and for the rest of your life, if you make it a daily habit. But high energy isn't the only thing a good breakfast can give you. Make a healthy morning meal a daily habit, and you'll likely be adding years to your life.

Breakfast might help your heart by lowering cholesterol, a factor in circulatory disease. Researchers at St. Joseph's University in Philadelphia looked at the breakfast habits of 12,000 people and found that those who ate cereal—any cereal—for breakfast had the lowest cholesterol levels, while breakfast skippers had the highest.

"We've known that one of the worst things you can do for proper nutrient intake is skip breakfast. But now we have new evidence that people who eat a breakfast including cereal have lower cholesterol," says John Stanton, Ph.D., the study's author and director of the Food, Nutrition and Health Research Institute at St. Joseph's University.

Along with high cholesterol, another cause of circulatory disease is blood clots, sticky plugs that block arteries. The clots are formed from platelets, the tiny, disk-shaped parts of blood that are responsible for normal clotting (like when you cut yourself) but can go into overdrive and become more like Krazy Glue than Scotch tape.

Researchers at the Memorial University of Newfoundland in St. John's

Breakfast in a Box—Healthful Cereals

With about a zillion kinds of cereal to pick from, choosing is confusing. Your best bet for breakfast is to find a cereal you like that has plenty of fiber and nutrients but not a lot of fat, calories, sugar or sodium. Look for adult choices on the top shelf in most supermarket cereal aisles and check out the options below. Nutritional values shown are for single servings; check the side of the cereal box for the serving size.

Cereals	Fiber (g.)	Calories	Fat (g.)	Sugar (g.)	Sodium (mg.)
All-Bran (original)	10	80	1	5	280
Cheerios (original)	3	110	2	1	280
Common Sense Oat Bran	4	110	1	6	270
Cracklin' Oat Bran	6	230	8	18	180
Fiber One	14	60	1	0	140
Frosted Mini-Wheats	6	190	1	12	0
Grape-Nuts	5	200	0	7	350
Healthy Valley Organic Amaranth Flakes	4	100	0	8	10
Kellogg's Complete Bran Flakes	5	100	0.5	6	230

looked at the effect of breakfast on platelets. They found that morning levels of the factor that makes platelets sticky were much higher in people who didn't eat breakfast.

Scientists already know that most heart attacks and strokes occur in the morning. Eating breakfast may be an important protection, says George Fodor, M.D., professor of clinical epidemiology at Memorial University who led the study. "It is definitely prudent and important to have breakfast every morning," he says.

Eat to Lose Weight

If you've been watching your waistline expand with the years, breakfast is your ally in that battle, too.

Breakfast appears to act as a wake-up call for your body's metabolism, stim-

Cereals	Fiber (g.)	Calories	Fat (g.)	Sugar (g.)	Sodium (mg.)
Kellogg's Corn Flakes	1	110	0	2	330
Kenmei Rice Bran	1	110	1	4	250
Multi Bran Chex	7	220	2	11	320
Nabisco 100% Bran	8	80	0.5	7	120
Nut & Honey Crunch	0	120	2	10	200
Oat Bran O's	3	110	0	7	10
100% Whole Grain Wheat Chex	5	190	1	5	390
Product 19	1	110	0	3	330
Quaker Oat Bran High Oat Fiber	6	150	3	1	0
Raisin Nut Bran	5	210	4.5	15	260
Rice Chex	0	120	0	2	230
Rice Krispies	1	110	0	3	360
Special K	1	110	0	3	250
Total (original)	3	100	0.5	5	200
Wheaties	3	110	1	4	210

ulating it to burn more calories. A study conducted by Wayne Callaway, M.D., associate professor of medicine at George Washington University in Washington, D.C., found that breakfast eaters had metabolic rates 3 to 4 percent above average, while breakfast skippers had sluggish rates, 4 to 5 percent below average. That means that in the course of a year, breakfast skippers will "conserve" 10 to 15 pounds of body fat, explains Dr. Callaway.

Eating breakfast can also help you to control your hunger and, when you do get hungry, to choose the right low-fat foods. A study at Vanderbilt University in Nashville led by David Schlundt, Ph.D., clinical psychologist and assistant professor of psychology, found that people who ate breakfast chose fewer high-fat foods and more healthy high-carbohydrate foods and more successfully fought off their cravings for late-day, unhealthy snacks than did those who didn't eat a morning meal.

Shifts in brain chemistry throughout the day make us more likely to crave fats as the hour gets later, explains Dr. Callaway. Most of us wake up craving carbohydrates rather than fats. "It's as if we were biologically programmed to eat a healthy breakfast," he says.

A healthy high-carbohydrate, low-fat breakfast will address more than your midlife battle of the bulge. Breakfast may also help protect you from developing gallstones, says James E. Everhart, M.D., a researcher with the Division of Digestive Diseases and Nutrition at the National Institute of Diabetes and Digestive and Kidney Diseases in Bethesda, Maryland. People who skip breakfast are essentially undergoing a short-term fast, and fasting has been shown to increase the risk of gallbladder disease.

What if all your stomach's had in it before noon for the past three decades is coffee the consistency of axle grease? Relax, we're not giving up on you. Read on for how to ease into the breakfast habit.

Sunrise Solutions

You may have noticed we haven't mentioned platters of buttered eggs and rashers of bacon. Sorry, but a Paul Bunyan breakfast can have the opposite effect on a man: Instead of giving you the heart of a lumberjack, high calories plus high fat can add up with age to an artery-plugging mess. Here's how to do breakfast right.

Just do it. You can get your body used to eating a healthy breakfast even if you've never eaten it in your life, says John Foreyt, Ph.D., director of the Nutrition Research Clinic at Baylor College of Medicine in Houston. "Eat breakfast, lunch and dinner for a week even if you have no appetite," he says. Within a week, it will start to feel like an old habit.

Avoid late-night snacks. Snacking at night will make you less hungry in the morning, says Robert Klesges, Ph.D., professor of psychology and preventive medicine at Memphis State University. And that, he says, starts a vicious circle: You have no appetite for breakfast, which makes you hungrier in the evening, which makes you snack more at night, he says.

Pour a bowlful. No matter what you eat for breakfast, make part of the meal cereal, says Dr. Stanton. Choose a brand that's low in fat and high in fiber and add some fresh fruit for extra flavor and nutrients.

Flip some flapjacks. Crave something hot from the griddle? There's nothing wrong with pancakes, Dr. Schlundt says, adding that pancakes are high in energy-boosting carbohydrates and low in fat if you make them without a lot of oil.

You can make enough for a week and freeze a single layer on a foil-lined tray. Then stack and wrap them tightly with wax paper or plastic wrap. Just stick two in a toaster oven; that's all it takes for a great breakfast.

Be a smooth operator. Smoothies are delicious, nutrition-packed breakfast drinks that take only a minute or so to make. Take one cut-up piece of fruit, 1 cup of nonfat yogurt (any flavor), ¼ cup of orange juice and a few ice cubes. Whip it all up in a blender and pour it into a glass—or even into your car mug.

Break away from bacon. "Nobody needs to eat meat at breakfast," says Dr. Schlundt. "Eat bread, cereal, juice or fruit, plus skim milk or low-fat yogurt instead.

"With these foods, it's really easy to get full in the morning, and their high carbohydrates are a really good source of energy."

Career Change

Sometimes It's Best to Move On

It used to be that you'd go to school, graduate, find a job and settle into a well-worn career path for the next 44 years until a gold watch told you to get lost. While this arrangement had a lot going for it in the way of security, it could also become something of a straitjacket, with no room to grow or change, no excitement. It was easy to feel trapped, bored, tired...old.

"It's true. If you're in a poorly fitting job and you feel trapped there, it can have a tremendously negative impact on your spirit, motivation and health," says Beverly Potter, Ph.D., lecturer, consultant and author of *Finding a Path with a Heart: How to Go from Burnout to Bliss*. "You actually start feeling fatigued, heavy and down. Your immune system is affected. Your level of general interest is affected. Everything slides."

Luckily, the times (and the careers), they are a-changin'. "You will find that today, most people are going to have four to five separate careers in their lifetime," says Charles Cates, Ph.D., general manager of EnterChange, a national outplacement firm with corporate headquarters in Atlanta. "And that's due not only to corporate downsizing causing forced career change. People today are more interested in finding work that's truly stimulating and satisfying."

And what satisfies you today may not ring your bell tomorrow. "Careers are part of growth, and you occasionally have to shed one like a skin to grow another that's more accommodating," says Patti Hulvershorn, director of Ability Potentials, a career counseling and aptitude measurement service in Alexandria, Virginia. "In fact, I see people getting the career change itch about once every ten years. It first happens between the ages of 28 and 30, then again at 38 to 40 and again between 48 and 50."

But before you rush out to trade in that tired old job for something new and invigorating, there's a lot of planning and self-examination that needs doing. Don't forgo a steady paycheck before you have a solid game plan.

A Career or Just a Job?

Some men have made complete career changes when a better alternative may have been to keep the career but change the job. It's sort of like killing a fly by hitting it with a Lexus.

It's classic. A schoolteacher stuck in a poor district becomes frustrated with the lack of educational funds, teaching materials and administrative support. So he quits and becomes a real estate agent. Fine, except that he loved teaching and the only real problem was the environment, not the career.

When potential career changers go to Dr. Cates, the first thing he looks at is whether the complaints stem from career problems or just problems with the work environment. "If the problem is a matter of personality clashes with the boss, the actual working conditions or the corporate culture, then the best move is to change bosses, change companies, change the whole environment you're working in," he says. "You have to be realistic. The easiest job change is a move to a similar company and a similar job at the same level and salary. And if the problem is one of work environment, this path can solve the situation much more easily than a total career change." But if you really dislike the work itself, then read on.

Making the Big Jump

Okay. You've been a corporate lawyer for ten years, and you are sick of it. You are bored, tired and as cranky as an 80-year-old man who just watched a neighborhood brat's baseball come through his living room window. No amount of fiddling with your current career is going to make you happy. It's time to burst out. But where do you start?

"The first thing to do is make sure you are not just running away from a career you don't like," says Dr. Potter. "Rather than being motivated by escape, you should be motivated by the idea of moving toward something positive—a goal, a dream, something you want."

The consequences of simply running away can be rather ironic. "I knew this man who loved airplanes so much that he became the general manager of an airport," recalls Dr. Potter. "But instead of spending his time around planes, he ended up dealing with labor disputes, lawsuits and bomb threats. He never got to see planes."

After going home night after night miserable and worn out, Dr. Potter's friend picked up his family, moved to California and took a job as a substitute teacher. "He liked teaching and eventually got his credentials to do it full-time," continues Dr. Potter. "But before he knew it, the school, having recognized his organizational skill, was putting him on committees. Then he was on the administrative staff. Finally, he was principal, and instead of teaching, he was handling teachers' strikes, lawsuits and everything else he had escaped only temporarily when he left the airport."

The lesson is, if you don't know what it is you want, you may go the long way around only to end up with what you didn't want in the first place. So here's how to find a direction and a game plan.

Take a good long look at what you like. "You have to ask yourself what parts of your current career you've enjoyed," says Dr. Cates. "And then also look at volunteer work and aspects of your social life that have provided you with satisfaction."

"What do you like to read when you don't have to read anything?" asks Hulvershorn. "What is your subject matter of choice when you read? What has been a continuing interest that you have maintained since you were young or an interest that went by the wayside because you were too busy to keep up with it?"

You're looking for experiences that give you a great deal of either pleasure or satisfaction. "Think of college and high school courses you loved," continues Hulvershorn. "And along those lines, papers you had to write in school that you thoroughly enjoyed researching. Hobbies that always intrigued you. Note the magazines you always pick up first at the dentist's office. Are they technical, financial or intellectual? What part of the newspaper do you read first? All these things can give you clues as to what really interests you."

Find a hook. "When you've found what you like, you've then got to find a hook," says Dr. Cates. "Something you've done in another area, be it volunteer work or professional, that will allow you to swing from your former career to the one you want."

According to Dr. Cates, most men approach career change a little starry-eyed and don't consider the fact that companies hire you for what you've done in the past and what you can do for them in the future. They really don't care how keen you are to embark on a new career. "You have to be able to make a case for yourself. You have to show them that despite your past career path, you are well suited for this new career."

And that means experience. "Get it any way you can," says Dr. Cates. "It may mean a low-paying apprenticeship in your off-hours; it may mean volunteer work. But you need to build a portfolio of experience."

Speak the lingo. Sometimes the ability to show pertinent experience may be no more difficult than presenting what you've done in a new light. Every industry has a language, and if you want to change careers, you'll need to take your past experience and rephrase it so that it seems pertinent to the new job. "For example, a high school teacher who wants to become an in-house corporate training director might describe past experience in terms of group motivation and training plans rather than lessons and curriculum," suggests Dr. Cates.

Explore opportunities in your company. It's possible that a new career may be available from within your own company. It's a possibility that shouldn't be ignored. "Whenever you work at a company for a period of time, you begin to build a power base," says Dr. Potter. "And I don't mean power in the sense of lording it over others. I mean power as the ability to accomplish and influence through your network of relationships and understanding of how things are done at your company. A power base is very valuable and not something to be thrown away lightly by leaving your company."

What Dr. Potter suggests, if possible, is a lateral move within your present organization, such as a move to another department or to a different position. "That way, you keep your power base and can expand on it by gaining knowledge of other areas of the company. In turn, this makes it easier for you to explore new possibilities, and it also makes you more valuable to the company and more likely to get challenging assignments."

Reshape your job. If you can't make a lateral leap, look for ways to expand your current position in the direction of your interests. "I tell people to look for unassigned problems," says Dr. Potter. "These are problems that don't belong to anyone. They are opportunities, and by solving them, they act as vehicles to get you where you want to go."

If, for example, you are a seasoned salesman but you think you might like to teach, perhaps you can volunteer to teach sales techniques to the rookies in your department. The boss might be thrilled to see you take on this new role.

Leave your company but take small steps. You're tired of being an accountant for a cracker company. And having inventoried all your hopes, dreams, values and dislikes, you now know that you want to be a movie director. Go for it, but slowly. "Changing careers in a competitive job market is not an easy thing to do," notes Hulvershorn. "Anything you can do to make your current skills work for you in gaining access to a new career is a big plus."

A good way to make a small step in the right direction is by changing industries without changing job functions. "Become an accountant for a motion picture company," suggests Hulvershorn. "It's easier to get things accomplished, make connections and learn the industry from the inside rather than by looking at want ads." From project accountant on a movie, you might move to associate producer, then executive producer, producer, and maybe someone would then give you a crack at directing.

Go back to school any way you can. When people go to Hulvershorn for a career makeover, it often requires that they go back to school. A lucky few can afford to hit the classroom full-time. Most cannot, and many end up viewing the need for additional school as an insurmountable stumbling block on the road to a new career.

"But what many people don't realize is that due to the increase in career changes, most universities are moving toward more flexible programs to accommodate professionals who haven't the time for the standard route," says Hulvershorn. "The first thing I try to get my clients to do is cut down on their hours or at least work out a flextime deal with their bosses. Maybe they go to school Tuesdays and Thursdays and put in makeup time in the office on Saturdays."

Some schools offer weekend programs where you head for the campus Friday night and come home on Sunday night. Others have correspondence courses. "There's always a way to do it, no matter how impossible it may seem at first," says Hulvershorn. "The important thing is to take the first step, and then you'll be surprised when you realize what you can do."

Think tangentially. "Large or small, the company you currently work for does not operate in a vacuum," notes Dr. Cates. "It has suppliers, and it has clients. The question you need to ask yourself is whether any of the companies currently doing business with your office has anything to offer with respect to your interests."

The advantages to this kind of thinking are many. "First, you speak the same language as these other companies, making it easier to find a possible position with them," says Dr. Cates. "Second, while they may or may not be personally familiar with you, they at least know your company, making you more than just an outsider from off the street."

Lead a Career-Change Lifestyle

With so many people changing careers, Hulvershorn advises getting used to the idea that you, too, may do some career hopping. So be prepared for it. Here are a few tips.

Find activities outside the office. "A hobby at 30 can become a full-blown career at 50," says Hulvershorn. "One of my clients was a stockbroker who happened to have a little farm on the side. He is now a full-time organic farmer. My advice is to constantly be growing through your outside interests in an active way that later can become something more."

Network like there's no tomorrow. "Those most successful in making career changes are those who maintain an elaborate network of people they know outside the industry," says Dr. Cates. "Cultivate contacts in the community, at the PTA or at your kid's sports league. That's how you get referred, and that's how you hear about opportunities an outsider would never know about."

Create a career change slush fund. Career change can be an expensive proposition. Tuition, downtime without pay, business start-up costs and relocation expenses can all be major roadblocks if you don't have ready cash. "I always tell people, especially young lawyers, to never live on their entire income," says Hulvershorn. "If you spend all your money and save none of it, you are basically denying yourself the freedom to explore new possibilities."

Hulvershorn suggests that people try not to expand their lifestyle expenses every time they get a raise. "Instead, put that money into an interest-bearing account that will buy you the freedom you'll need five years down the road when it's time for a change."

Be prepared. "Keep your résumé constantly up-to-date," says Dr. Cates. "And keep an eye on the want ads. This not only makes it easier to make the leap when the time is right, it gets you into a career change mind-set."

Never think it's too late for a career change. "People are always asking me if it's too late to make a career change," says Hulvershorn. Her reply is simple: "You're still breathing, aren't you?"

CHANGE AND ADAPTABILITY

Get Out of That Rut, Already

Imagine if you wore the same clothes to work, ate the same foods, talked to the same people about the same old things and watched the same TV programs day after day. Pretty boring, huh?

Sure, most of us don't get that deeply entrenched in our routines, but more than a few of us could use a booster shot of spontaneity and an occasional splash of change in our lives. For as much as we like routine, occasionally altering course can prevent us from feeling like life is passing us by.

"Staying flexible will keep you from falling into too many ruts," says William Rakowski, Ph.D., assistant professor of medical science at the Center for Gerontology and Health Care Research at Brown University in Providence, Rhode Island. "Leaving room in your life for new things certainly keeps a spark burning within you that helps keep you creative and motivated.

"On the other hand, it's far too easy to say to yourself that you can't change your life because you're getting old," says Dr. Rakowski. "What you're really telling yourself when you say something like that is the future is locked into place and there's nothing you can do to change it. That could be a warning sign that you're giving up too much control of your life. Don't let stuffiness get the better of you."

Why We Resist Change

If you look at your daily life, it's probably very structured. "Most people have their alarms set at a certain time. They take the same route to work, see the same people, watch the same TV programs or listen to the same radio stations day after day," says John Putzier, a Pittsburgh management consultant who conducts seminars nationwide on the importance of change and adaptability. "That's not necessarily bad, because routine is comfortable, and most people do like feeling comfortable in their lives. But as a result, it makes it more difficult for them to adapt to change."

To illustrate his point, Putzier often asks his seminar participants to trade seats with another person in the room. "They don't want to do it. You can't believe the resistance that people have to doing something that simple. In a matter of 30 minutes, they've established their turf. They literally think 'This is my seat, and I'm not going to give it up,' " Putzier says. "I ask them 'If you can't handle this, how do you think you're going to react when somebody comes in and changes your job or expects you to do something in your life differently?' "

So why do we stubbornly cling to old routines? Lack of self-esteem is one of the major roadblocks to change, says Sidney B. Simon, Ed.D., counselor and professor emeritus of psychological education at the University of Massachusetts at Amherst and author of *Getting Unstuck: Breaking Through Your Barriers to Change*. A man, for example, may not believe that he is good enough to have what he really wants, or he may think he doesn't have the skills or willpower to change.

Other men's resolve withers away because they don't get support from family or friends, or they are perfectionists who avoid making a change because they are waiting for an ideal moment or situation that will never occur, Dr. Simon says.

But fear of losing control—which can be experienced as loss of finances, status or respect—is, by far, the most common reason that men resist change. "Fear can be paralyzing. It keeps us stuck in our old ways," says Susan Olson, Ph.D., director of psychological services at the Southwest Bariatric Nutrition Center in Tempe, Arizona. "As we age, we begin to realize that life is bigger than we are and we don't have control over a lot of things. So we start to treasure our little routines and convince ourselves that we are safe within those limits."

Overcoming the Barriers

"That old saying isn't true; an old dog can be taught new tricks, but you have to want to learn," Dr. Olson says. "We can change our thoughts. We can change our actions. We can change our relationships. We don't have to be stuck within our boundaries if they no longer serve us.

"Change doesn't occur overnight," Dr. Olson says. "But if you're persistent, you can learn plenty of ways to limber up your mental flexibility." Here's how.

Tune in. Reprogram your car radio with new stations that you don't regularly listen to. Listen to the new stations—and none of the old ones—for a minimum of three weeks. "It's a mundane thing, but it teaches you to always be on the lookout for ways to break away from your habits and become comfortable with change. Get into the habit of not getting into habits," Putzier says.

Have a few laughs. Take a moment each day to laugh at yourself and the world around you, Dr. Olson suggests. Laughter will help you enjoy your day and open up creative ways of seeing the world.

Make the stars shine on you. "Make a schedule of your daily activities and put a star next to activities you like and a check by activities you don't enjoy. Is there a balance? If not, maybe it's time to make some changes so you get some fun and excitement into your life," Dr. Olson says.

Break the rules. "Most of us have learned that if you have some free time, you should be doing something productive. But ask yourself 'Who wrote that rule in the first place?' " Dr. Olson says. "So if you've mowed the lawn every Sunday evening for the past 15 years, why not skip it one night and do something frivolous, like going to an amusement park?"

Be a leader of the pack. Break away from the crowd and try a sport that your friends say is crazy, like windsurfing. Who knows? You might start a trend. Go to a different type of movie than you've ever seen. "The point is, don't be a follower," Dr. Olson says. "Make your life a unique piece of art."

Do it her way for a day. "Many fights in relationships are over toilet paper and toothpaste," Dr. Olson says. "Why not relax your standards for a day and try it the other person's way? You might find out they had a better idea after all."

Walk a mile in their shoes. "If you have difficulty understanding another person's point of view, close your eyes and imagine that you're that person," says Rebecca Curtis, Ph.D., professor of psychology at Adelphi University in Garden City, New York, and author of *How People Change.* If you work with an egomaniac who can't stop bragging about his achievements, try to imagine what it's like to be him. "Once we start letting these feelings into our consciousness, we realize that we're all human, we all have insecurities and we all have the potential to express them in many different ways," Dr. Curtis says.

Never say "can't." Every time you say you can't do something, write it down. Then beside it, write down the same statement, but this time change "I can't" to "I won't." " 'I can't' is a crippling statement. It takes control out of your hands. 'I won't' makes you realize you're making a choice," Dr. Olson says. "So if you say 'I can't go back to school,' try changing that to 'I won't go back to school because I'm too old.' Suddenly, that empowers you—who really says you're too old?—and you might decide to enroll in some night classes."

Know what friends are for. If you're trying to change an attitude or break a habit, tell a friend or relative about it. Ask that person to point out any time you fall into your old patterns, Dr. Curtis suggests.

Stop, look, listen. When you feel that you're making a judgment, stop and ask yourself if you've considered all viewpoints. Do you really have enough information to make a reasonable conclusion, or are you making a decision based on your biases? "Listen to at least one other person who has a different viewpoint of the situation than you do. You might discover she has a point," says Dorothy Booth, Ph.D., assistant professor in the School of Nursing at the University of Michigan in Ann Arbor.

Plan to act. No change is long-lasting unless you have a plan, Dr. Simon says. So on a sheet of paper, draw a four-column chart. Label the four sections "Do," "Get," "Be" and "Act." In the "Do" column, write down a goal, such as "I want to accept changes in my job." Under "Get," jot down the benefits of achieving that goal, such as "less stress" or "My boss will appreciate my cooperation." In the next column, write down a one-word description of how you'll have to be to reach your goal—in this case, "open-minded." In the last column, list the actions you'll have to take, such as "I need to write a computer program to keep track of the new information my supervisor wants me to gather now." Writing down your plan will make it more likely that you'll follow through on it. "That list is so important that I'd laminate it and carry it in my wallet instead of money," Dr. Simon says.

Forget perfection. Many men who are rigid avoid making decisions, because they fear making the wrong choice. "In their minds, a decision is all good or all bad," Dr. Olson says. If you feel that way, try making a small decision that doesn't feel perfect, like buying a magazine you've never read before. Chances are the world won't end if you don't like it. Try on the habit of congratulating yourself each time you make a "shades of gray" decision. This will help keep you focused away from perfection.

CONFIDENCE
AND SELF-ESTEEM

Stomach In, Chest Out

What do you make of that guy you peer at first thing every morning in the bathroom mirror? Do you see a man who is aging with dignity and grace, a rugged yet sophisticated guy whom women can't help but notice and other men can't help but admire? Or do you see a balding, battle-weary veteran of life whose stomach is too big and whose wallet is too small?

As we men age, funny things can happen to our self-esteem (our appreciation and acceptance of our inner worth) and our confidence (the faith we have in our abilities and talents). For some men, confidence and self-esteem can plummet at the first signs of a potbelly or a sky-bound hairline.

"Our culture places an extremely high premium on youth," says Bonnie Jacobson, Ph.D., director of the Institute for Psychological Change in New York City. "If you use youth as the only benchmark of how good you are, you will inevitably experience feelings of worthlessness and doubt as you show more signs of aging."

But confidence and self-esteem really aren't built on age or appearance. They're a product of attitude. For many men, confidence and self-esteem grow with every passing year.

When allowed to thrive, confidence and self-esteem can turn back the clock. The confident, self-assured man radiates with a youthful strength and energy, says Thomas Tutko, Ph.D., professor of psychology at San Jose State University in San Jose, California. The self-confident man is also more likely to respect and take care of his body by eating right, getting exercise and avoiding harmful things like cigarettes, drugs and booze.

Confidence and self-esteem are also good for our heads. They provide a buffer against anxiety. They relieve feelings of hopelessness, guilt and inadequacy. They give us the courage to fulfill our dreams. And they give us a willingness to try new things and widen our worlds, says Dr. Tutko.

Best of all, confidence and self-esteem are self-perpetuating; the benefits we derive from them tend to boomerang and bolster what we have. In general, the stronger our feelings of confidence and self-esteem, the more satisfied we are with life. And that gives us the power not only to survive but to embrace life.

Fame and Fortune

It's hard to talk of self-esteem and confidence except as a package deal. "A person with high self-esteem has a good picture of himself, and that invariably inspires confidence," says Dr. Tutko. "Likewise, a strong belief in your abilities, and the positive attitude that comes with it, will boost your feelings of self-esteem."

Where do these feelings come from?

According to a study by Robert A. Josephs, Ph.D., and his associates at the University of Texas at Austin, men and women derive confidence and self-esteem from very different places. While a woman's feelings of self-worth are more tied up with her relationships with others, a man's feelings of self-worth are more likely linked to his achievements, attributes and abilities.

That's not to say that the more successful you are, the higher your self-esteem. "Think of all the celebrities and rock stars who have the adoration of millions, have won all kinds of awards and have every kind of wealth, yet they still commit suicide or can't get through a day without drugs," says psychologist Nathaniel Branden, Ph.D., head of the Branden Institute for Self-Esteem in Beverly Hills and author of *The Six Pillars of Self-Esteem*.

Obviously, a man's self-esteem relates to more than fame and fortune. In fact, says Dr. Branden, the man with really solid self-esteem has a sense of self that transcends money and status.

Dr. Jacobson calls it inward vision. "Rather than looking to his peers for approval and status, a man develops a 'positive self-centeredness' and focuses his vision inward," she says. "The only standards he needs to live up to are those that he establishes, and the only person he needs to please is himself."

Hold Your Head High

If you feel that your confidence and self-esteem could use a boost, that's probably a sign that they could. Here's what the experts recommend.

Build your biceps. Can working out improve your self-esteem? It sure can. In one study at the State University of New York College at Brockport, 57 people were divided up into two groups: One group lifted weights for 16 weeks, while the other group completed a physical education theory course. Guess which group wound up with the lifted spirits?

Merrill J. Melnick, Ph.D., the sports sociologist who led the study, explains why the exercise group fared better: "You may see yourself as inferior if you're un-happy with your physical self." By building a little muscle and losing a little fat, he says, you can improve your feelings about your body and yourself.

Gag your internal critic. Guys with low self-esteem tend to hear a little voice in their heads. It says "You can't," "You're weak" and "You're worthless." When-ever your critical inner voice begins putting you down, silence it immediately, says Dr. Jacobson. Be aware of the times it's most likely to appear, such as when you're feeling down. Acknowledge that it's trying to hurt you. Then counter its arguments with assertions to the contrary. Tell yourself over and over that you are strong, ca-pable and worthy until the voice goes away. The same rules apply for external critics, too. "You have to take away the power of other people by learning to accept yourself on your own terms," she says.

Take a personal inventory. "Instead of dwelling on our shortcomings, we need to draw satisfaction from the things we have and can do well," says Stanley Teitelbaum, Ph.D., a clinical psychologist in private practice in New York City. To do this, list all your achievements, activities, traits and strengths on one side of a piece of paper. Then list your weaknesses, negative traits and things you wish you could change about yourself on the other side. You may be surprised to learn just how many pluses you have in your favor. And this alone can make you feel remark-ably good about yourself. Then for long-term confidence and self-esteem, work on accentuating your positives and eliminating your negatives.

Set up a hierarchy of goals. Setting up unrealistic goals for yourself is sure to lead to failure, which can take a toll on your self-esteem. "Reaching for a goal is great, but you must learn to crawl before you can walk," says Dr. Tutko. Suppose you have a goal of bowling a 300 game—a worthy goal, but somewhat unrealistic if your average is, say, 58. Instead of shooting for your ultimate goal, concentrate on reaching plateaus: 100, 150, 200, 250, then 300. "Find success on one level first, then try to transfer it up to the next," he says.

Specialize in something. Are you a jack-of-all-trades and master of none? Are you involved with so many tasks that you can't give adequate attention to any? Spreading yourself too thin only sets you up for disappointment, says Dr. Tutko. Find two or three things in life that you really enjoy—be it playing the clarinet, working with computers or cross-country skiing—and focus most of your energies on them. It's better to be successful at a few things than to fail at many.

Pursue what you love. The easiest way to lose faith in yourself is to get trapped doing something that you dislike or that others tell you "you're supposed to do," says Dr. Tutko. Rather than wallow in a career or activity that makes you miserable or that you attempt halfheartedly, seek out those things that really turn you on and pursue them with gusto. You're more likely to do them well, which will have a positive effect on your psyche.

Be of service. Lending your time and talents to help your community or people in need boosts confidence and self-esteem in many ways, says Dr. Ja-cobson. Foremost, it gives you a wonderful feeling of accomplishment and rein-forces your belief that you are useful and worthwhile.

How's Your Confidence and Self-Esteem?

Do you think highly of yourself, or do you see yourself as over the hill and going headlong into the valley of antiquity? It seems like a simple question, but it's not, says Thomas Tutko, Ph.D., professor of psychology at San Jose State University in San Jose, California. Many men are vaguely aware that they have some kind of problem in their lives, but they can't quite put a handle on it.

Warning Signs of Low Self-Esteem

• You are obsessed with your faults, foibles and mistakes and criticize yourself for them.
• You often let others put you down.
• You frequently try new clothes, diets or gimmicks to make yourself more attractive or acceptable to others.
• You value the judgments and opinions of other people more than your own.
• You frequently compare yourself and your accomplishments with others.
• You feel devastated by negative criticism.
• You become easily disillusioned.

Warning Signs of Low Self-Confidence

• Your daily routine rarely changes.
• You shy away from new challenges and uncomfortable situations.
• You rarely try things a second time.
• You always choose the safe over the risky.
• You measure success solely in terms of winning or acquiring.
• You can't express your inner wants and desires.
• You make up excuses for not doing things or to rationalize why things are the way they are.

Seek out positive people. The last thing you need in your life when your self-confidence is flagging is bores who criticize or find fault with you. Instead, surround yourself with people who look for the good in you. Invariably, those are people who themselves have high levels of confidence and self-esteem. "People with high self-esteem and confidence aren't quick to judge or put down others," says Dr. Jacobson. "They have a lot of love and encouragement to give, and their attitudes toward life can rub off on you."

Reward yourself. Stroke your confidence and self-esteem by doing something nice for yourself whenever you do something well, says Dr. Tutko. Congratulate yourself or treat yourself to a little gift. This reinforces your faith in yourself and gives the value of your accomplishment more weight.

Act your age. "Some people mistakenly believe that if they purchase all the external trappings of youth, it will enhance the way they feel about themselves," says Dr. Teitelbaum. "The truth is, you can't restore youth by buying a Porsche or dressing like a teenager."

Be *your* best, not *the* best. Competitive sports are a great way to enhance your confidence and self-esteem. But if you consider beating opponents and winning trophies the only measures of success, your confidence and self-esteem are already on shaky ground. "Playing sports can be fantastic, but only if you do it for the sheer love of it and for the exploration of being the best you possibly can," says Dr. Tutko.

Don't fear failure. View failure not as an evil but as an opportunity for a new success, says Daniel Wegner, Ph.D., professor of psychology at the University of Virginia in Charlottesville. "Life is a trial-and-error process, and we don't make any progress if we don't take chances in the face of failure," he says. "In the grand scheme of things, most of the actual 'failures' we will experience are not nearly as harmful as the damage we do to ourselves when we obsess and worry about our failures yet to come."

Deflate your worries. Silencing your inner critic isn't always easy. Sometimes you can just slam the door on him; other times he puts up a fight. Sometimes the more you try to suppress unwanted thoughts and anxieties, the more likely you are to become obsessed by them, says Dr. Wegner. Instead of wasting energy suppressing unhappy thoughts, try giving in to them for a little bit. Schedule daily 30-minute "worry sessions" to get them out of your system; then get on with enjoying life.

Get your kicks. Did you ever consider learning a martial art? As professor of psychology and director of the martial arts program at Wake Forest University in Winston-Salem, North Carolina, Charles L. Richman, Ph.D., strongly endorses the attitude-enhancing effects of martial arts. Like other sports, martial arts will build you up and improve your body image, which by itself can improve your self-esteem, he says. They also tend to emphasize discipline and control. "When you combine this disciplined thinking with the mastering of new skills and the realization that you can defend yourself from physical attack, you experience an amazing transformation in both confidence and self-esteem," says Dr. Richman. Check your Yellow Pages or newspaper for schools in your area.

COSMETIC DENTISTRY

Take Your Mouth In for an Overhaul

Let's be blunt. Who's she gonna kiss—Beau, the guy with the White Cliffs of Dover teeth? Or you, the guy with stains all over his choppers?

If your teeth aren't what they once were, don't despair. Cosmetic dentistry can take years off your smile. A cosmetic dentist can remove the stains that reveal lifetime habits of coffee and cigarettes. If you've lost teeth along the way, he can replace them. He can fix chips and cracks and build up surfaces to counteract the wear that comes from decades of chomping ice or gnawing steak.

It's all about looking young, fit and healthy instead of down in the mouth. And today's cosmetic dentistry doesn't mean a jaw full of teeth that look like Chiclets. Results can be so natural that no one will ever know your secret. Here's how it's done.

Whitening: Getting Back the Gleam

By the time you reach your mid-thirties, that pearly smile that melted your mother's heart has dimmed. Teeth tend to yellow over the years as tiny cracks in the enamel soak up stains from coffee, tea, wine, tobacco and food dyes. Fortunately, these age-related stains bleach away very well, says Stephen Sylvan, D.M.D., associate professor of dentistry at the State University of New York at Stony Brook and a dentist in New York City.

Your dentist can offer two good bleaching alternatives.

At-home bleaching takes commitment, but it's a simple process. Your dentist sends you home with a custom-fitted mold that resembles a boxer's mouthguard and a bottle of buffered peroxide gel. You fill the mold with the gel and wear it for three hours daily (usually after dinner or overnight) for two weeks. The cost of the procedure ranges from $150 to $500 for either your uppers or your lowers. (Many people bleach just the uppers, since they show most.)

If you want faster results or dislike wearing the mold, you can ask your dentist for an in-office bleaching. He places a rubber dam over your teeth to protect the gums and applies a stronger peroxide solution that is activated by five to ten minutes under a high-intensity light. After two to four sessions a few weeks apart, for about $200 a visit, your teeth should shine, says Dr. Sylvan. The treatment is painless, but some people have slight tooth sensitivity for a few days afterward. You can renew the bleaching once a year.

Dr. Sylvan points out that there are also over-the-counter bleaching products available, but he doesn't recommend them. They can be too abrasive on teeth and too harsh on gums, and their effectiveness is questionable, he says.

Veneers: Jackets for Your Teeth

Severe stains—like those you got from taking the antibiotic tetracycline as a kid—may need more than bleaching. That's where veneers come in. Ultra-thin porcelain veneers can camouflage not only badly stained teeth but chipped and poorly spaced ones as well.

Veneers are eggshell-thin pieces of porcelain, but they're hardly delicate. They are carved, colored and custom-shaped to the teeth they'll cover and then are attached to the teeth by a process called bonding. The underside of the veneer and surface of the tooth are "etched"—painted with a mild acid that microscopically roughens the surface. Then the surfaces are fused with a type of resin that hardens under a high-intensity light. There's no pain involved, so the process can often be accomplished without the need for anesthetic.

"The bonding of the veneer is so strong that the porcelain becomes an integral part of the tooth," says George Freedman, D.D.S., director of the programs in postgraduate esthetic dentistry at Case Western Reserve University in Cleveland and Baylor College of Dentistry in Dallas.

Making the veneer look natural is an art, says Dr. Freedman. "We can create a whole variety of true-to-life shades and even do a gradient of natural-looking colors on a single tooth. You really can't tell a veneer from a natural tooth, even close up."

Veneers can also be made slightly longer or wider than a tooth to fill in small gaps or make for a better smile. Prices for veneers range greatly—from $350 to $2,500, depending on the area of the country you live in or the severity of your dental problem. But they can last more than ten years, depending on how well you take care of them.

Crowns and Bridges: The Big Guns

Even a veneer may not be able to fix severely decayed, misshapen or badly positioned teeth. That's where dentists need to bring in the heavy weapons—crowns and bridges. Where a veneer is a very thin covering, a crown (or cap) is thicker and heavier and requires grinding down the tooth it will be attached to. A crown is made from porcelain, metal or a combination of the two and then cemented onto a tooth. A bridge is two or more connected crowns.

You and your dentist will need to decide between all porcelain and porcelain over metal. Porcelain usually looks more natural when there's no metal behind it, but you may need the metal base for back teeth, where the pressure from chewing is greater, says Irwin Smigel, D.D.S., president of the American Society for Dental Aesthetics. And some new porcelains are so good that they look convincing even over metal. "It used to be that the metal backing always made the crown look artificial," says Barry G. Dale, D.M.D., a cosmetic and general dentist in private practice in Englewood, New Jersey. "But the new porcelains provide close to lifelike quality."

What's the procedure like? Well, first your dentist numbs your gums with an anesthetic, then grinds down about 1½ millimeters of your tooth (otherwise, you'd have something fatter than the original tooth, which would look out of place and could irritate the gum). During a second visit, he cements the custom-shaped crown or crowns into place.

Are You Big Enough for Braces?

Braces aren't just kid stuff anymore. "They are appropriate for people of almost any age," says Mervin W. Graham, D.D.S., a Denver orthodontist in private practice whose oldest patient with braces is 65.

But at any age, braces work the same way. Here's how, according to Dr. Graham: The braces' tightened wires and rubber band elastics push on your teeth. Bone on one side of a tooth's root breaks down, allowing the tooth to move. And bone builds up on the other side of the tooth, ensuring that it will fit snugly into its new home.

The process starts with a fitting, after which you'll need to visit your orthodontist for regular adjustments. Your teeth will be somewhat sore for a few days after each visit. Depending on how much your teeth are misaligned, the time you'll need to wear your braces can vary from one to several years.

The price of braces will depend on the severity of the correction but can range from $1,800 to $4,500. If you decide to make the investment, don't worry—nobody will call you Metalmouth. When you were a kid, braces meant good-size stainless steel straps and bands around each tooth. But these days, you can be fitted with tiny brackets made from steel or even nearly invisible tooth-colored porcelain, says Dr. Graham.

Implants—Dentures That Don't Budge

You need a partial or complete denture to fill in your missing teeth, but you gag at the thought. You'd feel like your grandfather. How about new, natural-looking teeth that are permanently attached to your jaw?

They're dental implants. "Implants, because they're fixed in your mouth, are akin to having your own teeth," says Albert Guckes, D.D.S., deputy clinical director of the National Institute of Dental Research in Bethesda, Maryland. Here's how they work.

A tiny metal cylinder made from lightweight titanium, the same metal used for replacement hips, is surgically placed into your jawbone. Then a thin metal post is screwed into the cylinder. This part of the procedure, usually done under local anesthesia, will leave your mouth sore and swollen for about a week.

The next part of the procedure takes place about six months later. By then, bone has grown tightly around the metal cylinder. It's in rock-solid. Your new artificial tooth is mounted onto the metal post.

For each implant post, you'll pay between $750 and $1,500. Then you ante up for the replacement teeth—usually an additional $1,000 each. That's a lot of loot. But given that implants can last up to 20 years, you may consider them a worthwhile investment, Dr. Guckes says.

Crowns cost between $450 and $1,000 each and last 10 to 15 years.

How will your mouth feel with a crown in place? "It's a foreign body, so it's natural that the bite may feel a little strange," Dr. Smigel says. If after a week you still have discomfort, check with your dentist to have the fit adjusted.

Dentist Shopping

Needless to say, any cosmetic procedure is going to be only as good as the dentist who does it. You might ask a friend who has undergone cosmetic dental procedures for his recommendations.

Or you could contact the American Society for Dental Aesthetics (ASDA). "Dentists applying for membership present before-and-after cases before the society's board," says Diana Okula, ASDA secretary. "And they're judged not only on how good the results are functionally but also on how the results look."

Write to the ASDA at 635 Madison Avenue, New York, NY 10022. Enclose a self-addressed, stamped envelope, and they'll send you a list of recommended dentists in your area.

COSMETIC SURGERY

More Men Are Opting for a Nip and Tuck

You'd be surprised who gets cosmetic surgery these days. We all know about actors, and executives with salaries in the stratosphere, but would you believe construction workers? Athletes? One of your office buddies?

Plastic surgeons report that men—all sorts of men—make up increasingly large portions of their practices. For many of these men, the motivation is the same: They want to look younger.

If you're concerned about aging and the thought of going under the knife doesn't deter you, the technology is out there. Surgical techniques have been refined and simplified, and most cosmetic procedures involve a lot less trauma than they used to.

Most of today's cosmetic surgery is performed on an outpatient basis. You're home the same day and often to work after a couple of days. Sometimes local anesthesia is all that's needed, or tranquilizers plus a local anesthesia to put you in "twilight sleep"—a sort of dozy fog you barely remember afterward. Recovery times are shorter than they used to be, but they can vary widely depending on the individual, the surgeon and the procedure.

Don't Rush

Before you plan your before-and-after photos, a quick word about what you don't want cosmetic surgery for. You don't want it for just a few fine lines or moderate sun damage. For these, a dermatologist can offer you a variety of effective treatments, including chemical peels, wrinkle-filling injections and the prescription cream tretinoin (Retin-A).

But there are larger changes that happen to men and their bodies as the years go by. Wrinkles may become furrows, jowls may form, apple cheeks can go from boyish to lean to sunken, and of course, there are often love handles. Blame these changes on gravity, years of sun exposure, inactivity or genes from your Uncle Harry who looked like a geriatric bulldog at age 35.

Whatever your desired change, surgery is a serious undertaking and should never be treated as a whim. "For certain guys, surgery would never be right. There's no going back on it," says Alan Matarasso, M.D., a plastic surgeon at the Manhattan Eye, Ear and Throat Hospital in New York City. Of course, for other guys it could be just the ticket to newfound youthfulness. Here's a hand to holly look at the options.

Reshaping a Face

The newest facial plastic surgery techniques won't leave you wearing the tight, stretched-looking mask that Hollywood made famous. A good surgeon won't promise miraculous results, either, or decades off your looks. But he will offer you very natural-looking, subtle corrections for many age-related changes. Friends will remark how well rested you look—like you just took a long vacation.

Forehead lift. A forehead lift smooths a slouching brow and also eases deep crow's-feet and frown lines, says Dr. Matarasso. "This procedure is virtually painless," he says. "All stitches are hidden in the hairline, and though you may have swelling along the cheeks and some bruising, you could go back to work in as early as 48 hours."

Blepharoplasty. If you have that nothin'-but-a-hound-dog look, the change is dramatic when a surgeon removes fatty pouches under the eyes and tightens saggy upper lids with a procedure called blepharoplasty. Through minimal incisions hidden in the natural creases of the lids, the surgeon removes the fat and trims away excess skin. The result is a firmer, younger-looking, less tired-appearing eye area, says Dr. Matarasso.

Rhinoplasty. Your nose changes as you age, says Dr. Matarasso. It can droop a little toward the upper lip, thicken or get more bulbous. Nowadays most nose repairs (rhinoplasties) are done without the classic fracture, and the results are masculine and natural rather than the piggy-looking, scooped-out look of yore. The bottom third of the cartilage is delicately sculpted during the surgery, and the skin redrapes over it, he says.

Implants. Ever seen a long-distance runner in his thirties who looks 50? That's because marathon athletes can metabolize the fat in the face, or "the stuffing that gives the contour," says Geoffrey Tobias, M.D., a plastic surgeon at Mount Sinai School of Medicine of the City University of New York, in New York City. If you're looking haggard rather than fit, solid silicone implants can also be used to fill out hollow cheeks, he says. An implant can be inserted from small incisions within the mouth. "These implants don't contain the liquid silicone used in women's breast implants that has caused some problems in the past," Dr. Tobias says.

Upper face-lift. How would you look with an upper face-lift? "Look in the

Choosing a Plastic Surgeon

The first thing you should get from a surgeon is a realistic appraisal, says Michael Sachs, M.D., a plastic surgeon in private practice in New York City. "Cosmetic surgery can improve your appearance and help you make the most of your assets, but it won't cure an ailing relationship or get you a better job," he says.

Although the best reference is often from a friend who has already had the procedure you're contemplating, there are other steps you can take to find a reliable surgeon, says Alan Matarasso, M.D., a plastic surgeon at the Manhattan Eye, Ear and Throat Hospital in New York City. He recommends calling a county or state medical society or nearby teaching hospital and asking them to refer you to a surgeon or surgeons in your area certified by the American Society of Plastic and Reconstructive Surgeons. Or you can write this organization yourself at 444 East Algonquin Road, Arlington Heights, IL 60005.

Dr. Sachs recommends that you start with these basic questions at your first appointment.

What's my problem? Can the doctor pinpoint what specifically is causing you to look older than you'd like?

How will this procedure help? Exactly what's involved in the procedure the doctor is recommending? What steps will be followed, and how long will it take? What kind of anesthesia and pain relief will be offered?

Will I have a noticeable scar? Will there be any visible scars left behind after the healing process is over?

How risky is it? What could go wrong? How likely are any complications?

What will I look like afterward? Can the doctor give you a realistic idea of what this surgery will do for you?

What's it going to cost? Will your insurance pay for part of it? How much will the total bill be?

If you have lingering questions, don't hesitate to ask for a second appointment, says Dr. Matarasso. "And watch out for slick promoters," he says. "Chances are they're not out for your benefit."

mirror, put your index fingers by your sideburns, your thumbs by the corners of your jaw, and tug up and back a little," says Dr. Matarasso. Fat beneath the skin is removed by liposuction—a technique that actually vacuums out fat from under the skin—and sagging skin and muscle beneath are tightened. "In the past, they'd tighten only the skin, which gave that masklike stretched look," says Dr. Matarasso. "Now face-lifts are customized to each person's anatomy."

Lower face-lift. What man wouldn't hate it when his Dick Tracy jawline turns into Turkey Joe's? Or when a few too many double-chocolate scoops leave him with a double chin or a neck that hangs over his shirt collar? For a lower face-lift, a plastic surgeon firms up the neck by tightening cords of muscle and removes fat to resculpt the chin to a firm right-angle shape, says Dr. Matarasso. "Stitches are hidden behind the ear. Some people just have the neck lift, and some do both the neck and face," he says.

Trimming Those Love Handles

While you're down for the count under a general anesthetic or local anesthesia, the surgeon makes a small incision in your belly or groin. Next he inserts a blunt-tipped tube. With vigorous movements, he guides the tube back and forth under the skin over your belly or waistline. The tube is hooked up to vacuum that can suck out up to four pounds of fat.

That's liposuction. It sounds great, but liposuction is far from an instant weight loss plan. Removing large amounts of fat has limitations. It's ideally performed on people who are at or near their normal range in body weight and who have pockets of stubborn flab that remain despite diet and exercise, says Dr. Matarasso.

After the surgery, you're put into a stretchy, girdlelike garment that you wear under your clothes for two to four weeks to keep swelling down and your skin smooth while it contracts to its new foundation. This procedure can be performed on a Friday, and the patient can return to work on a Monday, says Dr. Matarasso. In most patients, the discoloration subsides in about two weeks, and the swelling completely disappears in about six months.

When fat cells are sucked away, they're gone for good. If you think that liposuction will let you pack in the beer and burgers unfazed, though, think again. Excess calories will still be stored in fat cells somewhere else in your body, and you could find yourself in the same dilemma elsewhere.

Are you up for liposuction? You'll be a better candidate if you're in good health and under age 50, when your skin is more pliable and elastic, surgeons say.

CREATIVITY

Liberating a Potent Force

The bluebird house sits in the middle of your worktable, perfectly calibrated to meet the needs of a small, vulnerable family of baby birds. You've designed the house so that the hole is too small for a squirrel but large enough for a baby bluebird, who will need to sit on the edge, ruffle its wings and check out the world before it takes off. You've also sanded any rough spots or edges so that the birds cannot be harmed.

And you've thoughtfully constructed the house so that one wall can swing open for "spring cleaning" after the birds have flown.

Yeah, you did it for your kid. But the fact is that it was your creativity that produced the house—your careful consideration of the birds' needs, your planning and design, your construction of something from nothing.

Many of us think of creativity only in connection with writing symphonies, directing a play or sculpting fountains. But it's actually something we use every day to solve problems, invent products, develop new technologies and, yes, even build birdhouses. Because creativity, experts agree, is simply the act of making, inventing or producing. And using our creativity is as necessary as breathing.

"I call everyday creativity mindfulness—when we focus on the process of inventing as opposed to the outcome. This everyday creativity or mindfulness is actually good for one's health and well-being," explains Ellen J. Langer, Ph.D., professor of psychology at Harvard University in Cambridge, Massachusetts, and author of *Mindfulness*.

It's so essential to our existence that the newness, surprise and variety provided by our creativity actually fuel our will to live. Dr. Langer's research with the elderly has shown that when the elderly are encouraged to be creative or mindful, as she says, they actually live longer and happier lives. "When we don't keep our minds active, the mind and body gradually turn themselves off," says Dr. Langer.

Creativity Killers

Some days creativity flows through your body and out into the world without effort. Other days it's as though the flow is blocked by an impenetrable wall.

"Creativity is a fragile commodity that can be suppressed or impaired much easier than it can be turned on," says Teresa Amabile, Ph.D., professor of psychology at Brandeis University in Waltham, Massachusetts.

But you can prevent interfering with its flow by avoiding these creativity killers.

People who say your ideas will never work. Constructive criticism is one thing, but the knee-jerk reaction of a skeptic to almost anything— "It won't work"—is not constructive criticism.

Drugs and alcohol. There is no good scientific evidence that creativity can be chemically enhanced. In the long run, these substances have the potential to destroy your creative abilities far more than they could possibly enhance them.

Material motivation. According to Dr. Amabile, most creative motivation comes from within, but extrinsic motivators—like money, fame, awards and acceptance—can severely dampen our creative powers.

Keeping score. The pressure of having to score points, meet certain standards or live up to others' expectations can seriously stifle your creative abilities, says Dr. Amabile. Ultimately, the most important judge you have to please is yourself, she says.

Creating in a crowd. How creative could you be if you knew your teacher, boss or the whole world was looking over your shoulder every minute? Dr. Amabile's research has shown that such environments can stifle creativity. Try to work in a setting that will put some distance between you and a pair of penetrating eyes.

Too little time. The ticking of the clock, the rigidity of a schedule or the finality of a rapidly approaching deadline can hinder the evolution of a great idea, says Dr. Amabile. Try working at a comfortable, even pace.

In other words, when we stop creating, we stop enjoying life, and there's less life to enjoy.

Fortunately, the ability to create remains virtually intact all our lives, although the actual number of certain types of products we might create—the number of paintings, gardens or sculptures—may decline as we get older.

"Creative productivity generally peaks at age 30 for math, science, poetry and anything that requires abstract thinking," says Carolyn Adams-Price, Ph.D., assistant professor of psychology at Mississippi State University in Starkville. "For history, philosophy, writing and anything that requires a lot of knowledge, it generally peaks at 60."

But it's only the number of creative products that declines, not the ability to create or the quality of what's produced, emphasizes Dr. Adams-Price.

If a poet wrote 100 poems a year at his peak age of 30, for example, he may produce only 10 a year at 60. But because the quality of his work remains unchanged, his chances for a Pulitzer Prize are the same at both ages.

Sharpening Your Creative Edge

Historically, men have had a distinct advantage over women when it comes to getting help in developing their creativity.

Studies show that more often than not, society has been quicker to provide men with educational possibilities, admission to professional societies and other specialized training to stimulate their creativity. Studies show, too, that teachers have more readily tended to reinforce creative behavior in boys while expecting girls to be well behaved and eager to follow the rules. Experts have also suggested that our culture's encouragement of a boy's natural assertiveness, dominance, ego and risk taking—in everything from football to physics—could perhaps help young men to develop the drive, single-mindedness and persistence necessary to pursue their own creative visions in a culture often hostile to creativity.

How can you liberate every ounce of creativity within? All it takes is a single idea and a desire to explore. Here's how to get started.

Consider the waffle cone. Necessity is the father of invention. Ask yourself: "What could the world really use right now? Creative alternatives to nursing homes for the elderly? Ways to capitalize on the talent of retired individuals?" Often the first step requires merely identifying a problem, says Dr. Langer. From there your ideas can branch off in hundreds of different directions.

One way to come up with good ideas is to think up many ideas without judging them. Then simply choose the good ones, says Dr. Langer. Alone or in a group, scribble out an idea on a sheet of paper. Then drawing inspiration from the first idea, jot down as many related ideas as possible. Compile a laundry list of ideas, go through it carefully and pull out the ones you like best. Discard the others.

"Sometimes a great idea is merely taking an older idea and turning it on its head," says Gabriele Rico, Ph.D., professor of English and creative arts at San Jose State University in San Jose, California, and author of *Pain and Possibility*. For example, ice cream was once served on top of a flat waffle. But some innovative thinker chose to fold that waffle into a funnel, and voilà! The world had its first waffle cone.

Don't Go Away Mad . . .

Eccentricity is not uncommon among creative geniuses. Accounts of emotionally disturbed writers, poets, composers, scientists and philosophers are easy to find in history books. We could start with Vincent van Gogh, Franz Kafka, Eugene O'Neill, Ernest Hemingway, Charles Darwin and Ezra Pound, but the list goes on and on.

Does this mean that highly creative people are more likely to be mad than the rest of us? It's an intriguing question. But despite the best efforts of science, the answer is still not clear.

In a study of more than 1,000 men and women conducted at the University of Kentucky in Lexington, researcher Arnold M. Ludwig, M.D., found that poets, writers, artists, musicians and others in creative professions were more likely to exhibit a tendency toward madness than people who were public officials, businessmen and military officers and in supposedly less creative jobs.

Those in the theater demonstrated higher rates of alcohol and drug abuse, manic episodes, anxiety disorders and suicide attempts. Writers were more inclined toward depression and alcohol. Artists had more alcohol-related problems, depression, anxiety and adjustment difficulties. Musicians and composers were more likely to be depressed. Poets were more prone to alcohol and drug abuse, depression, mania, suicide and psychosis in general.

The tendency toward madness in creative people seems simple until you consider a couple of points, as Dr. Ludwig does in his study. First, the demands on those in the more creative professions may be more likely to aggravate already existing problems. If you were genetically predisposed to depression, for example, a career in the theater might push you over the edge into depression, while a career as a banker might not.

A second point is that since our culture expects its writers and artists to be weird and its military officers and bankers to be stable, professions such as music and art may simply attract people who are predisposed to excess, while professions such as banking and the military attract people who are more likely to want a more regulated life.

Jot down ideas and dreams. Great ideas can materialize and vanish in an instant, so many creative men keep a log or diary to record ideas that come to them throughout the day, says Dr. Rico. All you need is a small notebook that fits in your pocket or briefcase or even under your pillow, since dreams can be rich in creativity, too.

"The mind makes some of its most unique connections and associations while you are asleep," says Dr. Rico. So start the day off by scribbling what you remember of your dreams on a notepad.

Take another look at failures. Mistakes and unexpected results can yield the biggest rewards of all, says Dr. Langer. For example, a new glue developed by the 3M Company was thought to be a failure because it wasn't sticky enough. But when that glue was applied to a sheet of paper, it became one of the most innovative office products of all time: Post-it Notes. So the next time you have an apparent "bomb" on your hands, don't be so quick to condemn it. Instead, turn it around and look at it from another direction.

Think for yourself. "One of our society's drawbacks is that it encourages inhibition and blind conformity," says Dr. Langer. "We become afraid to look at the world from different perspectives to challenge established ideas."

Ever notice that in some business meetings, everyone waits for the Big Boss to speak? Then what do they do? Do they express their own unique ideas? Or do they follow the mental tracks laid down by the Big Boss and simply expand on his thinking?

To enhance creativity, we must be willing to unlearn many of the conventions we've spent a lifetime learning. A creative person should not be afraid to challenge ideas or to think in directions others may consider unorthodox.

Learn. If you've chosen to express your creativity in a particular medium such as paint or song, learn as much about the medium as possible, says Dr. Rico. Start slowly, practice in your medium regularly and gain familiarity with your strengths and weaknesses. As your knowledge and skill increase, your ability to manipulate your chosen medium to express your creativity will expand.

Improve on the best. Stimulate your own creativity by studying the work of some of the creative giants in your area of interest, says Dr. Rico. But don't be a copycat. Imitation is not creativity. Instead, use someone else's work to get yourself thinking in ways you never considered. Or take themes they've explored in their work, approach them from another angle and come up with something new.

Explore yourself. The creative man must be willing to delve into a wide range of deep-seated emotions, experiences and memories. "Older people often use their personal experience as a source of creativity," says Dr. Adams-Price.

Explore the world. Most of us draw inspiration and creative energy from the things around us: the sight of a sunset, the aroma of a flower, the sound of a train whistle, the touch of moss. "The more things we know, feel and experience about our world, the more creative we will be," says Dr. Rico.

FIBER

Keeping You Young Inside and Out

Mom always knew best. Okay, so maybe those accordion lessons didn't exactly come in handy. But everything else she made you do was right on the money. Like when she had you start your day with oatmeal. And when she packed your lunch with carrots and apples—what she used to call roughage.

Today, science has proven what Mom always said: There's something special about fruits, vegetables and grains that really does do a man's body good. And roughage is what nutritionists now call dietary fiber, one of the simplest and most potent weapons we have in our age-erasing arsenal.

Fiber is a frontline warrior in the battle against heart disease, cancer, atherosclerosis, high cholesterol, high blood pressure, constipation, digestive problems, diabetes and even overweight. Get enough fiber, and your body will be healthier and will run like a well-oiled machine.

But most men don't get enough fiber. The recommended intake is at least 25 grams of fiber every day. "Most Americans, however, consume only about one-third of that total," says Diane Grabowski, R.D., nutrition educator at the Pritikin Longevity Center in Santa Monica, California.

A Natural Remedy

Fiber is a complex mixture of indigestible substances that make up the structural material of plants. It has very few calories and provides little food energy to the body. When we ingest it, it passes through our system without being broken down.

Fiber works its magic by carrying the bad stuff—like cholesterol, bile acids and other toxins—out of our system. And it comes in two basic forms: soluble, which dissolves in water, and insoluble, which doesn't. Most plant foods contain both types of fiber, though certain foods are richer in one or the other.

The coarser, insoluble fibers really live up to the word *roughage*. "They literally scour you out," says David Jenkins, M.D., Ph.D., director of the Clinical Nutrition and Risk Factor Modification Center at St. Michael's Hospital, University of Toronto. They absorb water, making stools softer, bulkier and easier to pass. This keeps food moving through the intestinal tract.

It also makes a natural remedy for ills such as constipation, irritable bowel syndrome, diverticulosis and hemorrhoids.

Soluble fibers act differently. Inside the body, they become gummy and sticky. As they move through the digestive tract, they pick up bile acids and other toxins, then haul them out of the body.

Squaring Off against Disease

Fiber plays a vital role in the offensive against heart disease and atherosclerosis. Studies show that a diet high in soluble fiber reduces blood levels of low-density lipoprotein (LDL) cholesterol, the so-called bad cholesterol. A study by Dr. Jenkins found that high intakes of soluble fiber continued to lower cholesterol even after dietary reductions of fat and cholesterol.

"Cholesterol builds up in our blood and clogs arteries if it is not excreted as bile acids from our digestive tract," says Dr. Jenkins. "When soluble fiber carries these substances out of the body, it draws cholesterol out of the bloodstream to be converted into more bile, which we continue to flush out of the body—as long as we regularly consume soluble fiber."

Other studies have shown that fiber is effective at lowering blood pressure, thereby reducing your risk of heart attack and stroke.

That's not all fiber can do. A high-fiber diet appears to lower your risk for colon and rectal cancer. It does this by diluting the concentration of bile acids and carcinogens and moving stools quickly through the intestines, decreasing the time the colon wall is in contact with carcinogens. Also, fiber increases the acidity of the colon, making it less hospitable to cancer-causing toxins.

Fiber can also help you better manage diabetes by controlling blood sugar and thus reducing the need for insulin. Fiber delays the emptying of the stomach, causing the sugars in your food to be absorbed more gradually.

A fiber-filled diet makes weight loss a lot easier, too, because it fills you up—meaning you're going to eat a lot less. Fibrous foods provide robust mouthfuls that must be chewed thoroughly, slowing down your eating time. And they tend to have fewer calories in every bite.

Bran: Where to Find a Lot of It

One surefire way to get a heap of fiber into your diet is by eating bran, the coarse outer layers of oats, wheat, rice and corn that contain the highest concentrations of fiber.

Consider oat bran, the bran that has received a lot of public attention. "What sets oat bran apart from other brans is that it is extremely high in a fiber called beta-glucan," says bran researcher Michael H. Davidson, M.D., medical director of the Chicago Center for Clinical Research at Rush-Presbyterian–St. Luke's Hospital. "Beta-glucan appears to be far more effective than other soluble fibers in lowering blood cholesterol levels."

How effective? Studies indicate that just two ounces of oat bran per day (a medium-size bowl) is enough to lower your LDL cholesterol 10 to 15 percent. The catch is that you have to eat oat bran daily; otherwise, your cholesterol levels will creep back up.

Wheat bran is jam-packed with insoluble fiber, so it's the bran of choice for people with digestive problems. This is probably the most common bran, found in most bran breakfast cereals and all whole-wheat products.

Rice, oat and corn bran are high in both soluble and insoluble fiber.

Unless your physician says otherwise, the best bran plan for most men is to get a smattering of each. This way, you'll get a healthy dose of soluble and insoluble fiber, not to mention some variety in your diet.

Getting your fill of bran is as easy as eating a bran breakfast cereal, a bran muffin or a whole-grain bread. But make sure you're always getting the goodness of the bran. "Refined grain products like white rice, white bread and most flour have had the fiber-rich bran removed in the milling process," says Grabowski. "Instant oatmeal, for example, has a lot less fiber than whole oats or pure oat bran."

Adding Fiber to Your Life

Making the commitment to a high-fiber diet is relatively easy. Here are some tips.

Ease into it. As great as fiber is, too much too fast can have some nasty side effects, including gas, bloating, diarrhea and cramps, says Dr. Jenkins. Start off your first week by increasing your intake by about five grams a day. Then take about a month to work up to the recommended level. From there, if your doctor says it's okay and if you feel no ill effects, you can increase your intake.

Don't dry out. We all know a high-fiber diet helps constipation, but if you don't get enough water, it can actually have an opposite effect and clog you up, says Dr. Jenkins. Drink eight to ten glasses of water a day.

Vary your sources. Doctors aren't certain what ratio of soluble to insoluble you should use when choosing your daily fiber sources, says Dr. Jenkins, so it's probably wise to get an even dose of both. The best way to do that is to eat a wide variety of fiber-rich foods throughout the day.

Go for the green. Brans and grains are not the only sources of fiber. "Don't forget your fresh fruits and vegetables," advises Grabowski. Legumes, beans, peas, salads and fruits can add a lot of that much-needed fiber to your diet. To get some extra fiber, select fruits that have edible seeds, such as strawberries and kiwis, suggests Grabowski.

(continued on page 422)

Getting Enough:
It's Easier Than You Think

Do 25 grams of fiber a day seem impossible to consume? Not if you know where to get them. Here's some help.

Food	Portion	Fiber (g.)
BREADS AND BREAD PRODUCTS		
Whole-wheat	1 slice	2.1
Pumpernickel	1 slice	1.9
English muffin	1	1.6
Rye	1 slice	1.6
Bagel	1	1.2
Waffle	1	0.8
White	1 slice	0.5
CEREALS		
All-Bran with Extra Fiber	½ cup	15.0
Fiber One	½ cup	14.0
Bran Buds	⅓ cup	11.0
All-Bran (original)	½ cup	10.0
Raisin Bran	1 cup	7.0
Fiberwise	⅔ cup	5.0
Grape-Nuts	½ cup	5.0
Common Sense Oat Bran	¾ cup	4.0
Cheerios (original)	1 cup	3.0
Frosted Bran	⅔ cup	3.0
Nutri-Grain Wheat	⅔ cup	3.0
Spoon Size Shredded Wheat	⅔ cup	3.0
Total (original)	¾ cup	3.0
Wheaties	1 cup	3.0
Puffed Rice	1 cup	1.2
Product 19	1 cup	1.0
Rice Krispies	1¼ cups	1.0
Special K	1 cup	1.0

Food	Portion	Fiber (g.)
FRUITS		
Strawberries, fresh	1 cup	3.9
Dates	5 medium	3.5
Orange	1	3.1
Apple, unpeeled	1	3.0
Applesauce	½ cup	1.9
Pineapple, canned	1 cup	1.9
Banana	1	1.8
Prunes	3 medium	1.8
Cantaloupe, cubed	1 cup	1.3
Grapes	1 cup	1.1
Orange juice	½ cup	0.1
LEGUMES AND BEANS		
Black-eyed peas, boiled	½ cup	8.3
Red kidney beans, canned	½ cup	7.9
Chick-peas, canned	½ cup	7.0
Pork and beans, canned	½ can	6.9
Lentils, dried, cooked	½ cup	5.2
Pinto beans, boiled	½ cup	3.4
VEGETABLES		
Brussels sprouts, cooked	½ cup	3.4
Peas, frozen	½ cup	2.4
Carrot, raw, 7½ in.	1	2.3
Broccoli, cooked	½ cup	2.0
Green beans, frozen	½ cup	1.8
Mushrooms, cooked	½ cup	1.7
Tomato	1 medium	1.6
Beets, canned	½ cup	1.4
Iceberg lettuce, shredded	1 cup	1.4
Corn, canned	½ cup	1.2
Celery, chopped	½ cup	1.0

Add a few sprinkles. "Fiber is easy to obtain in your diet if you include whole foods such as whole-wheat bread, beans, peas and fresh fruits and vegetables," says Grabowski. For additional fiber, pick up a box of oat bran at the grocery store and sprinkle it on yogurt, ice cream, fruit, cereal and salad. Use it in place of bread crumbs in meat loaf or stuffings or as a thickener for soups, stews and sauces. Or substitute oat bran for white flour in baked goods.

Read labels carefully. Don't assume that a product with the word *fiber*, *bran* or *oats* in its title necessarily has the fiber content you're looking for. Always check the nutritional information on the box or bag to see just how much fiber is available in each serving. "Also, look for the word *whole* to precede *grain* on the ingredient list," suggests Grabowski. "This way, you know nothing has been removed, and you are assured of getting the full benefit of the bran."

Avoid fiber pills. Fiber pills and drink mixes are a quick way to get more fiber, but most professionals don't recommend them, says Grabowski. They're expensive, and it takes several pills and drinks to equal the fiber content of a piece of fruit. Your best bet is to meet your fiber requirements by eating foods that are naturally rich in fiber.

Go whole. Slight changes in the way you eat can infuse your diet with fiber, says Grabowski. Instead of your morning glass of orange juice, try eating a whole piece of fruit, since almost all the fiber gets left behind in the juicing process. Serve whole brown rice instead of white. And if you're a meat-and-potatoes guy, substitute a baked potato with the skin in place of mashed spuds.

High fiber alone won't do. Many men think that eating fiber gives them a ticket to load up on fatty junk foods and snacks. Not so. "A high-fiber diet doesn't somehow neutralize or balance out other unhealthy eating habits," says Dr. Davidson. "Eating an extra candy bar or cheeseburger only makes it harder for fiber to do its job. Fiber will work only when used in conjunction with a low-fat, low-cholesterol diet and plenty of exercise."

FLUIDS

Life's Liquid Assets

Take two hydrogen atoms, stick them on an oxygen atom, and what do you get? Your old high school science fair project? No. A nuclear weapon? Uh-uh. Only the most abundant compound on earth. A vital nutrient. And a powerful age-erasing ally.

Congratulations, Professor. You have yourself some water. H_2O. A substance so simple, so common, so ordinary that it's easy to overlook how important it is.

For starters, water is present in every cell and tissue of your body and plays a vital role in almost every biological process from digestion to respiration to circulation. It transports nutrients throughout the body and carries harmful toxins and waste products out of the body. It regulates our body temperature. And it lubricates our joints and organs to keep them in working order.

Because water does so much, the body needs a constant fresh supply. "Water needs to continuously flow into, through and out of the body," says Diane Grabowski, R.D., a nutrition educator with the Pritikin Longevity Center in Santa Monica, California. "A minimum of two to three quarts is eliminated daily in our urine, sweat and breath, all of which must be replaced."

That's just to meet our minimal health needs. Getting plenty of water is essential for maintaining everything from youthful skin to strong muscles. "Consistently meeting your daily fluid needs makes all the organs in your body function better," says Grabowski. "It's a key ingredient if you want to look, feel and perform at your very best."

The Wonders of Water

Unless you're a camel, your body can go only about three days without a refill before the buzzards start picking on your parched corpse. But don't think that dehydration occurs only when you're as dry as the Sahara. You can technically be dehydrated even if your internal fluid levels dip just a bit below normal.

423

Ordinarily, this is no problem, because your sense of thirst will holler "Hey, pal! How about something to drink?" But sometimes your thirst-detecting powers are thrown off by other factors, such as hot weather, high altitude, exercise—and your age. Yes, while it isn't always obvious, our thirst sensitivity begins to diminish as we age.

When you become dehydrated, you lose not only water but also valuable electrolytes—essential minerals like potassium and sodium—which can leave you feeling especially tapped out. The feeling is like a hangover; you're achy, drained and feeling out of it. "When your body gets even a little low on fluids, physical performance and brain power can hit the skids," says Miriam Nelson, Ph.D., a research scientist and exercise physiologist in the Human Physiology Laboratory at the U.S. Department of Agriculture Human Nutrition Research Center on Aging at Tufts University in Boston. "Long before you experience the sensation of thirst, your body can produce symptoms like fatigue, dizziness, headache and flushed skin. All these conditions are caused by an increase in body temperature."

Frequent or long-term dehydration can really take a toll, causing irregular heartbeat, an unsteady gait, difficulty swallowing and shortness of breath. Extreme cases of dehydration can produce shriveled skin and lips.

Meeting Your Fluid Needs

You don't have to limit yourself to plain water, though. Experts recommend that we need to consume six to eight eight-ounce glasses of liquid a day. This can mean six to eight glasses of water, milk, juices, broths or other beverages.

"Heavier people require more, so a good rule is to try to drink about one-half ounce for each pound of body weight," says Grabowski. If you weigh 200 pounds, that comes out to 12½ eight-ounce glasses per day. You'll also need more if you're dieting, living in a hot or dry environment or sick with fever, vomiting or diarrhea, all of which can deplete your body's fluid reserves.

It's not hard to make fluids a part of your day. Here's how.

Start with a swig. Drink a glass of water after you wake up. It'll get you off to a good start, since your body has gone for hours without fresh fluids during your sleep, says Grabowski. And your morning coffee, though stimulating, can be dehydrating, because caffeine is a diuretic.

Drink steadily. If you guzzle your entire daily intake at once, you'll probably feel bloated, and you'll definitely excrete more, because your body can't hold that much new fluid at once, says Grabowski. Take frequent water breaks—about one every hour or two—so you're constantly hydrated. Drink even more if it's hot or humid or if your eyes, mouth or skin feels dry.

Don't skip meals. Much of your daily fluid intake comes during meals. Eat plenty of water-rich foods such as fruits and vegetables and always have water or another beverage with your meal, says Grabowski.

Say no to alcohol and caffeine. Booze, beer, coffee, tea and colas have a

Dehydration Warning Signs

Dehydration can sneak up on you. You could be dangerously dry and not even know it. Keep an eye out for these warnings.

Early Signs

- Dizziness, fatigue
- Weakness, headache
- Flushed skin
- Dry mouth
- Loss of appetite

Advanced Signs

- Blurred vision, hearing loss
- Difficulty swallowing
- Dry, hot skin
- Rapid pulse, shortness of breath
- Unsteady gait
- Extremely frequent urination (especially if you haven't been drinking fluids and the urine is cloudy and deep yellow)

diuretic effect—that is, they encourage fluid excretion. These beverages may quench your thirst initially, but they ultimately draw fluids out.

Avoid water-sapping foods. Salty foods can leave you feeling parched, because they draw water out of your system, says Grabowski. If you must have these foods, limit your intake and drink plenty of liquids.

Be careful with laxatives. Frequent laxative use can draw an enormous amount of water from the body and disrupt the normal function of your digestive and elimination systems. These shouldn't be taken on a regular basis unless you're under a doctor's care, Grabowski says.

Save the pulp. Home juicing machines provide a great means for getting your daily fluids, says Grabowski. But some of these gadgets completely separate the juice from the fruit or vegetable pulp, the part that contains the greatest concentration of fiber as well as additional nutrients and water. Make sure your juice concoctions contain a lot of that good pulp.

Men, Exercise and Fluids

The amount of water we sweat away when we exercise or play sports can be enormous, especially if it's extremely hot or humid. As much as two quarts an hour can be lost, says Dr. Nelson. Besides seriously jeopardizing your performance, such losses can take you into the dehydration danger zone. Heat and humidity accelerate the process. That's why active men need to pay close attention to their fluid needs. Keep these tips in mind.

Imbibe before, during and after. Prepare for sweat loss by drinking 8 to 20 ounces of water an hour before your workout, says Dr. Nelson. "Body size and the temperature of where you will be exercising affect the amount of water that you should drink. The larger you are and the hotter it will be, the more you need." However, don't overdose on water; this will result in poor performance, warns Dr. Nelson. Symptoms of too much water intake include a bloated feeling and stomach cramps. As you exercise, try to drink up to ½ to ¾ cup of water every ten minutes. Afterward, help yourself by drinking more water.

Step on a scale. How much should you drink after exercise? Weighing yourself before and after exercise will give you an idea of how much fluid you lose when you work out. Here's a handy formula: If you lose half a pound while exercising, drink at least eight fluid ounces afterward.

Drink beyond your thirst. Even if your immediate thirst feels quenched, your body's fluid reserves may not be adequately refilled, says Dr. Nelson. Play it safe and take a few additional slurps. A few minutes later, drink some more, and so on for about an hour afterward.

Keep it cool. Cool water will lower your body temperature faster than warm water. It's also dispersed much faster to the body, Dr. Nelson says.

Acclimate. If you come out of an air-conditioned building and try jogging five miles, the shock to your system will draw more water from your body than if you slowly accustom yourself to the outdoor heat, Dr. Nelson says.

Shield yourself from the sun. Direct sunlight on a hot summer day will dry you like a raisin, says Dr. Nelson. If you exercise in the heat and sun, wear a hat and light, loose-fitting clothing that breathes and lets in cool air. Dr. Nelson says frequent breaks aren't necessary if you feel fine. "If you feel dizzy or disoriented, stop exercising immediately," he warns. Find some shade and fluids to help cool your body temperature.

Ease into shape. If you've been out of action for a while and decide to resume an exercise regimen, you'll sweat more than guys who are in better shape. Start your workout program slowly, get used to exercising and gradually increase the intensity. This will go a long way in helping your body to regulate its fluids and body temperature, says Dr. Nelson.

Use sport drinks sparingly. Sport drinks, which are rich in the electrolytes that we lose when we sweat, are often touted for their replenishing abilities, and many of them do make excellent fluid sources. But you certainly don't need a sports drink for every workout. "After a workout or if you need a pick-me-up during a game, they can be a big help, but they are no more effective than water, which is what your body is really thirsty for," says Dr. Nelson. The only time these drinks have an advantage over water is if you have just come off an extremely draining workout, such as a marathon or a two-hour football game in the hot sun. Then you may need an immediate electrolyte boost.

FORGIVENESS

Practice It, or You May Be Sorry

Ask a typical guy about the shortest person to ever play professional baseball, and he'll chew your ear off about three-foot-seven Eddie Gaedel of the 1951 St. Louis Browns. But ask him to discuss his feelings, and he makes a monk seem like a blabbermouth.

Let's face it: Some of us aren't exactly great at expressing ourselves—unless, of course, you consider punching a wall in a fit of rage a valid form of communication. And when it comes to dropping a grudge, many men would just as soon willingly ask for directions or admit a fondness for Fabio.

"It's because of the way that many men are raised," says Sidney B. Simon, Ed.D., a counselor and professor emeritus of psychological education at the University of Massachusetts at Amherst. "As boys, we're raised to hold everything in—that 'big boys don't cry.' And we're taught that expressing our feelings is a sign of weakness. So when we grow into men and become angry or hurt, we tend to hold it all in—including the grudges. Many men have trouble with forgiveness. And as a result, they die earlier."

How Grudges Hurt You

Do you plan to hold a grudge against someone until your dying day? You may not have to wait as long as you thought. Men who are hesitant to forgive are more likely to die from heart disease than those who better roll with life's punches, according to research by leading scientists, including Redford B. Williams, M.D., director of the Behavioral Medicine Research Center and professor of psychiatry at Duke University Medical Center in Durham, North Carolina.

"But the damage isn't just to your heart," says Dr. Williams, who pioneered research on the link between heart disease and the Type A personality and wrote *Anger Kills*. "People prone to traits associated with an unwillingness to forgive are at a higher risk of dying from all causes."

In fact, a tendency to hold resentment and an inability to forgive have even been linked with an increased risk of cancer, according to O. Carl Simonton, M.D., director of Simon Cancer Counseling Center in Pacific Palisades, California, and co-author of *Getting Well Again*. Experts believe that the stress related to holding grudges may also trigger or aggravate higher levels of headache, backache, ulcers, wrinkles, even a weakened immune system and higher rates of colds, flu and other infectious diseases.

"There's no question that holding on to grievances and unforgiving thoughts can age you," says Gerald G. Jampolsky, M.D., founder of the Center for Attitudinal Healing in Tiburón, California, and the author of nine books on relationships, including *Love Is Letting Go of Fear* and *Good-Bye to Guilt: Releasing Fear through Forgiveness*. "Besides the depression and anxiety it causes, it can also lead to a host of other physical problems that take the zip and zest out of your life.

"The good news is, when you forgive, you can wipe the slate clean and sometimes maybe even reverse some of the damage done."

Overcoming the Wimp Factor

When you let go of a grudge, you also release the anxiety, stress and anger that eat away at you and cause these illnesses. But in order to do this and feel better, you have to make some changes in your manly state of thinking and overcome what Dr. Simon calls the wimp factor.

"In our society, we're programmed to be macho, Rocky-like protectors and providers," says Dr. Simon, who with his wife, Suzanne Simon, wrote *Forgiveness: How to Make Peace with Your Past and Get On with Your Life*. "We fear that if we show any weakness—like not giving some guy the finger when he cuts us off in traffic—we will somehow lose our manhood. Men resist appearing to be a wimp in any form."

In other words, you flip him the bird. And he curses back. And you tailgate. And he rides the brakes, so you can't pass. And the next thing you know, you're at work, consumed with thoughts of revenge toward a motorist you'll probably never see again. And if you're like most guys, your rage continues.

"Most men are less likely to forgive than women—especially for the small things," Dr. Simon adds. "So they carry around more grudges. A woman will whine about her resentment, but at least she's addressing it. A man who is angry for one reason will just go home and kick the dog."

Who Are You Really Hurting?

When you realize that holding a grudge isn't doing anything for you other than making your blood boil, you're halfway there. "Once you give up the notion of revenge, you make a conscious decision to save yourself from thinking about your hurt all the time," says Dr. Williams. "And when you do that, you feel better—emotionally and physically."

Robert Enright, Ph.D., educational psychologist and professor of human development at the University of Wisconsin–Madison who has researched forgiveness and its effect on mental health, says when you forgive, there is a change for the better in mind and body. When you think of what's eating you, for instance, it can raise your blood pressure, says Dr. Enright. "But when you forgive, there can be a drop in blood pressure."

Psychologically, forgiveness raises your self-esteem and lowers anxiety and depression. "And I guess you could say that people with high self-esteem tend to take better care of themselves, so they feel better," Dr. Enright adds. Perhaps you'll look and act younger.

What Forgiveness Isn't

So if forgiveness is so great, why are we so lousy at it? Probably because most guys don't understand what forgiveness is really about. It's not being a wuss or turning the other cheek so that it can get slapped. You don't have to "play nice" with the subject of your rage.

"You can forgive without feeling like a sucker by trying to understand the other's vulnerability," says Dr. Enright. Consider the co-worker who is so insecure about his own abilities that he must capitalize off yours. Or that the guy who mugged you didn't know who you were—you just happened to be in the wrong place at the wrong time.

Voilà! This is the beginning of forgiveness. No playing nice-nice or making kissy-face with people you hate. Heck, you don't have to offer forgiveness directly to people who hurt you, says Dr. Simon. For example, what do you do if the person is already dead? Forgiveness doesn't have to be face-to-face.

Here's how to master the art of forgiving.

Choose to be happy, not right. "It's important to have peace of mind as our only goal and to recognize that the attachment to anger doesn't really bring peace," says Dr. Jampolsky. The first step is willingness to forgive.

It's important to ask ourselves if we want to be happy or right, and it's important not to make others wrong and ourselves right. "When we recognize that holding on to unforgiving thoughts is really a decision to suffer, it makes it easier for us to have a desire to forgive, let go and heal the past. When we forgive, the other person doesn't have to change at all. It's just a matter of changing our own thoughts and attitudes. To forgive does not mean you have to agree with the behavior."

Think in the present. Kids live for the present, not dwelling on the past or worrying about the future. And that's good advice for adults trying to come to grips with their hurt. "When you're four years old and a friend takes your toy, you swear you'll hate that kid forever and never play with him again. Meanwhile, ten minutes later, you're out playing together like nothing happened," says Dr. Jampolsky. "We have much to learn from children. If you're angry about something that occurred in the past, ask yourself what that anger is doing for you today. If it's not improving your life—and anger rarely does—then don't dwell on it. Choose to let go of your attachment to anger. The people who feel less burdened by age are those who are in their eighties and nineties with what I call celestial amnesia; they live for the present."

Ask what's really bugging you. Sometimes the source of your resentment can be deep in your emotional well, hidden even from you—until some minor thing sets you off. "When we get uptight about the smaller things that happen each day, we are really getting upset about something deeper that we might never have forgiven," says Dr. Simon. So ask yourself about the root of your anger and try to come to grips with it.

One way to do this is to get your feelings down on paper, says James Pennebaker, Ph.D., a psychologist at Southern Methodist University in Dallas and author of *Opening Up: The Healing Power of Confiding in Others.* Simply write down your feelings—how you feel rather than just reporting that you feel bad. If you do this for about 20 minutes a day, this "diary" can help you focus your resentment, so you'll be better able to forgive.

Get a helping hand. Strong-but-silent types that we are, many guys prefer to deal with their feelings solo—which usually means not dealing with them. "Men in particular can benefit from group support, since they're usually more likely to seek another football game rather than seek someone to share their feelings with," says Dr. Simon. "I'm a big believer in men's support groups—giving men help in coming to terms with forgiveness." By discussing your feelings with other people, you get other opinions, which always helps. But if you feel foolish sharing your feelings, don't feel you have to.

Take action. Resentment often results from being a victim—of a crime, broken heart or some other situation where you felt powerless. In these instances, sometimes the person you need to forgive is yourself. Taking action against unfair treatment can be the first step. If your car mechanic treats you like an idiot, for instance, ask him if he wants to keep your business. If your girlfriend dumps you, let her go—she wouldn't have been happy in the long run anyway (and neither would you). If your boss is being unfair, talk with him or send out résumés.

Positive confrontation may not solve your problem, but you'll feel better letting others know that you're no patsy. "The best way is to simply tell the person how you feel, logically and without too much emotion," says Dr. Enright. "Simply say 'You upset me by such-and-such, and I wanted to let you know how I felt about it.' "

FRIENDSHIP

Try a Little Buddy Therapy

Peter and Robert, good friends for several years, took a trip to a remote island surrounded by furious tides in the Bay of Fundy. Their official mission was to help Peter's elderly father get his summer house in shape. But the real reason Robert tagged along was to escape the rat race of his New York City ad agency.

He and Peter had little idle time, but when they did, they talked about outboard motors, tides and how long you'd live if you fell in the 38°F water. The work got done, they had a lot of fun, and the days passed happily.

"How was the North Country?" Robert's wife, Lynn, asked when he returned. She'd spent the week with Peter's wife, Teresa, on a separate vacation to a Long Island resort where there was nothing to do but lie in the sun, take walks and read.

"Wonderful," he said. "How was Long Island?"

"Gosh, we talked for hours and hours. It seemed like we'd never stop. I told her every secret I'd ever had. She's such a wonderful friend. Did you and Peter talk about personal things?" she asked.

Robert had to think about it for a moment. "Not really," he said.

This story reflects the fact that men tend to "do" things together while women tend to "share" things, notably their feelings and needs. But while they might have different ways of going about it, men and women get the same thing from their relationships: longer, more healthy lives.

What It Does for You

"Friendship has a profound effect on your physical well-being," says Eugene Kennedy, Ph.D., professor of psychology at Loyola University of Chicago. "Having good relationships improves health and lifts depressions. You don't necessarily need drugs or medical treatment to accomplish this—just friends."

Make Yourself Likable

Likability is a talent. And like any talent, it can be honed, says Arthur Wassmer Ph.D., a psychologist in private practice in Kirkland, Washington, and author of *Making Contact*. Here are a few tips that will make you liked by all but the most miserable people when you meet them.

- Break the ice with questions like "Where are you from?" or "Are you enjoying the party?"
- Be an active listener.
- Ask questions.
- Reveal your feelings and experiences.
- Pay a compliment.

And perhaps one of the greatest health benefits of friendship is the youthfulness of extended life—of extra years of enjoyment and satisfaction.

One of the first studies linking relationships and longevity took place in Alameda County, California. Researchers there found that over a nine-year period, the people with the strongest social and community ties were the least likely to die. Not surprisingly, the most isolated people had the highest death rate.

Three more studies have duplicated these findings: In each study, people who were isolated were three to five times more likely to die than people who had intimate relationships.

Redford B. Williams, M.D., director of the Behavioral Research Center and professor of psychiatry at Duke University Medical Center in Durham, North Carolina, sees a definite connection between friendship and longevity. His team followed 1,368 heart disease patients for nine years. They discovered that just being married (even if it was a bad marriage) or having a good friend was a predictor of who lived and who died after a heart attack.

"What we found," says Dr. Williams, "was that those patients with neither a spouse nor a friend were three times more likely to die than those involved in a caring relationship."

Shoulder-to-Shoulder vs. Face-to-Face

Younger men often have as many buddies as women, although these friendships are usually less intimate than the female variety. There's a saying that women speak face-to-face and men speak shoulder-to-shoulder; men are more likely to play sports or work on cars than sit down and have a heart-to-heart talk.

But male friendships aren't flawed. Somewhere between greasing axles and throwing footballs, men have their emotional needs met.

Unfortunately, as we get older and friends become more important in keeping us youthful, women tend to develop more friendships while men develop fewer. That's not because men get crotchety or keep telling the same dull jokes (though you might want to keep an eye on those tendencies). Rather, it's because men often aren't as socially flexible as they could be.

"Men's friendships are traditionally with people they meet at work," says Paul Wright, Ph.D., professor of psychology at the University of North Dakota in Grand Forks. "Work offers you a common interest to base your friendship on." The problem with work relationships is that they tend to last only as long as the job lasts. And these days, that's not forever.

You Reap What You Sow

Friends don't spring up like wildflowers. They have to be cultivated like roses. And like roses, they'll keep blooming and growing as long as you nourish them. Here's how to take advantage of the age-erasing benefits of lasting relationships.

Be a friend for life. Friendships don't happen overnight. They require exchanges of trust and confidence that can develop only over time. You have to maintain and nourish your friends by showing genuine and continuing interest

Friendly Body Language

In his work with shy people, Arthur Wassmer, Ph.D., a psychologist in private practice in Kirkland, Washington, and author of *Making Contact*, learned that the way you move is just as important as what you say when you're trying to make friends. He offers these six tips for how to present yourself in a social situation. Combine the first letter of each tip to form the word *SOFTEN*, and you'll find it easy to remember Dr. Wassmer's advice. These tips will make you appear open and inviting to people you meet.

*S*mile
*O*pen posture (don't cross your arms)
*F*orward (lean toward, not away from, the person)
*T*ouch (just a light touch on the shoulder or arm)
*E*ye contact
*N*od in agreement

A Man's Best Friends

Rufus is nothing if not consistent. Every time you come in the door, he greets you like an incredibly important and wonderful person whom he's missed intensely. Before you know it, your jacket's covered with fur, and your vocabulary is reduced to things like "Roofa-roof, wattapooch."

So what if the dog does in your dignity? He has also eased your stress level and lowered your blood pressure.

Numerous studies have shown that dogs and other pets boost health and longevity. One study of 5,741 people in Melbourne, Australia, showed that pet owners had lower levels of blood pressure and cholesterol than non-owners—even when both groups had the same heart-harming habits, like smoking or a high-fat diet.

In another study, a group of 96 heart attack survivors were studied for a year after they were released from the University of Maryland School of Medicine's coronary care unit in Baltimore. The researchers found that more pet owners were still alive a year later than those without pets to go home to. Here, too, the results held firm even after researchers accounted for the patients' individual differences in heart damage and other medical problems. Studies have also shown that people with dogs have milder cardiovascular reactions to stress, which may play a role in protecting them from heart disease to start with.

Although all sorts of companion animals have been shown to have therapeutic effects, dogs do seem to have an edge, particularly in providing comfort and support to older people. A study at the School of Public Health at the University of California, Los Angeles, showed that recently bereaved elderly people who didn't own pets saw their doctors 16 percent more than pet owners and 20 percent more than dog owners. Dog owners saw their doctors less partly because they reported greater feelings of attachment to their pets. The researchers think that another factor in dogs' healing companionship is that they often take their owners for health-promoting walks.

How about a feathered friend? A few studies suggest the possibility of some increased risk of lung cancer for those living with a pet bird, possibly due to lung-damaging fungus spores that spread to the air from bird droppings. But other researchers say the connection is not as strong as originally was reported.

The choice is yours—whether you walk a dog, stroke a cat or talk to a budgie, you're getting love, easing stress and bolstering your heart health. So what's a little shedding and drooling?

in them. Don't just say "How are you?" Say it and really listen to the response. And then tell them truly how you are doing.

Try new activities. Often you attract friends to the extent you are doing things they are interested in, says Michael Cunningham, Ph.D., professor of psychology at the University of Louisville in Louisville, Kentucky. "Be willing to try new activities that will put you in contact with people who might turn out to be good friends," he says.

Be open and real. "Friendship depends on sharing and responding to each other," says Dr. Kennedy. "There's no formula for making friends. The real requirement is just being human and showing who you are to someone else."

Many men have the idea that revealing themselves is a tremendous risk, that they might face ridicule, says Arthur Wassmer, Ph.D., a psychologist in private practice in Kirkland, Washington, and author of *Making Contact*. In reality, he says, you're almost never going to get a bad response from someone when you try to be genuine and open with something personal. The fear of ridicule, he adds, often comes from low self-esteem.

Ask for what you need. Just because you tell someone your problems doesn't mean you'll get the emotional support you need, says Dr. Cunningham. You must ask for the type of support you need. If you want someone to help solve a problem, say so. But if you'd prefer that your friend just commiserate, let him know that, too.

Find a group of sympathetic people. It's a peculiar catch-22, but people who are lonely and needy have the most trouble making friends. Their neediness can scare others off. Dr. Cunningham says people develop "social allergies" to needy people and can become wary, tired and irritated with them. That's why it helps to look for friends among people who understand what you're going through. If you are a grieving widower, a recovering addict, depressed or otherwise feeling alienated and alone, look into self-help or 12-step groups in your area. There's bound to be one for you. Joining one of these groups can help you deal with your problems and become less needy and thus more attractive to others.

Have female buddies. Try having simple nonsexual friendships with women you like. Sometimes men feel more comfortable expressing their feelings to a woman than to a man.

Reach out and fax someone. These days, people are so busy that it can be difficult to find time for friends. But there are always telephones, faxes and old-fashioned letters. You don't have to have constant direct contact to maintain a good friendship.

Don't put all your eggs in one basket. Often married men rely on their wives for the majority of their emotional needs. This can be dangerous. What if she gets tired of listening to you talk about your problems? Or what if you're suddenly widowed and left without anyone to turn to? You'll suddenly be lonely and isolated, and you will probably feel a lot older in a short period of time. It would be wiser to spread your emotional needs around to various people.

GOALS

Mapping Your Route to Vitality

After your first hit in Little League, you wanted to nail a homer. After you landed your first job, you wanted a promotion. After you got married, you wanted kids.

You've had goals all your life. Each time you accomplish a meaningful task, you feel a surge of pride and boyish exuberance. Like most men, you find goals essential. They keep you feeling younger and moving forward.

"Goals sustain a man's sense of well-being and purpose. It's just natural to feel better about yourself and feel worthwhile if you're being productive in some way," says Barry Rovner, M.D., a geriatric psychiatrist at the Thomas Jefferson Medical Center in Philadelphia. "It's this basic: Like your heart needs blood, your mind needs to have a focus or a goal. People without goals feel lost and adrift."

They Do a Body Good

All of us have goals, including the mundane ones like getting to work on time. In any given week, the average guy is fulfilling dozens of different goals that may include reaching a sales quota at work, getting home in time to see his son's soccer game or taking his wife out for an anniversary dinner, says Paul Karoly, Ph.D., professor of psychology at Arizona State University in Tempe.

"We all have the same general desire in life, and that is to get from point A to point B," Dr. Karoly says. "At the core, that means having goals and learning to navigate toward them. Studies indicate that people who have reasonable goals are more satisfied with life and feel better about themselves."

Goals can also help you keep your mind and body in peak condition, says Dennis Gersten, M.D., a psychiatrist in San Diego and publisher of *Atlantis: The Imagery Newsletter*. "If you don't have goals, what happens? You won't be motivated to maintain your health and keep up your body," he says. "Your life won't have meaning, and you won't feel complete. So having goals makes you whole spiritually, physically and emotionally. And being whole can make you healthier and relieve stress."

Goals prevent boredom, and that's important, because boredom can put you at higher risk for disease, says Howard Friedman, Ph.D., professor of psychology and community medicine at the University of California, Riverside, and author of *The Self-Healing Personality*.

"Something's going on there, but we really don't know how it all fits together," Dr. Friedman says. "It may be that when you feel challenged by a goal, it triggers a psychophysiological process in the body. Or it could be that people who have goals do other positive things like eat better and exercise more."

In addition, some researchers speculate that difficult but achievable goals may be more invigorating than goals that are perceived as easy or impossible.

"If you see the task as either easy or impossible, then you have no motivation," Dr. Karoly says. "If you see it as reasonably possible, then it's worth your while to try it." Your heart may beat faster, and you may feel more energetic.

A Goal or Just a Dream?

Imagine you want to drive from New York City to Los Angeles. But when you get in the car, you don't have a road map, and the highway has no signs. So you'd have no way of knowing how far you'd traveled or if you were going in the right direction. That's what it's like to have a dream or vision without goals.

Goals are the road maps and highway signs that help you stay on course so that you can fulfill your dreams, says Marilee C. Goldberg, Ph.D., a psychotherapist in private practice in Lambertville, New Jersey, who specializes in cognitive and behavior therapy. Dreams or visions are often difficult to fulfill simply because they're vague. Goals are specific.

"People get confused about the distinction between goals and visions, and that sets them up for failure," Dr. Goldberg says. "Saying 'I want to be popular' is a vision, not a goal. That statement has no criteria to measure if you're making progress and is impossible to fulfill. A goal would be 'I'm going to phone ten people and ask them to play golf with me, and I won't stop trying until one of them says yes.' You can measure that. You'll definitely know if you made the phone calls and whether someone said yes."

Mapping Your Strategy

Your goals don't need to be grandiose or spectacular to energize you, Dr. Gersten says. But whether you're trying to spend more time with your family, organize a softball team or raise $1 million to build a new community center, the more carefully you shape your goals, the more likely your dreams will be transformed into reality. Here's how.

Write 'em down. Committing your goals to paper will make them more tangible to you, says Dr. Friedman. Keep your list in a conspicuous place and check off your goals as you achieve them. Be sure to include a mixture of easy goals that will encourage you, such as reading the newspaper every day, and several more difficult ones that will challenge you, like increasing your productivity at work 10 percent.

Do first things first. After you list your goals, decide which ones are most important to you and start working on them. "People often do the least important things first, and the things that are really important to them never get done," Dr. Friedman says.

Be picky. Try not to spread yourself too thin. If you have more goals than you can realistically accomplish, that can drain your energy and make you feel discouraged and depressed. It's better to have one or two well-defined goals that are meaningful to you than a dozen less important ones, Dr. Friedman says.

Get real. Goals not only need to be specific, they should be realistic, Dr. Goldberg says. If you say you're never going to watch television again, that's probably not realistic, because goals that include absolute words like "always" or "never" seldom are achievable. A more specific and reasonable goal might be to limit your viewing to no more than two hours of television each evening.

Love your goal. Choose goals that you feel passionate about, and you'll be more likely to follow through on them, Dr. Gersten says. So if you start collecting stamps but your heart really isn't in it, you're probably not going to stick with it. But if you're a devoted baseball fan, odds are you'll be more successful if you start collecting baseball cards, autographs or other memorabilia.

Make it uplifting. Instead of concentrating on what you don't want, create a goal that expresses what you do want, Dr. Gersten says. Positive goals are more pleasurable and more effective than negative ones. If you say, for example, "I'm not going to eat hamburgers anymore," you're focusing your attention on a negative goal. That goal can actually make hamburgers more tempting. A better goal would be "I'm going to eat a more balanced diet that includes more vegetables, fruits and grains. Then if I want an occasional hamburger as a treat, I can have one without feeling guilty."

Do it for you. A goal that is torturous to achieve or jeopardizes your health isn't worthwhile. "In effect, some men will say 'I'll kill myself to do this thing,'" says Dr. Goldberg. "You have to take your well-being into account no matter what your goal is. So if you want to plant a garden but you have a sore back, forcing yourself to get down on your knees and do it is a poor idea. If it's really that important to you, ask a friend or pay someone to do it."

Set deadlines. Without time lines to nudge us along, many of us would never reach our goals. "Setting a deadline doesn't mean that you're bad if you don't make it," Dr. Goldberg says. "But a deadline does give you a point in time to shoot for. Then if you haven't accomplished everything you'd planned when time is up, forgive yourself, re-evaluate your plan and reset your time line."

Divide and conquer. Chopping down your goal into several intermediate steps will make it seem less overwhelming and more achievable, Dr. Goldberg says. If you want to set aside $2,500 over the next two years for a fishing trip to Scotland, you're probably going to have a harder time saving the money if you set your sights on getting the whole amount than if you find ways to save $3.50 a day or $24 a week.

Involve your friends. If you tell a friend about your goal or, better yet, get him to help you work on it, you'll be more motivated to stick to it, Dr. Friedman says.

Find an idol. If someone you admire has achieved a goal similar to yours, use that person for inspiration, Dr. Gersten says. Take a moment each day to imagine the thrill of achieving what he did.

But don't compete. You should learn from the success of others, but you shouldn't set out to outdo them. "If you're a songwriter, you should study the works of the great pop artists, but you shouldn't feel like you need to sell more recordings than Billy Joel to be a success," Dr. Gersten says. "You'll be less stressed and more creative if you try to be the best that you can be rather than trying to be the best in the world."

Let go of your ego. Prepare yourself for rejection and criticism. In fact, you should welcome it, because criticism can help you focus your goal. "When you begin working on a goal that is important to you, you should put your ego aside and let people chop your work up," Dr. Gersten says. "For example, I'm writing a book, so I gave it to six friends and asked them to tear it apart. Then I paid an editor to do the same thing. As a result, I had to completely reorganize the manuscript. But if you want to successfully reach your goal, you have to open yourself up to criticism like that."

Forget perfection. If you think you have to do something perfectly, you'll probably never achieve your goals. Remember, you don't have to do something perfectly. "You want to do your very best, but your goal shouldn't be to perfection," Dr. Gersten says.

Keep your perspective. Goals are fine, but if they interfere with your work, family or social life, you could be headed for trouble, according to Brian Little, Ph.D., professor of psychology at Carleton University in Ottawa, Ontario. "Your goal might be to lose 20 pounds, so you begin jogging for an hour every morning," he says. "But unless you talk to your wife, you might not realize that she enjoys talking to you during that hour, because it's the one time of the day that you can be alone together before the kids get up. So your goals not only have to fit your needs, they also have to be timely and fair and take the needs of others you care about into consideration." In this case, instead of jogging for an hour, perhaps you could compromise and do it for 30 minutes twice a day.

Envision success. Imagine that you've already achieved your goal and people are praising your effort. It may motivate you to accomplish the goal and do it well. "I imagine the book that I'm writing is at the top of the *New York Times* best-seller list, and that makes me want to create the best book that I can," Dr. Gersten says.

Treat yourself. Give yourself rewards such as baseball tickets, a new compact disc or a cold beer when you complete a goal, no matter how small, Dr. Goldberg suggests. It serves as an incentive to set and accomplish new tasks. And don't forget to give yourself a pat on the back.

Update your goals. "It's important to reassess your goals every six months or so, because circumstances may have changed, and some goals may not fit your needs anymore," Dr. Goldberg says. If that's the case, don't hang on to it. Let it fade away and then choose something else that is important to you now.

HONESTY

It's the Right Thing to Do

It's Monday morning, and the boss is boiling. The computer crashed over the weekend and killed the Borkburger files, wiping out six days' worth of work.

You're the guy who botched it. You meant to make backup copies Friday but got tied up on a long-distance phone call and forgot. What do you say?

A. "I cannot tell a lie, Boss. I did it."

B. "I wasn't even here on Friday, Boss. I wonder how this could have happened?"

C. "I cannot tell a lie, Boss. Smith over there did it."

Go for A—the truth—for your health's sake. Honesty is more than just the best policy. It's a great anti-aging prescription, too. Leveling with your friends, business associates, spouse and especially yourself can wipe out stress and worry, help you sleep easier at night, strengthen relationships and restore your self-confidence.

"The bottom line about honesty is that it makes you feel better," says psychologist Nathaniel Branden, Ph.D., head of the Branden Institute for Self-Esteem in Beverly Hills and author of *The Six Pillars of Self-Esteem*. "When you tell the truth, you respect yourself, and you strengthen your self-esteem."

That doesn't mean you should constantly blurt out exactly what's on your mind. Such relentless honesty can lead to strained friendships and angry, revenge-minded colleagues, according to Michael W. Mercer, Ph.D., an industrial psychologist, president of the Mercer Group in Chicago and author of *How Winners Do It: High Impact People Skills for Your Career Success*.

"But once you establish that you are honest, people will respond positively," Dr. Mercer says. "They'll begin to value your opinion, because what you say is what you mean."

441

Unraveling the Yarns

Everyone knows a guy like Frankie "The Forger" Sharkington, voted Most Likely to Be Lying at Any Given Moment by his high school classmates. Through the years you watched Frankie progress from "The dog ate it, Teacher," to "You're the only one for me, Baby," to "I swear it was that way when I got here, Boss." Last time you saw him, he was sitting at a bar telling a group of guys how he would be playing second base for the Dodgers right now if it weren't for those sniper wounds he got in Desert Storm.

Dr. Mercer says some people feel the urge to fudge a little to make their lives seem a little more important. The problem is that once they start, it's tough to stop adding new layers of lies. Pretty soon they're like Frankie the Forger, telling one person one thing, the next guy something else and their bosses something else again.

The result? Dr. Mercer says these people build giant expectations, promising themselves and other people things they're not capable of delivering. They try to be something they simply cannot be—perfect. That disappoints both them and their acquaintances; they start feeling lousy about themselves and fret all the time about who's going to find them out.

"It's a whole lot easier on everyone to just tell the truth," Dr. Branden says. "That way, you don't ever have to remember what you said the night before or two months before." And others learn what you're all about.

Truth Serums

It sounds so simple: Tell the truth. But experts say that doing the George Washington thing takes commitment and a fair amount of courage. If you want to add more honesty to your life, try these truthful tips.

Take responsibility. Honesty comes from within. It's an open expression of how you feel, of what you think. And Dr. Branden says it's best to express yourself that way.

"Remember: Your opinions and feelings count," he says. Dr. Branden also says it's a good idea to tell people the truth in the first person. Say "I need to tell you about something that's bothering me" or "This is how I feel about what's been happening in our relationship."

These "I" phrases serve two purposes, according to Dr. Branden. First, they're a signal to the other person that you're talking from your heart. It's much more intimate to say "I'm worried about your drinking" than to say "You're making a fool out of yourself by drinking so much."

Second, "I" phrases are a form of self-affirmation. By talking openly about your feelings, in the first person, you're telling yourself that your thoughts matter. "It's an excellent way to build self-esteem," Dr. Branden says.

Make honesty a goal. "Resolve to tell the truth, starting now," Dr. Branden says. "It may seem scary at first, but the sooner you begin, the better."

Start small. Let your buddy at work know that his report could use a little polish. Tell your wife that the joy is gone from her chicken salad surprise.

Soon you'll feel better about sharing deeper feelings with friends and lovers—which is why they're friends and lovers in the first place.

Clear the decks. Mom thinks you've been going to church every Sunday for the past 13 years. But you wouldn't know Pastor Peterson from the parish plumber. Tell Ma the truth. She might be a little ticked at first, but Dr. Branden

---

Fact and Tact

Your girlfriend meets you for dinner dressed in the most hideous outfit you have ever seen. "Do you like it?" she asks with a smile. What do you say?

A. "That is the most hideous outfit I have ever seen."
B. "That is the most gorgeous outfit I have ever seen."
C. "I have never seen an outfit quite like that."

This requires a little discussion. B is out because it's just untrue. A is risky. You might end up wearing a glass of water or hurting her beyond the point of reconciliation. C may seem like a gutless cop-out, but is it really?

"It's important to be honest. But be honest and tactful," says Michael W. Mercer, Ph.D., an industrial psychologist, president of the Mercer Group in Chicago and author of *How Winners Do It: High Impact People Skills For Your Career Success.*

Sometimes zapping a friend with a bolt of truth can lead to hard feelings, Dr. Mercer says. Some people can handle more bluntness than others. "You need to figure out who you can tell the truth to flat out and who you have to handle with care," he says.

For more sensitive types, Dr. Mercer suggests using vague phrases like "You have a point," "That's quite an idea/dress/report/golf swing" and "I've been listening to you, and you may be right." That gives you a little room to dodge, to start a conversation without putting the other person on the defensive.

Once you've shown people respect and won their trust, Dr. Mercer says you can work up to your point more easily. "There's no sense making someone angry with unnecessary bluntness," he says. "You'll never be able to communicate that way, whether you're completely honest or not."

says it will relieve the pressure of always having to lie to her. Ultimately, he says, it will probably strengthen your relationship.

Dr. Mercer offers a basic rule: If a fib from the past still bothers you, come clean about it. Try an opening line like this: "I told you something in the past that wasn't true. I really value our relationship, so I want to set it straight." Telling someone you care about them first will soften the blow, Dr. Mercer says.

Know your limits. Everyone wants to be liked. But sometimes the desire for approval makes you commit to things you can't possibly do. Don't spread yourself too thin trying to please the world, Dr. Mercer says. And never promise to complete a task that you have neither the time nor the expertise to handle.

"You're better off telling someone to hire an expert than claiming that you can fix a roof or rewire a circuit," Dr. Mercer says. "That's only going to cause problems later when the roof still leaks or the electricity shorts out."

Accentuate the positive. Remember that honesty is a positive emotion. Being honest doesn't mean only telling people what you dislike about them, Dr. Branden says. Tell them what you like—their hairstyle, their work, the way they can hit to the opposite field.

Be a little easier on yourself. You aren't J. Paul Getty, but that doesn't mean you're a failure. "Admit that you have strengths as well as weaknesses," Dr. Mercer says. "See yourself in a positive way, and it will become a lot easier to always tell the truth."

HUMOR

Go For a Yuk a Day

I'm at the age where food has taken the place of sex. In fact, I've just had a mirror put over my kitchen table.

—*Rodney Dangerfield*

Remember Joey Blutoni's tenth birthday party? You know, the one where his mom tripped on the living room carpet and dumped vanilla fudge ice cream all over Stevey Doyle's buzz-cut head? Sure, it was low humor. But you and your buddies laughed so hard that the fruit punch you were drinking blew right out your little noses.

These days, your sense of humor is probably a tad more refined, partly because you've discovered that blowing club soda out your nose hurts like hell. Still, laughing like a little kid now and then can be a great way to keep yourself young. Humor is one of the most potent age erasers around, capable of relaxing your body, easing your mind, relieving stress and boosting your creativity and problem-solving abilities.

"A sense of humor is not a cure-all or end-all for healthy living," says Joel Goodman, Ed.D., director of the Humor Project in Saratoga Springs, New York. "But it's a tool you should keep in your toolbox. It's a great way to beat stress and worry, and it can really make you feel better about life. And the best part of all is that you can do it for yourself."

Happy Mind, Happy Body

Money can't buy happiness . . . but then, happiness can't buy government-insured CDs.

—*Bruce Willis*

When something strikes your brain as funny, your body responds with a laugh. That simple, involuntary action has tremendous short-term benefits, says

445

psychiatrist William F. Fry, M.D., associate clinical professor emeritus at Stanford University School of Medicine in Stanford, California. You flex, then relax, 15 facial muscles plus dozens of others all over your body. Your pulse and respiration increase briefly, oxygenating your blood. And your brain experiences a decrease in pain perception, possibly associated with the production of pain-killing, pleasure-giving chemicals called endorphins.

There's some evidence that laughter can spur your immune system, increasing the activity of lymphocytes and other "killer cells" (antibodies) and possibly raising disease-fighting immunoglobulin A levels in your bloodstream, according to Kathleen Dillon, Ph.D., a psychologist and professor at Western New England College in Springfield, Massachusetts. Prolonged laughter may even provide you with a very mild aerobic workout—not enough to replace exercise, but hey, every little bit helps.

By the time you're done laughing, your body is calmer, your brain is clearer, and you may even discover that your headache or stiff neck has disappeared. Research shows that you might be capable of solving problems that seemed impossible just a few grumpy moments before. Not bad for half a minute's work—if you can call watching the Three Stooges work.

Laughing It Off

Nyuk, nyuk, nyuk.

—*Curly Howard*

The long-term effects of humor are harder to measure. The late author Norman Cousins credited humor with helping him beat a potentially fatal connective tissue disease. After his diagnosis, Cousins holed up in a hotel room, watched funny videos and movies, read funny books, laughed like crazy—and staged a stunning recovery.

Despite Cousins's success story, experts say that humor by itself won't cure disease or make you live longer. Still, many doctors have started working humor into treatments for everyone from cancer patients to people undergoing psychotherapy. "I think that when used judiciously, it can indeed help with recovery," Dr. Fry says. "If nothing else, it makes the patient feel better for short periods of time."

Even if you're the picture of physical health, a well-honed sense of humor can boost your self-esteem—and maybe even make you more popular. "Humor can help you deal with unpleasant or difficult circumstances," Dr. Goodman says. "If you're able to laugh at yourself or a difficult situation, you're probably going to cope better and feel better in the long run."

Experts say a sense of humor is clearly a desirable trait, one that guys look for in friends—and that women look for in men.

Oh, and one other thing: Don't worry about developing laugh lines on your face. You're going to get some wrinkles no matter what you do with your mug, be it frowning or squinting or laughing. And specialists like Karen Burke, M.D., a dermatologist in private practice in New York City, say "positive" wrinkles like laugh lines give your face character.

Honing Your Funny Bone

I don't want to achieve immortality through my work. I want to achieve it through not dying.

Woody Allen

Dear old Mrs. Stonyface. You remember her—the Creature Teacher from third grade, the one whose idea of funny was two hours of detention. Well, this may be hard to believe, but even she had the potential to develop a sense of humor.

"Everyone can laugh," Dr. Goodman says. "The trick is to work on your humor so that you can use it to your advantage." So how do you go about honing your funny bone? Experts offer these tips.

Focus on funny stuff. Look for humor in everyday life. It might help, Dr. Goodman says, to pretend you're Allen Funt of "Candid Camera" for a few minutes each day. "Act like you're carrying around a video camera," he says. "Look for people doing funny things, or animals or children or anything that might make you laugh. The more you look for humor, the more you'll find it."

Take a kid's-eye view. Buried under a pile of paperwork? Think of how silly a seven-year-old would find it. Dr. Goodman says you should try picturing how most stressful adult situations would look to a kid. Bills to pay? Grass to mow? Tax forms to fill out? They all look a little less serious when seen with a childlike perspective.

Check your humor pulse. When it comes to laughter, it takes different jokes for different folks. Dr. Fry suggests spending a week or so to gauge your own sense of humor. Which comic strips make you laugh? Which movies? Which situations? Once you've figured it out, start a laugh library. Clip funny comics and stick them on your refrigerator door. Rent or buy funny movies or stand-up comic routines. Shoot home videos of your wacko dog chasing a boomerang.

Meet your laugh quota. Dr. Goodman suggests trying to get 15 laughs a day, even if you have to look for the humor. "There's no magic in the number," he says. "It just feels about right to me. If you manage to reach your humor quota, you're probably feeling pretty good about life."

Even if you don't particularly feel like laughing, give it a shot once in a while. The reflexes, the smile and the physiological changes your body will undergo just might make you feel better. You may even find yourself injecting humor into tense situations—a great tool everywhere from the boardroom to the bedroom.

How to Build a Laugh Library

Some days it's hard to work up a smile without a little outside help. That's when you need to check out a chuckle from your personal library of laughter.

"Everyone should have a collection," says Patch Adams, M.D., director of the Gesundheit Institute in Arlington, Virginia. "There are times when a funny book or movie can change your whole day."

Dr. Adams visits his patients while dressed like a gorilla, a dead French king and even Santa Claus. The nonprofit Gesundheit Institute has been around since 1971, and in that time Dr. Adams and others have treated more than 15,000 patients with humor therapy–styled medicine, helping them laugh themselves back to health. Dr. Adams has found that a humorous context helps prevent burnout and seems to affect the healing process in a positive way. Dr. Adams is so sold on the idea of humor and healing that he's pushing for construction of a "silly hospital" with hidden passages, slides and chutes and other decidedly un-medical features.

Dr. Adams has more than 12,000 items in his personal collection, including 1,500 cartoon books, scores of funny videos and dozens more comedy albums. Among his favorites:

- *Being There*, a movie starring the late Peter Sellers
- *The Search for Signs of Intelligent Life in the Universe*, a play and book by Jane Wagner and a movie starring Lily Tomlin
- Comic strips like "Calvin and Hobbes," "The Far Side," "Pogo" and "The Neighbors"
- Any books by Dave Barry or Lewis Grizzard
- Any classic video from slapstick artists like the Three Stooges and Jerry Lewis, plus all works by the Marx Brothers (try *Duck Soup*) and Monty Python (try *Monty Python's Life of Brian* or *Monty Python and the Holy Grail*)
- Comedy records from Woody Allen ("a great stand-up guy before he went into movies"), Jonathan Winters ("a true genius"), Lenny Bruce or Sid Caesar

Collecting comedy, especially on albums, can even be cost-effective, Dr. Adams says. He suggests checking out garage sales, where you're almost certain to encounter at least one 25-cent comedy album in every stack of records.

"And they've only been played three or four times, probably, so there's a lot of life left in them," he says.

Choose wisely. Laughter can be contagious. So can the plague. If you start cracking wise about women or races or nationalities, people will start avoiding you. "Pick subjects that will bring people together in good humor," Dr. Fry says. "And never single someone out. That will make that person withdraw—and could give him incentive to get back at you when you're most vulnerable."

Draw the line. Not everything is funny. And humor won't solve every dilemma. "There are times when you have to take things seriously," Dr. Goodman says. "Laughing at everything can be a form of avoidance. It helps to have a good attitude, sure, but there are certain times that we need to be sensible—like at funerals or in court or at important business meetings—and we need to consider if it will work for or against us."

IMMUNITY

Winning the War Within

Somewhere in your body, your immune system is tackling a virus, throwing bacteria for a loss, blitzing fungi or pouncing on parasites.

At its best, a healthy immune system is an aggressive age fighter that helps keep you feeling good, looking good and brimming with energy, says Terry Phillips, Ph.D., director of the immunogenetics and immunochemistry laboratories at George Washington University Medical Center in Washington, D.C.

"If the immune system is doing its job, and you have good health, you don't even think about it," Dr. Phillips says. "The best way to keep it that way is to do all the things that are going to keep it naturally strong, like exercising, eating right and coping with stress as best you can."

But as we age, our immune system, like an aging team of veteran football players, loses some of its all-star luster. This incredibly complex defensive unit gradually weakens and is less able to tackle invading organisms.

"The immune system certainly ages and clearly functions less optimally as we get older. We believe that loss of immune system function is related to the onset of cancer, autoimmune diseases like rheumatoid arthritis and the frequency and severity of infectious diseases. For a 27-year-old, for example, pneumonia is a nuisance, but for 70-year-old, it can be life-threatening," says Michael Osband, M.D., adjunct professor at Boston University School of Medicine.

A Look at the Star Players

The immune system actually consists of millions of cells that have many specialized roles. Some play generalized defense, while others are stimulated to act only in specific situations. Among the key players are B-cells and T-cells, which are types of white blood cells. B-cells hang out in the spleen and lymph nodes, lying in wait for specific invaders known as antigens. Once a B-cell recognizes an invader, it releases antibodies into the bloodstream. These Y-shaped proteins latch on to the antigen and tag it for destruction.

T-cells mature in the thymus—a small gland in the throat—and are one of the most important parts of the immune system. They are among the few cells in the body that can distinguish normal cells from foes like cancer cells, viruses, fungi and bacteria, says John Marchalonis, Ph.D., professor and chairman of the Department of Microbiology and Immunology at the University of Arizona College of Medicine in Tucson. How T-cells learn to do that is complicated. But basically, on the surface of each T-cell is a receptor, a chemical molecule that recognizes one of the ten million known antigens. So when a T-cell detects an antigen, it not only seeks out and attempts to destroy that antigen but also sends out signals to the other parts of the immune system that determine how aggressively the body will attack the invader.

"T-cells act like quarterbacks," Dr. Marchalonis says. "They tell the other parts of the immune system what the play is and what the formation will be."

T-cells can activate macrophages, amoeba-like cells that literally gobble up the intruder or signal the B-cells to crank up their production of antibodies.

A Slow Decline

The immune system reaches its prime just about the time that you enter puberty. Then the thymus begins to wither away, and your T-cell production and function drop considerably. Although you may continue to make T-cells throughout your life, these cells don't identify invaders and coordinate the defensive effort of the immune system as well as the ones produced when the thymus was at its peak, Dr. Osband says. Why the thymus shrinks remains a mystery, but some researchers suspect that the hormones that trigger puberty may also turn off the thymus.

"You generally don't make a lot of T-cells after the thymus goes away. The thymus is important, because that's where T-cells learn to recognize antigens," Dr. Osband says. "Clearly, that learning process doesn't stop when the thymus goes, but your T-cells are left to learn on their own. It's like trying to educate yourself by reading an encyclopedia instead of going to college."

Genetics and free radicals—chemically unstable oxygen molecules that cause havoc through the body—also contribute to the decline of the immune system, says Marguerite Kay, M.D., professor of microbiology and immunology at the University of Arizona College of Medicine.

In addition, some invaders like HIV (human immundeficiency virus, the virus that causes AIDS) attack the immune system directly and destroy it.

Keeping Your Immunity Strong

While some declines in immune power may be a natural part of aging, researchers including Dr. Phillips say that making just a few lifestyle changes can keep your immunity vigilant long into your life. "In the end," Dr. Phillips says, "it's how well we look after ourselves that decides how well our immune systems look after us." Here are some ways to boost your body's natural defenses.

Smother stress. Researchers have long suspected that stress suppresses the immune system, and emerging evidence supports that theory.

Researchers at Carnegie Mellon University in Pittsburgh, for example, gave cold viruses in the form of nasal drops to 400 volunteers. Placebo drops were given to 26 subjects. The researchers then identified stress levels in both groups and watched for new infections. The highly stressed volunteers ended up being twice as likely to develop colds as the low-stressed volunteers. None of the 26 people who received the placebo got a cold.

Scientists believe that steroids produced by the adrenal glands are released during stress and suppress the activity of immune system cells, Dr. Phillips says.

How you ease stress is an individual choice, but for starters, you could play with your kids or pet, participate in a hobby like gardening or woodworking, do meditation or yoga, watch a funny movie or TV program or just read an enjoyable book.

Get some Zzzz's. "Sleep is the repair shop for the immune system," Dr. Phillips says. During sleep, your brain and body rest, but your immune system doesn't. So it has less competition for the nutrients needed to strengthen your disease-fighting mechanisms. If you don't get enough rest, your immune system will suffer. In a study of 23 people, for example, researchers at the University of California, San Diego, School of Medicine found a 30 percent decrease in immune response after these people missed three or more hours of sleep in a night.

Try to get at least six to eight hours of sleep a night, Dr. Phillips suggests.

Stop smoking. Tobacco smoke contains formaldehyde, a chemical that can paralyze macrophages in the lungs and make you more susceptible to upper respiratory ailments, including colds and flus, Dr. Phillips says. So if you smoke, quit.

Sweat it out. Moderate exercise helps prevent bacteria from gathering in the lungs and strengthens the vigilance of the immune system by increasing circulation of antibodies in the blood, says William H. Adler, M.D., chief of clinical immunology at the National Institute on Aging in Baltimore. To keep your immune system at its best, do aerobic exercise like walking, jogging, swimming or bicycling at least 20 minutes a day as often as possible.

Eat, Drink and Be Immune

"The role of diet in immunity is very direct," says Jeffrey Blumberg, Ph.D., associate director of the U.S. Department of Agriculture Human Nutrition Research Center on Aging at Tufts University in Boston. "Specific nutrients play very particular roles in pushing immunity up and down."

Here's an A-to-zinc guide to some vitamins and minerals that could help keep your immunity in high gear as you get older.

Shooting Down the Sniffles

Your immune system is rawhide-tough, but every year you seem to attract the attention of the latest version of the flu bug. Yet all it takes to protect most people against the illness is a shot. In fact, an annual flu vaccination is probably the best health deal in town, says William H. Adler, M.D., chief of clinical immunology at the National Institute on Aging in Baltimore.

Don't wait to get immunized until everyone around you is hacking and coughing. That may be too late, since it takes at least two weeks for the vaccination to completely kick in. If possible, get your shot by early October. About one-third of the people who are vaccinated will still get the flu, though usually a much milder case than if they weren't protected at all. Expect to pay between $10 and $15. At some doctors' offices, you don't even need an appointment; you can just walk in, and a nurse will administer the vaccine on the spot.

Get on the A list. Vitamin A fortifies the top layer of skin against cracks through which invaders can enter and fights cancer tumors, possibly by boosting white blood cell activity. But since too much vitamin A can be toxic, it's probably a good idea to get your daily requirements from food rather than high-dose supplements, says Ranjit Chandra, M.D., research professor at Memorial University of Newfoundland in St. John's and director of the World Health Organization Center for Nutritional Immunology. The Recommended Dietary Allowance (RDA) is 1,000 micrograms retinol equivalents (or 5,000 IU). One medium sweet potato has more than double your daily needs of vitamin A. Other foods rich in vitamin A are liver, carrots, spinach, broccoli, lettuce, apricots and watermelon.

Boost your beta-carotene. An antioxidant, beta-carotene, which is converted to vitamin A in the body, also combats free radicals and may strengthen the immune system's ability to prevent cancer. Like vitamin A, beta-carotene is found in carrots, spinach, broccoli and lettuce. But unlike vitamin A, beta-carotene is not toxic and can be taken as a supplement with little danger. Dr. Osband suggests taking six to nine milligrams a day.

Don't forget B_6. "When older people were fed diets deficient in vitamin B_6, their immunity was lowered substantially," Dr. Blumberg says. "When their intake was then increased one step at a time, immunity gradually returned to normal—but only after intake of more than 1.6 milligrams was provided."

You can get the RDA of 2 milligrams of vitamin B_6 by eating two large bananas. Other good dietary sources are chicken, fish, liver, rice, avocados, walnuts, wheat germ and sunflower seeds. Vitamin B_6 can be toxic in very large doses (1,000 to 2,000 milligrams per day), Dr. Blumberg says.

Supercharge with C. From keeping viruses from multiplying to stimulating tumor-attacking cells, vitamin C gives almost every part of the immune system a boost, Dr. Blumberg says. Fruits and vegetables like oranges, strawberries, broccoli and red bell peppers are good sources of this nutrient. It appears that optimal dosages range from 500 to 1,000 milligrams a day, says Dr. Blumberg.

Do some D. Although scientists know that vitamin D is an immunity booster, they are mystified by its role. They do know that vitamin D is needed for strong bones, which is significant because immune system cells are formed in the bone marrow. Fortunately, most people get their fair share of vitamin D. (The RDA for vitamin D is five micrograms, or 200 IU, a day.) An eight-ounce glass of fortified milk has about 100 IU. It's also abundant in cheeses and oily fish such as herring, tuna and salmon. You can also get vitamin D from sunlight, since ultraviolet radiation triggers a vitamin D–making substance in the skin. In summer, about 10 to 15 minutes of sun a day will give you all the vitamin D you need. Vitamin D is toxic in large amounts, so doctors say it should never be taken in supplements.

Eat some E. A real powerhouse, vitamin E can boost your immunity across the board. In particular, it prevents free radical damage to cells, improves white blood cell activity and increases interleukin-2, a substance that promotes the growth of T-cells. It also turns off prostaglandin E_2, a naturally occurring substance that suppresses the immune system.

Vitamin E—also considered an antioxidant—can be found in oils, nuts and seeds, but it's difficult to get a health-promoting or immune-boosting dose through food alone, says Dr. Blumberg. Healthy diets generally provide only 20 IU a day. Optimal dosages appear to be from 100 to 400 IU a day, he says.

Ax the fat. In animal studies, a diet consisting of 40 percent of calories from fat—the typical American diet—had a detrimental influence on the immune system, says Dr. Chandra. So try to cut your fat consumption to 25 percent of calories or less.

To do it, use low-fat or nonfat dairy products, trim skin or visible fat from meats and eat no more than one three-ounce serving (about the size of a deck of cards) of poultry, fish or red meat a day. Be sure to eat at least six servings of grain products like breads, beans and rice and at least five servings of fruits and vegetables like apples, pears, broccoli and spinach daily.

Pump up your iron. Iron is a vital catalyst that helps your immune system nab intruders and corral renegade cells like cancer. Most men need about ten milligrams of iron a day. A dinner of a three-ounce broiled lean steak, a medium-size baked potato and a half-cup of peas provides more than seven milligrams. Other iron-rich foods are clams and oysters, pork, dark chicken meat, dried apricots and green leafy vegetables. But don't depend on iron supplements unless they are prescribed by a doctor. Too much iron can cause health problems such as constipation, skin discoloration, cirrhosis of the liver and diabetes.

Maximize your magnesium. Some studies suggest that magnesium deficiency can cause the immune system to run amok, attack normal cells in the body and trigger autoimmune diseases such as rheumatoid arthritis, Dr. Phillips says. Taking a magnesium supplement may be a good idea for men on water pills (diuretics) or high blood pressure drugs. Both make you lose this mineral. So does drinking excessive amounts of alcohol. The rest of us can get the RDA of 350 milligrams without supplements by regularly eating leafy vegetables, potatoes, whole grains, milk and seafood.

Stock up on selenium. This nutrient, an antioxidant that's a known cancer fighter, may be required to fire up your immune system's infection-fighting team. You should be getting plenty in your normal diet. The RDA of selenium for men is 70 micrograms, and you'll get 138 micrograms from a tuna sandwich alone. All fish, shellfish and whole-grain cereals and breads are selenium-rich. Very high doses can impair immune responses, however, so supplements should not exceed 200 micrograms a day, Dr. Chandra says.

Try zinc, the missing link. "Of all the minerals, zinc is probably the most important for maintaining immunity," Dr. Phillips says. A shortage can cause a drop in production of the white blood cells that surround and destroy microscopic invaders. Zinc also helps the body process vitamin D, another important nutrient that bolsters immunity. To get the RDA of 15 milligrams from your diet, eat lean red meat, oysters, milk, oats, whole grains, eggs and poultry. Avoid supplements providing more than 40 milligrams, Dr. Blumberg warns. Beyond these levels, zinc can actually slow down the immune system.

LEARNING

Knowledge as You Like It

How many times did you sit there in Mr. Grumpola's ninth-grade algebra class rolling your eyes, watching the clock and asking the same question that untold millions of high school students have pondered through the centuries: "Why am I learning this?" Decades later, you still haven't found a practical use for the quadratic equation.

Lucky for you, there's a different formula for learning now. You can learn what you want, when you want to. And, wonder of wonders, you might even enjoy it.

"It's one of the great things about being a grown-up," says Ronald Gross, chairman of the University Seminar on Innovation in Education at Columbia University in New York City and author of *Peak Learning: A Master Course in Learning How to Learn*. "When you were in school, you were pretty much told what to learn. Now you can pick your own topics and change whenever you feel like it. It gives you a great feeling of freedom."

Read the great philosophers. Learn how to fix your chain saw. Heck, bake your first apple crumb pie. It's like being a little boy again, discovering what makes the world spin or figuring out why the sky is blue. And you don't have to worry about pop quizzes, hall passes or final exams.

Flex That Brain

Let's start by debunking one of the great myths of aging. Yes, you are losing 50,000 to 100,000 irreplaceable brain cells a day. But it doesn't make a bit of difference, because you started with more than 100 billion. By the time you reach age 70, you'll still have 99 percent of your original total.

Experts say it's not the number of cells that counts, anyway. It's what you do with them. "The adage 'Use it or lose it' applies to the mind as well as the muscles," says Marian Diamond, Ph.D., professor of neurosciences in the Department of Integrated Biology at the University of California, Berkeley. Physical exercise makes muscles grow, and mental exercise makes the connections between brain cells grow.

"Studies show that the area in the brain devoted to word understanding is significantly larger in the average college graduate than in the average high school graduate," Dr. Diamond says. "Why? Because college graduates spend more time working with words."

So biologically speaking, there's no reason adults can't learn as well as children do. In fact, being an adult often makes learning easier. "You can put things in context," says Gross. "When you're learning something, like philosophy, you have years of experience that will help you see where things fit in. You never had that edge when you were young."

The key to learning is overcoming the notion that the whole process is boring—or scary. It doesn't have to be either. "Learning can be life's greatest joy," Gross says. "It's what makes humans human." And the part about being scared? "Why worry when you're doing it for yourself?" Gross asks. "Failing is not an issue. There's not going to be a test. Learn for the sake of learning, and you'll see how great you feel."

A Primer for Men

Ready to get started? Experts offer these tips.

Follow your dreams. What have you always wanted to learn? Gardening? Plumbing? Spanish? Gross says you should make a list—and don't worry about whether the items seem "important" enough. Remember, you're learning for yourself.

Pick one or two topics, save the rest for later and take it from there.

Do it your way. In school everyone learned the same way: by being quiet, listening to the teacher, going home and studying. Well, forget that.

People learn in different ways. Some do best in large groups. Some like to go off on their own. Others like to interact with one or two good friends, to share ideas.

How about you? Are you a morning person or a night person? Do you like seminars with lots of people or one-on-one sessions? Do you concentrate best with the radio playing softly in the background?

"How you learn plays a large part in what you learn," Gross says. "Figure out your own style and make yourself comfortable."

Don't overdo it. It's one thing to learn to play chopsticks. It's another to play Beethoven's Fifth Symphony. And it's yet another to play Beethoven's Fifth while cooking Cajun blackened fish like Paul Prudhomme and driving an Indy car like Mario Andretti.

In other words, take your time, or you may burn out on learning. "Too much stimulation loses its value," Dr. Diamond says. "By all means, enrich your

Are You a Grouper or a Stringer?

What's the best way to learn? Your way. If you like to read the end of a book first, great. If you like to juggle ten topics at once, super. Experts agree that following your own style is key to learning.

To see how you can learn best, take this quiz, developed by David Lewis and James Greene of the Mind Potential Study Group in London, England. Circle either a or b after each question.

1. When studying one unfamiliar subject, you:
   a. prefer to gather information from diverse topic areas.
   b. prefer to focus on one topic.
2. You would rather:
   a. know a little about a great many subjects.
   b. become an expert on just one subject.
3. When studying from a textbook, you:
   a. skip ahead and read chapters of special interest out of sequence.
   b. work systematically from one chapter to the next, not moving on until you have understood earlier material.
4. When asking people for information about a subject of interest, you:
   a. tend to ask broad questions that call for rather general answers.
   b. tend to ask narrow questions that demand specific answers.
5. When browsing in a library or bookstore, you:
   a. roam around looking at books on many different subjects.
   b. stay more or less in one place looking at books on just a couple of subjects.
6. You are best at remembering:
   a. general principles.
   b. specific facts.
7. When performing some tasks, you:
   a. like to have background information not strictly related to the work.
   b. prefer to concentrate only on strictly relevant information.

mental life and keep your brain active, but allow yourself adequate time to assimilate new information."

Change course. So you always wanted to build a model boat. And now you're halfway through the *Queen Mary*. But it's just not as much fun as you thought it would be.

8. You think that educators should:
    a. give students exposure to a wide range of subjects in college.
    b. ensure that students mainly acquire in-depth knowledge related to their specialties.
9. When on vacation, you would rather:
    a. spend a short amount of time in several places.
    b. stay in one place the whole time and get to know it well.
10. When learning something, you would rather:
    a. follow general guidelines.
    b. work with a detailed plan of action.
11. Do you agree that in addition to specialized knowledge, a person should know some math, art, physics, literature, psychology, politics, languages, biology, history and medicine? If you think people should study four or more of these subjects, score an a on this question.

If you marked six or more questions with an a, you're a grouper. If you answered six or more with a b, you're a stringer.

What does this mean? Groupers are "big picture" people who need to learn in an unstructured fashion, according to Ronald Gross, chairman of the University Seminar on Innovation in Education at Columbia University in New York City and author of *Peak Learning: A Master Course in Learning How to Learn*. You should hop right into a subject, read manuals from back to front if you feel like it and never be afraid to take on several tasks at once. And don't worry about the details at the beginning. You'll pick them up as needed.

Stringers are much more detail-oriented. They like to follow a plan or a structure that will take them logically through a subject. Gross suggests reading the tables of contents in several good books on your subject of choice. Develop a plan of attack. And make sure you have absorbed material before moving on.

Try something else. "There's no sense staying with something that isn't what you really want to learn," Gross says. "And there's certainly no shame in it. Just try something else instead."

There's one exception. Before you torpedo your dream ship, make sure it's for the right reason. Are you quitting because it's not interesting? Or are you having trouble with it because you're still learning the basics? A new task can involve some rough sailing. But riding out the storm has its rewards.

Challenge yourself. Do you play computer games only on settings that you can win easily? Then you're not challenging yourself. While pushing too hard inhibits learning, not going hard enough can be stifling, too. Gross says you should always leave another bridge for yourself to cross. "Proceed at your own pace, but always proceed," he says. If you reach a goal, bask in the victory. Then set another goal and go after it.

Don't be afraid to ask. What is it about guys that keeps us from asking for directions? If you're stuck on something, don't sit there and spin your wheels. If you are taking a class and don't understand, raise your hand. If you're not sure how hard to tighten an oil filter, call a garage and ask. Or consult your friendly librarian. (By the way, a library card is one of the most powerful learning tools around.) "Part of learning is knowing when to ask questions," Gross says. "Try to work things out for yourself. But you're not doing yourself any good if you reach a dead end and stay there."

LEISURE TIME

No Man Can Do without It

You work a 50-hour week, not including the commute. Come the weekend, you mow the lawn, sweep the walks, change the oil in your car, fix that leaky showerhead and run the kids to the mall. Before you know it, it's Monday morning again.

Whoa, you need time out. Leisure isn't a luxury, doctors say, it's a necessity.

Leisure plays an important role in your overall health and well-being, says Leslie Hartley Gise, M.D., associate professor of psychiatry at Mount Sinai Medical Center in New York City. If you don't give yourself time to unwind, she says, you begin to feel grouchy, fatigued, depressed and old. Over time, life without leisure can lead to ulcers, migraines, cardiovascular disease, high blood pressure and other physical ailments, she says.

On the other hand, a healthy dose of leisure can help keep you feeling zestful, energetic and young, says Howard Tinsley, Ph.D., professor of psychology at Southern Illinois University at Carbondale.

Saving Your Oil

One way to look at the importance of leisure is to imagine that your body has two types of fuel, says Walt Schafer, Ph.D., professor of sociology at California State University, Chico, and director of the Pacific Wellness Institute in Chico. Some of the fuel is like gasoline. It provides the quick bursts of energy we need for day-to-day living and can easily be replaced with rest and relaxation. But another type of fuel is like a slow-burning oil that keeps us going in times of illness and long periods of stress. This type is irreplaceable and is intended to last a lifetime.

"With adequate sleep, adequate time away from pressure and adequate play, we can replenish our 'gasoline' stores," Dr. Schafer says. "But if we don't, then we start tapping into our 'oil'—and that accelerates the aging process."

Learning to Play

Unfortunately, many guys simply haven't ever learned how to use their leisure time properly. To them, play is just another chore.

"Some men treat their leisure as if it were a job," Dr. Schafer says. "Their leisure is task-oriented, demand-oriented and packed with pressure to perform well. Instead of experiencing the joy and playfulness of leisure, they're putting themselves at risk of draining their energy reserves even further."

Ironically, the pressure from that approach to fun can create stress—the very thing that leisure is supposed to relieve. And experts suspect that stress siphons youthfulness from your body.

"We all want to feel useful. We all want to feel as if we're contributing. But if that's all you do, then you're short-changing yourself," says Jeanne Murrone, Ph.D., a clinical psychologist at the Center for Mental Health, a clinic affiliated with the Charlotte-Mecklenburg Hospital Authority in Charlotte, North Carolina. "Leisure is the time to renew yourself. Without that renewal time, you're going to burn out." So leisure time, when you don't have to do something perfectly but you do it just for the enjoyment of it, is probably just as necessary as sleeping, exercising and eating properly, says Dr. Murrone.

Finding Your Leisure

Of course, not all leisure activities are equal. The key to a healthy and rejuvenating leisure life is to participate in a variety of stimulating activities, says Jane M. Healy, Ph.D., an educational psychologist in Vail, Colorado, and author of *Endangered Minds: Why Our Children Don't Think and What We Can Do about It.* "Our minds are wired to look for new stuff. Without it, your life starts to disappear into a rut. Variety keeps us awake, attentive, coaxes our minds to work and keeps our brains growing through a lifetime."

Here are some tips that will help you make the most of your leisure time.

Keep a diary. For a week, write down what you're doing every 30 minutes, including things like showering, reading the newspaper and working, says Roger Mannell, Ph.D., a psychologist and chair of the Department of Recreation and Leisure Studies at the University of Waterloo in Waterloo, Ontario. At the end of the week, take a look at your diary and see how much time you spent working and how much free time you had. Is there a balance? Each day, rate your satisfaction with each leisure activity. Was tennis on Tuesday more fun than that party on Friday? You may find that you have more free time than you suspected. You may also find that you're filling your days with activities you don't find rewarding.

Make your own fun. What is leisure for one person is work for another. Know yourself. Make a list of your strengths and weaknesses, what you like to do and what you detest. Then make your leisure choice based on that list. "Gardening, for example, is fun for some people, but for others it's boring work," Dr.

Where Does Your Time Go?

Finding enough time in your life to play is an ongoing struggle. But you probably have a lot more free time than you think.

On average, Americans have about 41 hours of time a week when they're not working, doing household chores or sleeping, says William Danner of Leisure Trends, a Glastonbury, Connecticut, company that analyzes how Americans use their time. But because the number of leisure activities is expanding rapidly (who ever heard of windsurfing or bungee jumping 20 years ago?), the amount of time we can devote to any one activity is shrinking.

But one activity—watching television—is probably gobbling up much more of your leisure time than you might suspect. In fact, a Leisure Trends survey of over 5,000 people found that almost one in three of our free-time hours is spent anchored in front of the tube. That's a lot of hours that you could be doing more invigorating things, like walking, playing tennis or learning to dance.

Schafer says. "I do white-water kayaking, and I think it's joyful and great fun, but for others it might be terrifying."

Investigate your options. Leisure doesn't just happen. It sometimes requires a conscious effort and planning. Read the newspaper, scan the bulletin boards in your neighborhood supermarkets. Phone your local parks and recreation department and ask about outdoor trips, sports leagues and craft classes, suggests Patsy B. Edwards, a leisure counselor in private practice in Los Angeles. You can also explore your library, community college and church for new activities and educational opportunities.

Find a motivation that makes sense. Find a reason to make room in your life for leisure, says Carol Lassen, Ph.D., clinical professor of psychology at the University of Colorado School of Medicine in Denver. It might be as simple as telling yourself that you want to live longer or have a better relationship with your spouse or kids. But whatever it is, it has be something that is important to you. If it's not, says Dr. Lassen, then you're less likely to stick with it.

Set limits. It's important to draw boundaries between your work and home life. For example, avoid taking work home at night. "By doing that, you're letting both your employer and your family know that your leisure time is just as important to you as your job," Dr. Murrone says.

Make time to shift gears. Create a space at the end of your day—even if it is only 10 to 15 minutes—to be alone with your thoughts, so you can make the transition between work and home. Walking, reading the newspaper or listening to music could do it for you. For some guys, it's just a matter of changing into their informal clothes, says Dr. Lassen.

Be imperfect. Some men avoid doing certain types of leisure activities because they don't feel they can master them. "It's important to recognize that you don't have to do everything well," Dr. Murrone says. "Write a story but don't edit it, draw a picture as messy as you want. You don't have to win the golf tournament, you don't have win the race, you don't have to create a painting that is a masterpiece. It's really a matter not of how well you do but that you enjoy doing it."

Divide and conquer. Here's one way to make your leisure time more meaningful and slash your television viewing at the same time. Take a piece of paper and fold it in half lengthwise. As you watch television, write down every program you view and its length. You might be stunned by how much television you actually watch, says Leonard Jason, Ph.D., professor of clinical and community psychology at DePaul University in Chicago. On the other half of the page, jot down a list of activities (like learning to golf) you'd like to do in the next month or year. Think about how much better you'll feel about yourself if you start doing some of those things, and make a commitment to do them.

LOW-FAT FOODS

Lessen the Lard,
Lengthen Your Life

You know there's too much fat in your diet. You know that fat leads to more health-robbing problems than you can shake a stick of butter at. But you also know that cutting back on fat means giving up the good things every red-blooded American man loves: sizzling steaks, burgers and fries, ice cream, giant deli sandwiches slathered with mayo...

Give up all this for Special K and no-oil tuna? You'd rather trade a Porsche (if you had one) for a station wagon. So you stick with the fatty foods, figuring that if you're going to hell in a handbasket, there might as well be some onion rings in it.

Well, guess what, guys. You can have your cake and eat it, too. You can eat the foods you like, and eat a lot of them, and never feel like you're suffering from grease deficiency.

"It's a misconception that cutting back on fat means giving up all the foods we love," says Judy Dodd, R.D., former president of the American Dietetic Association and a food and nutrition adviser. "There are no bad foods, only bad eating habits, which are easy to change if you take things one step at a time."

Listen to Your Body

You're probably tired of hearing it: Eating a high-fat diet is committing suicide with a knife and fork. Hundreds of scientific studies have shown that getting too many of your calories from fat increases your risk for all kinds of killers—heart disease, high blood pressure, stroke, cancer and diabetes, to name the worst of them.

High-fat food can also doom you to a fate worse than death: impotence.

465

Eat a Lot Less to Live Longer

If you're a guy who thrives on self-denial and scorns high-fat delights, you might be a candidate for life in the Biosphere—or at least for a longer life, says Roy Walford, M.D., professor of pathology at the University of California, Los Angeles, and author of *The 120-Year Diet*.

Dr. Walford served as chief medical officer for Biosphere 2, a closed ecosystem in Arizona where for two years the resident scientists experienced an unexpected food shortage. On strict daily rations of 1,800 to 2,200 calories (instead of the normal 2,500 they expected, given their high levels of physical activity), they all lost weight and showed marked reductions in blood pressure and cholesterol.

Their daily fare was a modified fast, or very low calorie diet (VLCD). Some researchers define VLCDs as diets containing 800 calories or less per day. But others consider a low-fat, nutrient-packed diet of up to 1,800 calories per day for men or women to be a reasonable modified fast.

VLCDs have already been shown to increase life span and slow down almost all age-associated physical changes and diseases—in rats, says Edward J. Masoro, Ph.D., a physiologist and director of the Aging Research and Education Center of the University of Texas Health Science Center at San Antonio. But Dr. Masoro feels that a long-term modified fast is "unchartered" in humans and doubts that many people would adopt such a strict diet for life.

A study at the University of Utah in Salt Lake City showed that high-fat foods lower testosterone, the hormone that fuels your sex drive, says researcher Wayne Meikle, M.D. And every urologist and sex therapist knows that a fatty diet clogs all your arteries, including those that escort blood to your penis so you can have an erection. Does that 16-ounce steak seem a little less macho now?

But the most obvious consequence of a high-fat diet is right under your nose: your gut. "The fat you eat is more likely to become the fat you carry," says Robert Kushner, M.D., director of the Nutrition and Weight Control Clinic at the University of Chicago. "Fat contains about nine calories per gram, which is about twice as many calories as proteins and carbohydrates. And unlike proteins and carbohydrates, which are easily burned and metab-

But if you're eager to work out your iron will, here's how to do a VLCD safely.

Ask your doctor to help. No one should embark on a long-term fasting diet without medical supervision, experts say.

Know your history. If you are prone to gallstones, steer clear of VLCDs, says researcher James E. Everhart, M.D., of the Division of Digestive Diseases and Nutrition at the National Institute of Diabetes and Digestive and Kidney Diseases in Bethesda, Maryland. Studies have shown that up to 25 percent of people on VLCDs develop gallstones, he says.

Eat no junk. "A healthy modified fast has to be very high in nutrients, with no junk food," says Dr. Walford. There's simply no room for high-fat food or wasted calories.

Read Pritikin. Next to *The 120-Year Diet*, the diet closest to that of the Biosphere team is the Pritikin Longevity Center plan—largely vegetarian, high in fiber and with only 10 percent of its calories from fat, says Dr. Walford.

Swear off alcohol. The Biosphere results came from an alcohol-free modified fast, Dr. Walford says.

Take a vitamin and mineral supplement. "Take a multivitamin with at least the Recommended Dietary Allowance of everything to avoid deficiencies," says Dr. Walford. Additionally, the Biosphere team took 400 IU of vitamin E and 500 milligrams of vitamin C each day.

olized by the body, fatty foods burn slowly and are almost immediately stored in the fatty areas of the body."

The problem, says Dr. Kushner, is that our bodies store excess calories as fat cells. If we ate 100 calories of fat, almost all would be stored as fat cells. But in converting the same amount of carbohydrates or proteins to storage fat, your body would actually burn up about 20 percent of that total. In other words, fewer calories are converted to body fat when we eat carbs and proteins than when we eat fat alone.

In fact, a wealth of scientific research indicates that just a little less fat in your diet can lead to a trimmer, slimmer you. According to one study at Cornell University in Ithaca, New York, people on low-fat diets lose weight even when they don't try to restrict their total calories or the amount of food they eat. For 11 weeks, the 13 participants in this study merely reduced their fat intake to 20 to 25 percent of total calories and, in the process, lost weight at the rate of about one-half pound per week. Best of all, they experienced no hunger pangs, cravings or depression.

Studies also show that a low-fat diet reduces your risk of developing chronic disease. James W. Anderson, M.D., and researchers at the University of Kentucky in Lexington showed that adults 30 to 50 years old with moderately high levels of serum cholesterol (the artery-clogging substance that produces high blood pressure, heart disease and stroke) can lower their cholesterol levels by as much as 9 percent just by trimming their fat intake to 25 percent of total calories. What's more, when that low-fat diet is coupled with a high intake of soluble fiber (the fat-free substance found in oat bran and whole-grain products), serum cholesterol is reduced even further: a whopping 13 percent.

The bottom line: If health and longevity are among your goals, low-fat foods can help take you there.

Lean Facts

Don't get the idea that fat is all bad. It's a nutrient—as essential to keeping you alive as water or vitamin C.

It's only when we eat too much fat—which most men do—that trouble starts. "The typical American male gets as much as 40 percent of his calories from fat, which is far too much," says Diane Grabowski, R.D., nutrition educator at the Pritikin Longevity Center in Santa Monica, California. "That's much, much higher than the diets of other cultures. It's no coincidence that America also has a much higher incidence of heart disease and obesity than other nations in the world."

When nutritionists talk about dietary fat, they mean more than just that chunk of greasy suet on the edge of your steak. Fat is found in all kinds of foods—sometimes visible, sometimes hard to see. And the fat in the foods we eat really consists of several fat compounds called fatty acids. These fatty acids come in three main categories based on their chemical composition: saturated, monounsaturated and polyunsaturated.

Every fatty food contains these three fatty acids in different combinations. For example, animal fats, butter and tropical oils (like palm and coconut oil) have extremely high concentrations of saturated fats. Margarine, fish and certain cooking oils (like safflower and corn oil) contain mostly polyunsaturated fats. And other oils (like canola and olive oil), as well as avocados and certain nuts, consist mostly of monounsaturated fats.

Since all three types are equally fattening to our waistlines, fat watchers would do best to reduce their overall intake of each. But experts believe we should place special emphasis on eating fewer foods that are high in saturated fats. "Saturated fats tend to raise the level of cholesterol in the blood,

The Good, the Bad and the Lethal

This table lists the percentage of saturated and unsaturated fats in commonly used cooking oils and fats. (The percentages may not add up to 100 percent, since many of these fats have small amounts of other fatty substances.)

Oil/Fat	Saturated	Mono-unsaturated	Poly-unsaturated
11 TERRIFIC COOKING OILS AND FATS . . .			
Canola oil	7	60	30
Safflower oil	9	13	76
Walnut oil	9	23	65
Sunflower oil	11	20	67
Corn oil	13	25	59
Olive oil	14	76	9
Soybean oil	15	24	59
Peanut oil	17	47	32
Rice oil	19	42	38
Wheat germ oil	19	15	63
Margarine	20	48	32
. . . PLUS 7 TO AVOID			
Coconut oil	89	6	2
Butter	64	29	4
Palm oil	50	36	9
Lard	39	45	11
Chicken fat	30	45	20
Cottonseed oil	26	18	53
Vegetable shortening	25	45	20

which raises the risk of heart disease," says Grabowski.

Monounsaturated fats, on the other hand, do not seem to produce this rise in blood cholesterol levels, while studies have shown that polyunsaturated fats can actually lower your cholesterol count. That's why if you're going to be using oils in cooking or eating foods that do contain fat, you're much better off if those foods or oils contain mostly monounsaturated or polyunsaturated fats.

Low-Fat Superstars

Cutting fat shouldn't be an all-or-nothing affair. In fact, many of the foods you love are already low in fat. And others aren't so bad—as long as you don't eat them every day. Here are some definite choices that Grabowski recommends you include on your low-fat menu.

Potatoes and sweet potatoes. Spuds—of the baked variety—are a light and filling energy source. Just don't smother them with butter, sour cream or gravy.

Legumes. Beans, peas and lentils offer the same essential vitamins, minerals and proteins found in meats, but virtually none of the fat.

Fruits and vegetables. While there are a handful of fatty fruits and vegetables (like avocados and coconuts), most contain very little or no fat. Of those that do, most of the fat is of the monounsaturated or polyunsaturated type. Fruits and vegetables are also excellent sources of fiber, vitamins, minerals and carbohydrates.

Whole-grain breads and cereals, pastas and brown rice. These foods are virtually fat-free when left alone, so don't overdo it with butter and sauces. They're also our best sources for complex carbohydrates—the nutrients that give our bodies the most reliable, long-lasting form of energy—and fiber, which fights disease and aids digestion.

Fish and fowl. A low-fat menu doesn't mean you have to do without meat entirely. Fish, shellfish and poultry provide all the protein and minerals of red meats but not nearly as much fat.

Keeping the Flavor

You're more likely to win with a low-fat diet if you ease into it. "Look at what you're already eating and how you could eat the same foods with less fat," advises Susan Kayman, R.D., Dr.P.H., a dietitian and consultant with the Kaiser Permanente Medical Group in Oakland, California. Here are some suggestions.

Skip the greasy extras. A lot of the foods we eat are naturally low in fat until we heap them with extras like butter, dressings and creams. Your fat-reducing program can start by using fewer condiments and fatty add-ons. For example, using only a tablespoon of jam on your morning toast instead of butter will save you 100 calories of fat. Or try mustard on your sandwiches instead of mayo. "In a year's time, that'll make a big difference," Dr. Kayman says.

Season to perfection. Add herbs, spices or tomato or lemon juice to liven up less flavorful foods without adding fat, says Grabowski.

Choose low-fat cheese. Cheese is one of the most common fat boosters in a man's diet, says researcher Wayne Miller, Ph.D., director of the Indiana University Weight Loss Clinic in Bloomington. Most cheeses

Your Personal Goals

This chart shows you the maximum number of grams of fat you should be eating each day to both ensure that you're getting no more than 20 percent of your total calories from fat and maintain your current weight. If you're trying to lose weight, aim for the fat limit of your goal weight.

Your Weight (lbs.)	Calorie Intake	Fat Limit (g.)
130	1,800	40
140	2,000	44
150	2,100	46
160	2,200	49
170	2,400	53
180	2,500	55
190	2,700	60
200	2,800	62

average about 66 percent of calories from fat, but some shoot well into the 80 percent range. You can generally distinguish high- and low-fat varieties by their color, Dr. Miller says; white cheeses like mozzarella, Swiss, ricotta and Parmesan are lower in fat than yellow cheeses like Cheddar and American.

Cut down on milk. Switching from whole milk to 1 percent can substantially cut your fat intake: 1 percent milk gets 23 percent of its calories from fat, while whole milk gets 48 percent. For better results, choose skim milk; it has virtually no fat. If you have trouble getting used to the taste of skim or low-fat milk, Dr. Miller suggests you make the transition slowly, combining it with regular whole milk and gradually increasing the amount of skim or 1 percent in the mix.

Try low-fat versions of your favorites. "It's harder to totally swear off ice cream than to simply trade it for low-fat varieties or low-fat frozen yogurt," says Dr. Kayman. These days, with all the special low-fat and nonfat products available, finding healthy alternatives to favorite foods is easier than it's ever been. One study found that substituting fat-free products in just seven categories (cream cheese, sour cream, salad dressing, frozen desserts, processed cheese, baked sweets and cottage cheese) cut fat intake by 14 percent a day.

Lean toward leaner red meats. There's room for red meat in a low-fat diet if you make the right choices and eat it only two or three times a week, says Dodd. Best choices include cuts like London broil, eye of round steak and sirloin tip, which get less than 40 percent of their calories from fat. Keep portions to about three ounces (the size of a deck of cards), trim off all visible fat before cooking and prepare it by grilling, broiling or baking.

Try not to fry. Cutting back on fried foods will cut a load of fat from your diet. Cooking anything in oil, even lean poultry, boosts its fat content considerably, says Dr. Miller. According to the U.S. Department of Agriculture, the average breaded fried chicken sandwich at a fast-food joint has 15 grams more fat than a quarter-pound burger. Go for broiled or baked foods, he suggests.

Skin the bird. Chicken and turkey are already leaner alternatives to beef and pork, says Grabowski, but you make them even leaner if you peel off the skin before eating.

Fridge and skim. Grabowski recommends an easy way to make gravies and broths less fatty: After cooking, stick them in the refrigerator for several hours. Much of the fat will congeal and rise to the top, and all you have to do is skim it off with a spoon or a strainer. When you're ready to serve, just reheat or microwave.

Fill up when hunger strikes. By replacing fat with other filling, nutrient-dense foods, you can actually eat more and still lose pounds or maintain a healthy weight, says Annette Natow, R.D., Ph.D., of NRH Nutrition Consultants in Valley Stream, New York, and co-author of *The Fat Attack Plan*. Count on carbohydrates—pastas, cereals, breads, beans and most fresh vegetables and fruits—to fill you up without the fat. Most of these foods in their whole or unprocessed forms are also loaded with fiber, which binds with fat and speeds it from your system.

Beware fat wolves in sweet clothing. Many sugary foods are also high in fat. A chocolate bar, for example, gets most of its calories from fat, says Dr. Natow. Sweet cravings are often really fat cravings in disguise. If you want something sweet, try some fresh fruit or a bowl of sugared breakfast cereal with low-fat milk, she says. Or when you're cooking, use cocoa, which has less fat than baking chocolate.

Fat by the Numbers

By following the guidelines above, you should be able to cut your fat intake to about 30 percent of total calories, which is the government's official recommendation—an excellent start.

Still, many experts say the 30 percent goal doesn't go far enough. For example, Grabowski says the fat-fighting regimen at the Pritikin Center calls for reducing your intake to 10 percent of total calories.

Unfortunately, 10 percent is a pretty tough figure for most guys to stick with. Unless your doctor recommends that you cut back that much, a more realistic goal is around 25 percent. To achieve that, you'll need to closely monitor the amount of fat you're eating. "It's not enough to know that chips are bad," says Ron Goor, Ph.D., former coordinator of the National Cholesterol Education Program and co-author of *Choose to Lose Diet: A Food Lover's Guide to Permanent Weight Loss*. "You need to know how bad." Here's what you should do.

Make a fat budget. Knowing how much fat you can eat each day within the 25 percent limit is like having a salary, Dr. Goor says. "Once you know what you can afford, you can blow your budget on a double cheeseburger if you want, as long as you eat less fat for the rest of the day." Your budget is based on your total daily caloric intake.

Keep a food diary. Get hold of a fat- and calorie-counting guide (available at bookstores and supermarkets) and keep a record of all the food you eat for about three days, says Dr. Goor. This will give you a good idea of how your normal diet shapes up. It will heighten your awareness of what you put in your mouth, making you more likely to consider low-fat alternatives. And months from now, it will give you a way to measure your progress.

Read labels. Most packaged foods list their fat content per serving. You'll need to tally these numbers throughout the day keep a keen eye on portion sizes, which are often unrealistically small, Dr. Goor says. For example, the fat listing on a box of Oreos is for one cookie; if you eat six in a sitting, be sure to multiply accordingly.

Finding the Fat in Your Foods

This handy guide will give you a good idea of the kinds of foods you should make a part of your low-fat eating program and how many grams of fat each one contains.

Food	Portion	Fat (g.)
BREAD AND BREAD PRODUCTS		
Italian	1 slice	0.0
Melba toast	1 slice	0.0
Matzo	1 piece	0.3
Rice cake	1	0.3
Pita	1	0.6
Cracked wheat	1 slice	0.9
Mixed grain	1 slice	0.9
Rye	1 slice	0.9
White	1 slice	1.0
English muffin	1	1.1
Pumpernickel	1 slice	1.1
Tortilla, corn	1	1.1
Whole-wheat	1 slice	1.1
Oat bran	1 slice	1.2
Bagel	1	1.4
French	1 slice	1.4
Taco shell	1	2.2
CEREALS		
Wheat flakes	1 cup	0.0
Cornflakes	1 cup	0.1
Corn squares	1 cup	0.1
Puffed rice	1 cup	0.1
Puffed wheat	1 cup	0.1
Farina	1 cup	0.2
Shredded wheat	1 biscuit	0.3
Bran flakes	1 cup	0.7
Wheat germ, toasted	1 Tbsp.	0.8
Raisin bran	1 cup	1.0
Bran squares	1 cup	1.4
Oat rings	1 cup	1.5
Oatmeal, instant	1 package	1.7
Oatmeal, cooked	½ cup	2.4

Food	Portion	Fat (g.)
CHEESES		
Yogurt cheese	1 oz.	0.6
Cottage cheese, 1% fat	½ cup	1.2
Parmesan, grated	1 Tbsp.	1.9
American	1 oz.	2.0
Swiss, diet	1 oz.	2.0
Mozzarella, skim milk	1 oz.	4.5
Cottage cheese, 4% fat	½ cup	4.7
Blue cheese	1 oz.	4.9
Ricotta, part skim	¼ cup	4.9
Monterey Jack, light	1 oz.	6.0
Feta	1 oz.	6.1
CHICKEN		
Breast, no skin, roasted	3½ oz.	3.5
Thigh, no skin, roasted	1 small	5.7
Chicken roll, light meat	3½ oz.	7.3
Breast, with skin, roasted	3½ oz.	7.8
Leg, no skin, roasted	3½ oz.	8.0
Leg, no skin, stewed	3½ oz.	8.1
Breast, fried, floured	3½ oz.	8.8
Thigh, fried, floured	1 small	9.2
CONDIMENTS		
Horseradish, prepared	1 Tbsp.	0.0
Soy sauce, low-sodium	1 Tbsp.	0.0
Teriyaki sauce	1 Tbsp.	0.0
Worcestershire sauce	1 Tbsp.	0.0
Cranberry sauce	¼ cup	0.1
Ketchup	1 Tbsp.	0.1
Sweet relish	1 Tbsp.	0.1
Yellow mustard	1 Tbsp.	0.3
Brown mustard	1 Tbsp.	1.0
CRACKERS		
Rye wafers	1	0.0
Whole-wheat, low-sodium	1	0.0
Rye snacks	1	0.4

(continued)

Finding the Fat in Your Foods— Continued

Food	Portion	Fat (g.)
CRACKERS—CONTINUED		
Wheat snacks	1	0.4
Graham	1	0.5
DESSERTS		
Gelatin	½ cup	0.0
Angel food cake	1 slice	0.1
Vanilla wafer	1	0.6
Fig bar	1	1.0
Fruit-flavored frozen yogurt	½ cup	1.0
Vanilla pudding, sugar-free, 2% milk	½ cup	1.2
Gingersnap	1	1.6
Chocolate pudding, sugar-free, 2% milk	½ cup	1.9
Orange sherbet	½ cup	1.9
Chocolate/vanilla sandwich cookie	1	2.3
Chocolate chip cookie	1	2.7
Vanilla ice milk	1½ cup	2.8
Cupcake, no icing	1	3.0
Sponge cake	1 slice	3.1
Chocolate pudding	½ cup	4.0
Tapioca pudding	½ cup	4.0
Rice pudding with raisins	½ cup	4.1
Macaroon	1	4.5
Apple turnover	1 oz.	4.7
Brownie, chocolate icing	1	5.0
Cupcake, chocolate icing	1	5.0
Plain doughnut	1	5.8
Vanilla ice cream	1½ cup	7.2
Strawberry shortcake	1	8.9
EGGS		
White only, raw	1 large	0.0
Whole, raw	1 large	5.0

Food	Portion	Fat (g.)
FISH		
Anchovy, fillet, canned	1	0.4
Tuna, light, canned in water	3½ oz.	0.5
Cod, cooked	3½ oz.	0.9
Haddock, cooked	3½ oz.	0.9
Flounder, broiled	3½ oz.	1.5
Sole, broiled	3½ oz.	1.5
Halibut, broiled	3½ oz.	2.9
Rainbow trout, cooked	3½ oz.	4.3
Swordfish, cooked	3½ oz.	5.1
FRUITS		
Plums	2 small	0.0
Grapefruit	½ medium	0.1
Peach	1 medium	0.1
Casaba melon, cubed	1 cup	0.2
Figs	2 small	0.2
Honeydew melon, cubed	1 cup	0.2
Orange	1 medium	0.2
Papaya, sliced	1 cup	0.2
Apricot	2 small	0.3
Grapes	12	0.3
Kiwifruit	1 medium	0.3
Cantaloupe, cubed	1 cup	0.4
Dates	½ cup	0.4
Prunes	½ cup	0.4
Raisins	½ cup	0.4
Apple, unpeeled	1 medium	0.5
Banana	1 medium	0.6
Blueberries	1 cup	0.6
Mango	1 medium	0.6
Nectarine	1 medium	0.6
Strawberries	1 cup	0.6

(continued)

Finding the Fat in Your Foods— Continued

Food	Portion	Fat (g.)
FRUITS—CONTINUED		
Bartlett pear	1 medium	0.7
Pineapple chunks	1 cup	0.7
Watermelon chunks	1 cup	0.7
Cherries, sweet	12	0.8
GRAVIES AND SAUCES		
Chili sauce	¼ cup	0.0
Tomato sauce, canned	¼ cup	0.1
Barbecue sauce	¼ cup	1.2
Beef gravy, canned	¼ cup	1.2
Turkey gravy, canned	¼ cup	1.2
Taco sauce	¼ cup	1.4
Mushroom gravy, canned	¼ cup	1.6
Marinara sauce, canned	¼ cup	2.1
Spaghetti sauce, canned	¼ cup	3.0
Chicken gravy, canned	¼ cup	3.6
JUICES		
Cranberry	1 cup	0.1
Prune	1 cup	0.1
Grape	1 cup	0.2
Apple	1 cup	0.3
Orange	1 cup	0.5
LEGUMES AND BEANS		
Mung beans, sprouted	1 cup	0.2
Lima beans, boiled	1 cup	0.5
Lentils, boiled	1 cup	0.7
Navy beans, cooked	1 cup	1.0
Red kidney beans, canned	1 cup	1.0
Split peas, dried, cooked	1 cup	1.0
Pinto beans, boiled	1 cup	1.2
White beans, boiled	1 cup	1.2
Refried beans	1 cup	2.7
Garbanzo beans, canned	1 cup	4.6

Food	Portion	Fat (g.)
MEATS		
Canadian bacon	1 slice	2.0
Tenderloin pork roast	3½ oz.	4.8
Ham, extra lean	3½ oz.	5.5
Veal roast, shoulder and arm, lean	3½ oz.	5.8
Lamb chop, rib, lean, broiled	1	7.4
Leg of lamb, lean, roasted	3½ oz.	7.7
Veal, rib, lean, braised	3½ oz.	7.8
Ham roast, lean	3½ oz.	8.9
Roast beef, bottom, lean	3½ oz.	9.6
Pot roast, arm	3½ oz.	9.9
MILK AND MILK PRODUCTS		
Evaporated, skim	½ cup	0.3
Skim	1 cup	0.4
Nondairy creamer	1 Tbsp.	1.0
Nondairy whipped topping, frozen	1 Tbsp.	1.2
Half-and-half	1 Tbsp.	1.7
Buttermilk	1 cup	2.2
Low-fat, 1%	1 cup	2.6
Sour cream, imitation	1 Tbsp.	2.6
Cream, light	1 Tbsp.	2.9
Sour cream, cultured	1 Tbsp.	3.0
Low-fat, 2%	1 cup	4.7
Cream, heavy, whipping	1 Tbsp.	5.5
Whole	1 cup	8.2
MUFFINS		
Oat bran with raisins	1 small	3.0
Blueberry	1 small	4.0
Corn	1 small	4.0
Bran	1 small	5.1

(continued)

Finding the Fat in Your Foods—
Continued

Food	Portion	Fat (g.)
NUTS AND SEEDS		
Chestnuts, roasted	½ cup	0.9
Sesame seeds, roasted	1 Tbsp.	4.3
Pumpkin/squash seeds, roasted	½ cup	6.2
OILS AND FATS		
Low-calorie mayonnaise	1 tsp.	1.3
Diet margarine, corn	1 tsp.	1.9
Whipped butter	1 tsp.	2.4
Whipped margarine	1 tsp.	2.7
Regular mayonnaise	1 tsp.	3.7
Regular butter	1 tsp.	3.8
Soft margarine, corn or safflower	1 tsp.	3.8
Stick margarine, corn	1 tsp.	3.8
Olive oil	1 tsp.	4.5
Vegetable oil	1 tsp.	4.5
PASTAS AND GRAINS		
White rice, cooked	1 cup	0.0
Bulgur, cooked	1 cup	0.4
Macaroni, whole-wheat, cooked	1 cup	0.8
Spaghetti, cooked	1 cup	1.0
Spinach pasta, cooked	1 cup	1.3
Brown rice, cooked	1 cup	1.8
Egg noodles, cooked	1 cup	2.0
Spanish rice	1 cup	4.2
ROLLS AND BISCUITS		
Brown 'n' serve roll	1	2.0
Hard roll	1	2.0
Hamburger/hot dog bun	1	2.1
Biscuit	1 small	5.1
SHELLFISH		
Shrimp, cooked	3½ oz.	1.1
Scallops, steamed	3½ oz.	1.4
Clams, cooked	3½ oz.	5.8

Food	Portion	Fat (g.)
TURKEY		
Breast, no skin, roasted	3½ oz.	0.7
Turkey loaf, from breast	3½ oz.	1.6
Smoked	3½ oz.	3.9
Turkey ham, from thigh	3½ oz.	5.0
Dark meat, no skin	3 oz.	7.2
Turkey pastrami	3½ oz.	7.2
Turkey roll, light meat	3½ oz.	7.2
VEGETABLES		
Carrot, raw	1 medium	0.1
Celery	1 stalk	0.1
Romaine lettuce, shredded	1 cup	0.1
Sweet potato, baked	1 medium	0.1
Swiss chard, boiled	1 cup	0.1
Zucchini, boiled	1 cup	0.1
Butternut squash, baked	1 cup	0.2
Cauliflower, raw	1 cup	0.2
Potato, baked, peeled	1 medium	0.2
Spinach, raw, chopped	1 cup	0.2
Acorn squash, baked	1 cup	0.3
Mushrooms, raw	1 cup	0.3
Sweet pepper, raw	1 small	0.3
Tomato	1 medium	0.3
Broccoli, boiled	1 cup	0.4
Cabbage, boiled	1 cup	0.4
Green or waxed beans, boiled	1 cup	0.4
Asparagus, boiled	1 cup	0.6
Summer squash, boiled	1 cup	0.6
Brussels sprouts, boiled	1 cup	0.8
Corn, fresh, boiled	1 small ear	1.0
Onion ring, fried	1	2.7
French fried potatoes, frozen	10	4.4

MARRIAGE

It Could Be Life's Best Investment

The next time you see one of those bumper stickers that reads "I love being single," take a good look at the guy behind the wheel.

He may seem carefree and remind you of the joys of bachelorhood, when you could squeeze the toothpaste tube any way you pleased and leave the toilet seat up. But there's also a good chance that he'll be sneezing, coughing or wheezing. He's also more likely to be depressed, anxiety-ridden and stressed than you are, if you're married.

In fact, from the moment a guy says "I do," marriage can do wonders for his health and happiness, says Robert W. Levenson, Ph.D., a psychologist at the University of California, Berkeley.

Married men usually drink less, eat fewer junk foods and exercise more regularly. Your single buddies probably marvel that you seem more relaxed, have a better sex life and get sick less often than they do. Some may even think you look more youthful and are more energetic than when you were a wild and crazy guy.

"Clearly, a satisfying marriage can help you feel younger and more alive. It's good for your health, good for your longevity and can help you live a more productive and happier life," says Howard Markman, Ph.D., a University of Denver psychologist and co-author of *We Can Work It Out: Making Sense of Marital Conflict.*

Why a Wife Makes a Difference

Marriage—no matter if it's good or bad—is beneficial for men but not for women. Researchers are puzzled by that, but some, like Dr. Levenson, speculate that men in bad marriages save their health by detaching themselves emotionally from the relationship. They may stop listening to their wives, spend more time at work or immerse themselves in other activities. (Women in bad marriages work harder to heal the wounds, and that effort takes its toll on their well-being.)

But others suspect getting hitched simply enhances a guy's lifestyle.

"Marriage adds stability to men's lives," says Patrick McKenry, Ph.D., professor of family relations and human development at Ohio State University in Columbus. "Men gain a lot from marriage even if it is less than satisfactory. Marriage improves a man's nutrition. He gets companionship and emotional support, and he develops healthy routines and habits, such as getting regular physical exams."

Because women cook more often than men, for instance, men often adopt the diets of their wives, and that can be a healthy change. In Seattle, researchers at the Fred Hutchinson Cancer Research Center followed 188 men whose wives had switched to diets deriving less than 26 percent of their calories from fat. After a year, these men ate fewer calories, less cholesterol and less saturated fat than 100 men whose wives continued to prepare an average American diet that derived about 40 percent of its calories from fat. As you probably know, high-fat American diets have been linked to heart disease, stroke and cancer.

The Best Years of Your Life

A married man's inclination to live a healthy life pays off big time.

Researchers at the National Center for Health Statistics, for example, estimate that married men live an average of ten years longer than single men. In another study, researchers at the University of California, San Francisco, found that men in their forties and fifties who live alone or with someone other than a spouse are twice as likely to die in the next ten years as similarly aged married men. Other studies have shown that married men are far less likely to commit suicide.

Married men not only live longer, they're healthier. In a survey of 47,000 households, the National Center for Health Statistics found that married men were more likely to say their health is good or excellent than single, divorced or widowed men. Married men also were less likely to have chronic illness, were less prone to injury and disability and recovered more quickly from colds, flus and injuries than single men. Married men also said they had fewer sick days than divorced men.

Even if a married guy gets a serious ailment, he is more likely to seek treatment earlier and have a better chance of survival than a single man. After looking at 27,779 cancer cases, James Goodwin, M.D., director of the Center on Aging at the University of Texas Medical Branch at Galveston, concluded that married men had survival rates that were comparable to single men ten years younger.

"That was a rather striking finding," Dr. Goodwin says. "The treatments for cancer—chemotherapy and radiation—can make you feel very sick. So it just makes sense that having a supportive partner makes it easier for patients to cope."

The Stronger, the Better

While many researchers believe that even a rocky marriage can help keep you healthy, some evidence suggests you'll have more resilience against ill health if your union is strong and happy.

For example, men who suffered heart attacks and were able to talk openly and honestly with their wives about it reported better health and were much less likely to have chest pains or be readmitted to the hospital within a year following the attack, according to Vicki Helgeson, Ph.D., a psychologist at Carnegie Mellon University in Pittsburgh.

Men who are satisfied with their marriages are also 24 times less likely to suffer from major depression than men who are in troubled unions, says James Coyne, Ph.D., professor of psychology in the Departments of Family Practice and Psychiatry at the University of Michigan Medical School in Ann Arbor.

In addition, researchers at Ohio State University found that the more put-downs, sarcasm and other hostile words and gestures used by newlywed couples during a discussion of their marital conflicts, the more likely they would have higher blood pressure and weakened immune systems. No, a marital argument on Tuesday doesn't mean you'll get a cold on Wednesday. But these researchers believe that couples who consistently argue may be more susceptible to infection and disease.

Keeping It Solid

No marriage is like June and Ward Cleaver's in "Leave It to Beaver." Did you ever hear June yell at Ward for leaving the toilet seat up? You have your spats, your passion wavers, and sometimes boredom envelops you. Even the best relationships

Calling It Quits

Your relationship with your wife is colder than the Alaskan tundra. But is it time for you to split up?

"Ending a marriage is the psychological equivalent of cutting off your own arm or leg. It's going to hurt," says John Mirowsky, Ph.D., professor of sociology at Ohio State University in Columbus.

But there are some clear signs that it may be time to end your marriage. "If there is any one sign that it's time to pack it in, indifference—that feeling that you neither love nor hate your spouse—is that indication," says Martin Goldberg, M.D., psychiatrist and director of the Marriage Council of Philadelphia, a counseling service. "Hatred is often just a frustrated form of love. You have to care about someone to hate her. If you really don't care, that's a sizable warning."

Other signs that it may be time to leave are if your spouse is abusing drugs or alcohol or if the relationship is physically or emotionally abusive.

The Look of Love

When you look at your wife these days, do you see yourself staring back? It's a good possibility, particularly if you've been together a long time.

After closely examining the photographs of 12 couples who had been married for at least 25 years, a panel of observers at the University of Michigan in Ann Arbor concluded that facial features of couples do become more similar after years of living together.

Why? Couples tend to unconsciously mimic each other's facial expressions, says Robert Zajonc, Ph.D., professor of psychology at the University of Michigan. Over time, this mimicry reshapes the facial muscles and wrinkles so that their faces acquire many of the same features. Couples also tend to adopt the same hand gestures, body posture and gait, Dr. Zajonc says.

---

need occasional tune-ups. Here are some suggestions to keep the heart and soul of your marriage together.

Make the moment happen. If you don't schedule time together, it may never happen. Try to spend at least 20 minutes a day just talking with each other. "You exercise that much each day to keep your body in shape. You need to spend at least that much time keeping your marriage in shape, too," says Sherelynn Lehman, a licensed family, marriage and sex therapist in private practice in Cleveland.

Surprise her. "To keep the spark in the marriage alive, you need to be creative," says Ruth Rice, Ph.D., a psychologist in private practice in Dallas. Arrange occasional surprises like a weekend at a bed-and-breakfast, a hot air balloon ride or just a romantic card under her pillow.

Play together, stay together. Common interests and hobbies relieve boredom and are the glue that holds many good marriages together. "The couple that really enjoys doing things together, like traveling, golf or tennis, is going to have an advantage as they get into the later years of their marriage and they have more time on their hands," says Martin Goldberg, M.D., psychiatrist and director of the Marriage Council of Philadelphia, a counseling service.

Laugh it up. "Being able to be childlike and laugh together is important, because it means that you feel comfortable enough to allow yourselves to be vulnerable with each other," says Arlene Goldman, Ph.D., a psychologist and sex therapist on the faculty of the Family Institute of Philadelphia.

Listen until you hear her. If your wife feels frustrated because you seem to be tuning her out, stop, acknowledge that she may be right and take time to really listen to her, says Dennis Gersten, M.D., a psychiatrist in private practice in San Diego. Let her know you heard what she said by repeating her concern back to her: "I know it must be frustrating that I didn't paint the kitchen when I said I would." If that's not what she's upset about, then ask her to repeat it until you understand. "Say 'I'm really trying to understand your concern, but I don't seem to be getting it. Could you say it in a different way that might make it clearer to me?' " Dr. Gersten suggests.

Focus on your feelings. The surest way to start a fight, according to Dr. Goldman, is to say things like "You're wrong" or "I think you're being silly." Dr. Goldman adds, " 'You' statements are almost always thoughts and are usually hurtful." Instead, try saying "I feel anxious when I don't know where you are. One way you can help me cope with that feeling is to get a message to me, so I know where I can get in touch with you." That's much less challenging than "You're always late."

Change yourself first. Focus on working on your own faults rather than your spouse's, Dr. Markman suggests. You have more control over your own behavior than your wife's actions, and often when one person in a relationship starts making changes, the other will follow.

Start small. "Making big changes in a relationship is really the result of

Coping with a Cheatin' Heart

Your golfing buddy is the talk of the country club now that his love affair has burst his marriage at the seams. Fortunately, nothing like that could ever happen to your relationship, right?

"You can never be 100 percent certain that your marriage will be immune from affairs," says Sherelynn Lehman, a licensed family, marriage and sex therapist in Cleveland and author of *Love Me, Love Me Not: How to Survive Infidelity*. "You must woo your mate every day. You can't let down your guard, because believe me, there is someone out there who thinks your wife is the apple of his eye."

Men and women often begin affairs because they're bored or in search of sexual adventure, Lehman says. Maintaining good communication and keeping zest in your sex life are among the keys to preventing an affair. But an affair doesn't mean all is lost.

"A marriage rocked by an affair is like an egg that cracks. Although the crack will always be there, you can work around it. The marriage doesn't have to shatter, but counseling is essential," Lehman says.

Retying the Knot

You knew that more than half of all marriages end in divorce. But you were stunned and hurt when your union unraveled. Now here you are thinking about heading for the alter again.

In a sense that's good, because divorced men who remarry probably regain many of the health advantages of married men, including longer life expectancy, says Patrick McKenry, Ph.D., professor of family relations and human development at Ohio State University in Columbus.

But before you enter the chapel of love, you should ponder a few things that can increase your chances of a happy and lasting marriage this time around.

First, don't rush into a new marriage. "The way a lot of men try to adjust to divorce is to remarry," Dr. McKenry says. "I think a man needs to take some time—approximately one to two years—to adjust to living a single lifestyle and relearn how to take care of himself before he moves on to another serious relationship. He needs to assess what went wrong in his previous marriage, so the pattern won't be repeated."

Ask yourself what you expect out of marriage, suggests Joel Kahan, M.D., a psychiatrist at the Medical College of Georgia School of Medicine in Augusta who has studied multiple marriages. Many men, for instance, have difficulty dealing with intimacy. "If a man doesn't want or expect a strong, intimate relationship, then perhaps he shouldn't be married," Dr. Kahan says. "He'll need to work on that issue before he dives into another relationship."

Consider what went wrong in your last marriage and ask yourself if similar problems loom in your new relationship. "A huge number of men remarry women who are very much like their previous spouses. That's one of the most important things to avoid," says Sol Gordon, Ph.D., psychologist, professor emeritus at Syracuse University in Syracuse, New York, and author of *Why Love Is Not Enough*. If your new love has any bothersome traits that remind you of your ex-wife, ask yourself if you can cope better with them this time. If not, don't get married.

making a series of small changes," Dr. Markman says. "If you can say just one less critical thing to your spouse each day, you could be on your way to significant change."

Stop stinging each other. A sharp-tongued put-down in the middle of an argument may feel good, but the hurt of that one zinger will erase your last 20 acts of kindness from your wife's mind, Dr. Markman says. It's better to bite your tongue than to needlessly open a new wound.

Can the blame. Blaming your wife rather than acknowledging that you share some of the responsibility for a problem in your relationship increases the likelihood that you'll end up in divorce court, Dr. Markman says. To break out of that pattern, try telling your wife "I know we've been caught up in this pattern of criticizing each other at the drop of a hat lately, so I'm going to work on being less critical of you and trying to see you in a more positive light."

Divide housework fairly. If you or your wife is doing more than your share of the housework, that can cause resentment, Dr. Rice says. List everything you need to accomplish: cleaning, laundry, shopping, yard work, bill paying, home repairs. Then negotiate a fair division that includes an equal number of things that each of you enjoys doing and things you consider to be drudgery. If your budget allows it, consider hiring people to help you.

Let gadgets do it. If television is important to one of you but not the other, watching it may rob you of quality time together, Dr. Rice says. Get a VCR, tape the show and watch it later. If the telephone is constantly ringing, get an answering machine and screen your messages, so you can spend time with your spouse.

MASSAGE

Giving Age the Rub-Out

You're lying facedown on a low, cushioned table. Gunther is working you over good.

Rub-rub. Knead-knead. Chop-chop.

You arrived a cranky, creaky, aching mess. Too much exercise. Too much pressure. Too little sleep.

Stroke-stroke. Push-push. Tappity-tappity-tap.

But after 45 minutes of massage, Gunther has worked his age-erasing magic once again. Your back has stopped hurting. Your head has stopped pounding. And the thought of an after-dinner racquetball match doesn't seem so bad after all. You rise slowly from the table, sing praise to Gunther and leave what feels like 20 years of pain and worries behind.

"Nothing makes you feel more rejuvenated than a massage," says Madeline P. Rudy, a certified massage therapist with Massage Therapy in West Reading, Pennsylvania. "If you're looking for a way to put yourself back in sync and feel younger, there isn't a better thing out there."

Studies in Relaxation

Man has been rubbing sore muscles since the day he dragged his first woolly mammoth home for supper. But medical science has yet to figure out why massage feels so good.

"There's not a lot of research out there yet," says Tiffany Field, Ph.D., director of the Touch Research Institute at the University of Miami School of Medicine. The institute is the first organization in the country dedicated to studying massage's medical benefits.

Dr. Field says we have gained a few insights into the way massage works on

(continued on page 492)

Do-It-Yourself Massage

At first you were a little leery about getting a massage, being a macho guy and all that. The idea of lying on a table partially unclothed seemed a little, well, threatening.

But that was then. Now you can hardly wait for Gunther to work his magic. Your next appointment is in five days, but you need to shake out some kinks now. What can you do? Try some self-massage. All you need are a couple of tennis balls, a quiet corner and your own two hands.

Head

Take advantage of pressure points in your skull to relax your whole body. "There are two very significant acupressure points at the base of the skull on what's called the occipital ridge," says Robert DeIulio, Ed.D., a licensed psychologist and muscle therapist in private practice in Wellesley Hills, Massachusetts. "If you apply consistent pressure there, you can achieve total relaxation." Here's how. Put two tennis balls in a sock so that they touch each other and tie the end. Lie on your back on the floor and place the sock behind the upper neck so that the two balls touch the skull ridge that's right above the hollow spot. Stay like that for 20 minutes. Listen to soothing music, if you like. "Those acupressure points send messages down the spinal column to relax all the muscles," says Dr. DeIulio.

Face

Just touch your face. You don't need to knead it. With a very light touch, cup your cheeks and temples with your hands using no more pressure than the weight of a nickel. Hold your hands there for a minute. "The warmth of the hands relaxes the muscles and connective tissue, bringing on an overall sense of relief," Dr. DeIulio says.

Jaw

Pull the sides of your ears gently straight outward, then straight up, then straight down. Or with your index finger, press the tender spot next to your earlobe where it attaches to your head. Press and release, alternating ears, 10 to 15 times.

Torso

Get a quick boost by rubbing the area above your kidneys. That's at waist level where the tissue is still soft. Rub briskly with your fists in a circular motion. This will energize you, says Dr. DeIulio.

Feet

Few things on this earth feel as good as a foot massage. Here are a few winning techniques. After you try them out on one foot, switch feet and repeat.

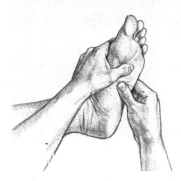

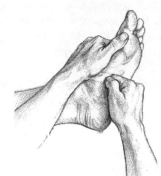

Make a fist and press your knuckles into the bottom of your foot, moving from your heel to your toes (left). Repeat five times.

Sit on a chair and place one foot on the opposite thigh (above). Rub oil or lotion onto your foot if you like. Apply pressure with your thumbs to the sole, working from the bottom of your arch to the top near your big toe. Repeat five times.

Hold your toes in one hand and bend them backward, holding them there for five to ten seconds (above). Then bend them in the opposite direction and hold for five to ten seconds. Repeat three times.

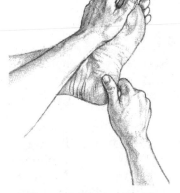

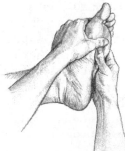

Press and roll your thumbs between the bones of the ball of your foot (left).

Massage each toe by holding it firmly and moving it from side to side (above). Extend each toe gently out and away from the ball of your foot. Then apply pressure to the areas between your toes.

a man's body, however. For one thing, it seems to restrict the body's release of cortisol, a hormone that plays a big role in triggering stress reactions. The less cortisol you produce, the less stress you may feel, Dr. Field says. Massage also has been shown to improve the deep, resting phase of sleep. And it may boost your production of serotonin, a hormone linked to positive mood changes and improved immunity, Dr. Field says.

In a Touch Research Institute study of medical faculty and staff, 15 minutes of daily massage appeared to lessen anxiety, make people more alert and increase the speed with which they could complete math problems. "The key to a better work force," Dr. Field says, "could be regular massage."

The institute is working on a series of 34 studies, involving hundreds of participants, that look at massage therapy's effects on everything from depression and high blood pressure to helping improve the immune function of males who've tested positive for HIV (human immunodeficiency virus, the virus that causes AIDS).

For now, some doctors say they need to know more about what massage can do before they start prescribing it as therapy.

"No one is willing to accept any nebulous explanation that involves the metaphors of energy, toxins, good vibes or any other poetic verse," says Larry Dossey, M.D., co-chairman of the Panel on Mind/Body Interventions, Office of Alternative Medicine at the National Institutes of Health in Bethesda, Maryland, and former chief of staff at Medical City Dallas Hospital in Dallas.

But that attitude may be changing. Many insurance companies now cover massage if a doctor orders it. And some massage therapists note that some of their best, most loyal clients are physicians.

Knead Some Advice?

If you're thinking about trying massage therapy, Rudy says you should be prepared to spend anywhere from $25 to $65 per session, with a typical session lasting about 50 to 55 minutes. Go as often as you like or can afford. For more guidance, follow these tips.

Choose your massage therapist wisely. There are massage "parlors" (wink, wink), and then there are places to get a legitimate massage. To find a reputable, qualified massage therapist, ask questions. "Look in the phone book," Rudy says. "Make sure they're a member of the American Massage Therapy Association (AMTA). Ask if they went to accredited schools to learn massage. And always avoid places that offer 'discreet billing.' That's a sign that they may not be on the up-and-up."

The AMTA has a customer referral service that will help you find a registered massage therapist in your area. Write the group at 820 Davis Street, Suite 100, Evanston, IL 60201.

Pick your pleasure. When it comes to massage, there really are different strokes for different folks. Swedish massage—with its kneading, rubbing and use of oils—is the method most people think of. But there's also shiatsu, or oriental massage, in which a therapist works pressure points along nerve pathways to relieve pain and stress (Rudy says some people may experience some discomfort with this method). There's specialized sports massage, which focuses on soothing overworked muscles and joints. And then there's a grab bag of techniques and sub-techniques like Rolfing, Feldenkrais, Trager, Alexander and Aston-Patterning, which promote everything from body lengthening to spine realignments to posture improvements.

"The key is to talk to therapists first," Rudy says. "You want to find someone whose specialty matches your needs. And you want to make sure they're legitimate."

Know when to say no. Massage isn't for everyone. AMTA guidelines say that people with phlebitis or other circulatory ailments, some forms of cancer or heart disease, infections or fevers should not use massage therapy. In most cases, avoid massage for about three days after suffering a fracture or serious sprain. If you have any doubts, ask your physician.

Don't push it. Massage is about relaxation. And let's face it: Some guys just aren't comfortable taking off their clothes for a Swedish massage.

"Only go as far as what feels right," Rudy says. "Maybe you'll have to work your way up to it. This is your special time. Enjoy it."

Therapists should be conscious of your feelings. They should cover parts of the body they're not working on. Private parts are always off limits. They shouldn't discuss intimate details of their lives or ask about yours. And they should respect your wishes. If they don't, find another massage therapist.

"The whole thing," Rudy says, "is about health and well-being and feeling better. If there's tension or pressure in a relationship, go somewhere else."

MEDICAL CHECKUPS

Avoid at Your Own Risk

Men will go to war, scale the most forbidding mountains, ride a raging rocket into space and drive overpowered cars around hairpin turns at speeds just short of the sound barrier. But let a doctor snap on just one little rubber glove...

Why men fear the doctor's office is hardly a mystery. First of all, no one likes being poked in profoundly private places. But even more dreadful is the annual parade of test results that tell you exactly what you've been trying to ignore: You're getting older. Your body—that once efficient machine built of granite and rocket fuel—is slowly turning to sand and molasses.

It makes it all the more ironic, then, to realize that one of the best ways of maintaining your body's youthful vigor and vibrant health is to do exactly what you've been putting off. By getting a regular checkup, you and your doctor can keep an eye out for developing problems and put a stop to them before they become serious.

But more importantly, the occasional doctor visit can give you both a chance to discuss certain lifestyle factors that can make the difference between a long and vigorous life and a short one plagued with problems you shouldn't have to face until you're 80 years old.

Choosing Dr. Right

Getting a checkup seems simple enough, but where it can quickly start to resemble the quest for the Holy Grail is when you start looking for a doctor. Who's qualified? What should you, as a smart consumer, be looking for?

"Basically, anyone who holds himself out by training and practice as a primary care physician should be fully qualified to take care of checkups for normal, healthy adults," says Douglas Kamerow, M.D., director of the Clinical Preventive Services Staff for the Office of Disease Prevention and Health Promotion in the U.S. Public Health Service in Washington, D.C. "But in my opinion, there are really only two groups that are qualified by their training to do so—general internists and family physicians."

A quick look in the phone book should net you a fair selection of these fairest of all primary care givers. But the selection process does not end with your finger, the Yellow Pages and a fast game of eeny meeny miny mo. "Set up a get-acquainted visit," says Kenneth Goldberg, M.D., founder and director of the Male Health Center in Dallas and author of *How Men Can Live as Long as Women: Seven Steps to a Longer and Better Life*. "Many M.D.'s will be happy to give you a short introduction without charging you."

In that short amount of time, there are a couple of things you can check on. "Diplomas don't mean what they once did," says Dr. Goldberg. "All medical schools are fully accredited, and the vast majority offer a quality education. Board certification, however, can be one sign of a competent doctor, because it means that he or she fulfilled certain residency training and took examinations of some type to be qualified by peers."

You may also want to ask whether the doctor takes continuing medical education (CME) courses. "Medicine advances so rapidly that a physician has to read constantly and participate in postgraduate training to keep up," says Dr. Goldberg. "A good doctor attends two or three CME courses each year. When you ask about CME courses, you'll also get a hint of the doctor's area of specialization. After all, you're not looking for an obstetrician."

If the training is there and you seem to get along, schedule a checkup and continue your assessment in the examination room. "Does the doctor listen well?" asks Dr. Goldberg. "You're in the market for a partner, not someone who dictates care. The doctor should want to hear from you. That means undivided attention. No interruptions and no impatient hand on the doorknob."

Healthy lifestyle education is one of the most important things that happens at a checkup and one of the most important sources of education to help you stay young and healthy. Does your doctor explain and educate? "The word *physician* means teacher, and a good doctor is a good teacher," says Dr. Goldberg. "Your doctor should speak a language you can understand, and he should enjoy helping you understand."

Preparing for Your Checkup

Sherlock Holmes may have been able to get to the truth based on the murkiest of clues, but your doctor needs clear information. You can best supply that information by doing a little homework before your visit.

Keep a food log. When it comes to health habits, the weakest information tends to surround diet. How often do you really notice what you eat throughout

How Often Should You Go?

The annual physical. When most men think of a checkup, they tend to picture a yearly barrage of pokes, prods and needle pricks that are done like clockwork whether they are needed or not. This has a lot to do with tradition.

Back in 1922, the American Medical Association (AMA) first endorsed the annual examination of healthy people, and for many years after it was standard practice. "It was only in 1983 that the AMA withdrew support for this concept," says Douglas Kamerow, M.D., director of the Clinical Preventive Services Staff for the Office of Disease Prevention and Health Promotion in the U.S. Public Health Service in Washington, D.C.

In this brave new world of checkups, the current medical wisdom is that for healthy people, a more tailored program of preventive services can be effective. In layman's terms, this means fewer checkups will do just as well as the time-honored annual physical.

If you have no serious ailments that need increased monitoring, most experts advise you to touch base with your primary care physician every three to five years from ages 30 to 39, every two to three years from 40 to 49 and, past 50, every year. That's not too much to ask.

the day? That mid-morning candy bar, a bag of chips in the car. It all adds up, but it's easily forgettable when making a report on your eating habits to your doctor. And what in reality is not the healthiest of eating habits suddenly becomes squeaky clean in the doctor's office.

"If you know you're going in for your checkup and plan on discussing diet, it's not a bad idea to keep a precise food log for a week beforehand," suggests Dr. Kamerow. "Don't change your eating habits, just keep track of them. It's the little forgettable things like snacks that add up to a lot of dietary fat, and it's these things that you'll need to focus on when talking to your doctor."

Get to know your family tree. Coming up with a complete family history of illnesses will also require a little attention and, depending on what you discover, may affect the types of tests you'll need at a checkup. "People with a family history of certain health problems may be at greater risk of developing them, and it's reasonable to screen these people more regularly or earlier for these diseases," says Dr. Kamerow.

"Talk to your parents, grandparents and siblings about what ails them and what ailed those who may already have passed on," suggests Dr. Goldberg.

"Granted, it's not easy to probe into such delicate matters with an aging grandfather, but your success depends on your being tactful but firm and letting him know just why this is so important to you."

While there may well be hundreds of diseases that may be passed along genetically, there are, in fact, only a few that you really need to be concerned with. "Studies at Johns Hopkins University have shown that a man whose father has had prostate cancer is at $2^1/_2$ times the risk for developing the disease himself," says Dr. Goldberg. "And if both his father and grandfather had it, the risk jumps to nine times."

Testicular cancer is another hereditary pitfall. "Research in Great Britain has shown that men whose fathers have had cancer of the testicles are at four times the risk of developing it themselves," notes Dr. Goldberg. "And the genetic tie appears even stronger between brothers. When one has the disease, the risk to the other is nearly ten times the normal rate."

"You also want to search in your family tree for very rare forms of inherited colon cancer," says Dr. Kamerow. "If there is a history of it, you definitely need to test for it sooner."

And the final one to really watch for is heart disease. "If you have a father or grandfather who had a heart attack in his forties, that would be good to know about, because you might want to spend more time talking to your doctor about your cholesterol and other factors that might elevate your risk," suggests Dr. Kamerow.

Prepare your files. You'll want to make sure your doctor has records from any other physicians you may have visited. You'll also want to inform him of any medications you are taking and any problems that you feel you may be experiencing because of them. You may also want to prepare a list of current health complaints complete with symptoms and dates if possible. "This is especially a must for those patients who seem to suffer from examination room amnesia," says Dr. Goldberg.

What a Checkup Checks Out

You've picked the doc and done your homework, and now you're cooling your heels in the waiting room listening to a Muzak version of "Eleanor Rigby." What lies in wait for you beyond the smiling nurse? Or more to the point, what should happen in the examination room to make for a perfect checkup?

"Working from the head down, your physician should check your body thoroughly," says Dr. Goldberg. He says your doctor should do the following.

• Check the eyes for acuity, voids or dark or black spots in your field of vision and damage from high blood pressure.
• Peer and whisper into the ears, checking for infection and hearing problems.
• Inspect the tongue and gums for signs of oral cancer.

• Listen to the neck for bruits, abnormal sounds that can indicate a clogged artery.
• Examine your skin from head to toe for signs of skin cancer, especially your face, ears, shoulders and the backs of your hands.
• Listen to your chest for heart sounds and lung congestion, crackles or wheezes.
• Probe the abdomen for liver size, kidney and spleen problems and abnormal masses.
• Massage the areas in the neck, armpits and groin for signs of lymph node swelling.
• Check the abdomen and groin for hernia.
• Examine your testicles and penis for cancer or other abnormalities, including warts or sores.
• Tap your arms, knees and toes for reflexes.
• Check your muscle strength for signs of weakness by moving your arms and legs.
• Prick your arms and legs for signs of nerve damage.

What else might you expect?

"Blood pressure should be measured at checkups every one to three years regardless of age," says Dr. Kamerow. "And height and weight should also be noted. It's also not a bad idea to do a non-fasting total blood cholesterol screening, and this is especially needed if there is a history of heart disease in the family."

Outside of those standard tests, not much changes between the ages of 30 and 49 unless there are other risk factors involved. If you are not in a monogamous relationship, for example, you might want to be screened regularly for sexually transmitted diseases, suggests Dr. Kamerow.

When it comes to the more exotic blood and urine tests, electrocardiograms and x-rays, the U.S. Preventive Services Task Force (of which Dr. Kamerow is staff director) does not routinely recommend them for healthy patients.

The only place that there is some hubbub is in the area of rectal examinations and prostate-specific antigen (PSA) tests. "We don't recommend rectal examination," says Dr. Kamerow, "but some groups feel that starting at age 40, this should be a routine part of the checkup."

Dr. Goldberg is part of the "pro" group. "Beginning at age 40, every man should have a digital rectal exam every year. It's the first line in detecting prostate cancer, which is the second leading cancer in men," he says. At age 50, Dr. Goldberg also recommends screening for PSA. "It's produced exclusively by the prostate gland, so it's a sensitive marker for prostate cancer and other prostate problems," says Dr. Goldberg. "After age 50, your blood should be analyzed for PSA once a year. And if you have hereditary risk factors, you should start at 40."

Taking the Doc's Advice Home

Take a deep breath and relax. The poking and prodding are behind you. Now it's time to direct the hard light of science onto your lifestyle. "Outside of the few tests and shots you should get, the most important thing that can be done at a checkup is to team up with the doctor and take stock of your health habits," states Dr. Kamerow firmly. The big four topics are exercise, sexual practices, diet and vices such as smoking and drinking, he says. "Poor habits in these areas contribute mightily to the leading causes of disease and death in this country, and yet they are the very things we cannot test for or fix with medicine."

If you smoke, team up with your doctor on ways to quit. The same goes for recreational drugs, excessive use of medications such as sedatives and diet pills and alcohol abuse. If you are the fast-and-easy type when it comes to sex, have a sobering conversation on safe sex as well as the potential dangers involved in bed hopping. Diet? Haul out that food diary and go over it in detail. And as for exercise, ask your doctor for tips to incorporate physical activity into your daily routine.

If you think that all this is taking up too much of your doctor's valuable time, forget it. "The most important thing that goes on at a checkup is the counseling and the activity that the patient then does because of that counseling," says Dr. Kamerow. "Doctors are beginning to realize that the most healing thing they can do is provide information and motivation."

And the most important thing you can do for your continued health and vigor is take advantage of that information and motivation.

OPTIMISM

How Hope Builds Health

Two men, an optimist and a pessimist, are strolling down the sidewalk in the sleet. They each have holes in their galoshes, and icy water is starting to creep into their wing tips.

"Hmm," the optimist says to himself. "Got a hole there, so I'll drop by the shoe shop tomorrow."

"Of course there's a hole in my galoshes," the pessimist mutters, sloshing along. "Everything always goes wrong for me. I can't even pick out galoshes right."

Other things being relatively equal, which of these men is more likely to live a longer, healthier life? It's the optimist. Here's why.

A Matter of Interpretation

Optimism is not about ignoring what's real but about becoming aware of your thoughts about why things happen, according to Martin Seligman, Ph.D., professor of psychology and director of clinical training at the University of Pennsylvania in Philadelphia and author of *Learned Optimism*. "And there's a good chance that optimism may keep you healthier during the course of middle age and old age."

What's really at the heart of optimism, Dr. Seligman says, is how you explain negative experiences to yourself. When something bad happens to a pessimist, he's likely to descend into a dark cloud of worry in which he believes "It's all my fault, it's permanent, and everything is ruined."

The optimist's explanation? "It was bad luck, it will pass, and I'll handle it differently next time because I learn from my experiences." With this kind of reasoning, the optimist feels a greater sense of control over his future—and his health.

Comeback Power

Optimism can give a man real comeback power as he grows older. "Research has shown that optimistic attitudes and beliefs are associated with fewer illnesses and quicker recovery from illness," says Christopher Peterson, Ph.D., professor of psychology at the University of Michigan in Ann Arbor and author of *Health and Optimism*.

In one study, Dr. Peterson took 99 mentally and physically healthy male students from Harvard University in Cambridge, Massachusetts, evaluated how these men explained negative events in their lives and then tracked their health over the next 35 years. The men who were pessimistic in their twenties were 30 percent more likely to be in poor health two and three decades later, with the strongest negative effects of pessimism showing up when the men were 35 to 50.

Although the researchers aren't certain how optimism works, they speculate that optimists may choose healthier lifestyles and take more advantage of social supports such as family and friendship.

And optimistic men are more likely to feel that they can take charge of their health and not just passively slide down the slope to old age, Dr. Peterson says.

"You're not going to find an 85-year-old with a smiley button who looks 20," says Dr. Peterson. But optimists do tend to show the effects of taking better care of themselves. "They sleep better, don't drink or smoke as much, exercise regularly and are more free from depression," he says. "Optimistic people believe they can control events in their lives, and they make an effort to do so."

So optimists are more likely to live longer and age more gently. If you're fatalistic and believe there's nothing you can do to slow down the aging process, you may be less motivated to stay away from age-accelerating habits, Dr. Peterson says. But optimists tend to make healthier choices.

"And when optimists do fall ill," Dr. Peterson says, "they go to the doctor and shut down and rest, believing this will make a difference. They stay home, drink fluids and follow the doctor's advice. They allow themselves to heal."

Pessimism's Punch

Optimism's negative sibling, pessimism, may also short-circuit your body's resistance to illness, set you up for heart disease and even shorten your life, researchers say.

Pessimism may weaken the immune system. That's the finding of researchers from Yale University in New Haven, Connecticut, the University of Pennsylvania in Philadelphia and the Prince of Wales Hospital in Sydney, Australia. They interviewed 26 men and women to find out what kind of explanations they gave for their health problems and then tested their immune cell activity. The pessimists had higher levels of T-suppressor cells, which interfere with the action of cells that boost immunity. The researchers don't know the

When Pessimism Pays Off

Although extreme pessimism never does anybody any good, some jobs call for a steady dose of realism. And in these fields, moderate pessimism may spell success, says Martin Seligman, Ph.D., professor of psychology and director of clinical training at the University of Pennsylvania in Philadelphia and author of *Learned Optimism*.

Moderate pessimists do well in these areas, Dr. Seligman says.

- Design and safety engineering
- Technical and cost estimating
- Contract negotiation
- Financial control and accounting
- Law (but not litigation)
- Business administration
- Statistics
- Technical writing
- Quality control
- Personnel and industrial relations management

When do you need to be a die-hard optimist? In sales, brokering, public relations, acting, fund-raising, creative jobs, highly competitive jobs and high-burnout jobs, an optimistic outlook is a must, he says.

exact mechanics of how pessimism inhibits immunity, but they do think it might be an important risk factor in immune-related diseases.

But your immune system isn't the only part of the body that's victimized by your feeling like a victim. Dr. Seligman describes pessimism as a kind of depression—and one study shows that a heavy heart is more prone to heart disease.

Researchers at the Centers for Disease Control and Prevention in Atlanta tracked the health and attitudes of 2,832 adults for 12 years. They found that those with the most negative and hopeless attitudes were at greater risk of developing heart disease.

If you're feeling grim, you might even expect an early visit from the Grim Reaper.

Researchers at the Center for Gerontology and Health Care Research at Brown University in Providence, Rhode Island, studied the responses of 1,390 older men and women to questions about their daily lives and the problems of aging. Those who believed their problems were the inevitable result of aging had a 16 percent higher death rate over the next four years than those who believed their problems were due to specific, treatable conditions.

"People who are saying their problems are just due to age are saying 'I have something that's not really treatable,' " says William Rakowski, Ph.D., assistant professor of medical science and co-author of the study. "Whereas, the optimists—people who say it's a specific, treatable condition—are saying 'I can do something about it.' "

It's Never Too Late to Cheer Up

You can learn to cultivate a more upbeat attitude, and it's never too late to start, says Dr. Seligman. "I'm a born pessimist myself, so I've had to learn these techniques, and I use them every day," he says.

Pick positive pals. Look at your friends' attitudes, says Dr. Peterson. "Optimism and pessimism are both contagious states," he says. "So to 'catch' optimism, associate as much as possible with positive people."

Negotiate with naysayers. Likewise, you can't be the only optimist in a family of pessimists, Dr. Peterson says. You're likely to cave in, go numb under the onslaught and become a pessimist yourself. So if it's a family member who spouts negativity all day long, try saying "It really drives me crazy when you talk like this. Can we be negative once a week instead?"

Take credit. There's no need to belittle your triumphs with "I was just lucky," says Dr. Peterson. Instead, you can say to yourself "I worked really hard, I did a good job, and I'm proud of myself," he says. That's the optimistic way of thinking about good events that you brought about by your own efforts.

Be realistic. But never give up. Optimism doesn't mean you don't look at life head-on, Dr. Rakowski says. "Be realistic about what's happened in your life: 'Yes, I've had it tough,' 'I was a victim of circumstance there,' 'That was my fault,' 'That wasn't,' 'I did this well.' " And then use optimism to resolve that, in spite of it all. Tell yourself "With effort, initiative and good luck, I will still have good things to look forward to," he says.

Make the best of it. Some men face a great deal of adversity and still call themselves optimists, Dr. Rakowski says. Why? "When you're optimistic, you're also believing 'I can make the most of what I have,' " he says. "Sometimes you need to redefine your objectives and let go of an initial expectation. Then your basic objective is still to make the most of what you have."

Don't confuse belief with fact. It's essential to realize that your beliefs are just that—beliefs, Dr. Seligman says. If a business rival said to you "You're a lousy manager, and you'll never make it in this market," you'd know to ignore his insult. But what about the perpetual put-downs that you tell yourself? ("I can't find a parking place. I'm such a loser.") They can be just as baseless as an enemy's bad-mouthing, only it's bad thinking—a mental reflex you don't have to find convincing. "Check out the accuracy of your reflexive beliefs and argue with yourself," he says.

Learn your optimism ABC. Three things happen when you face a tough situation, says Dr. Seligman, and ABC is a good way to remember the pattern. You respond to *a*dversity with a *b*elief, which determines the *c*onsequence. For example, you're on the phone trying to make a sale, and your first caller hangs up on you—adversity. When you respond to the adversity with an optimistic belief—"Oh well, that's one no out of the way. It brings me closer to the yes"—the likely consequence is that you'll feel relaxed and energetic. Compare that with a knee-jerk negative belief ("I'll never get any better at this"), which produces an equally negative consequence (you feel lousy about yourself).

Just say no. There are lots of specific techniques to stop negative thoughts that just won't leave you be, says Dr. Seligman. Smack your palm on your desk and say—loudly—"Stop!" Or put a rubber band around your wrist and snap it every time you have the thought. (One wag says this helps you "snap out of it.") Or write down the thought and set aside a time to think it over later. These techniques can stop a bout of pessimism before it starts.

Give back. If painful circumstances have made you unhappy, doing what you can to help others may give you a more optimistic view, says Dr. Rakowski. Whether you do volunteer work or simply offer to listen to a friend's troubles, you can find a way to give. There's a real sense of fulfillment in giving that can lift you out of your pain, he says.

Get help for depression. "If you're a real pessimist, odds are you're fairly depressed," says Dr. Peterson. "It's a good bet that undergoing therapy for depression will make you healthier and improve your life." Cognitive behavioral therapy, during which you learn to challenge defeatist ways of thinking, is particularly helpful in turning depression around, he says.

Chronically unhappy people do a running negative commentary on their lives that they're often not aware of, he says. A therapist can teach you ways to divert yourself when you get in these moods. These techniques may not reduce the frequency of episodes of depression you have but will shorten them, he says. And in some cases, a prescription for antidepressant medication may help.

RELAXATION

A Powerful Ally against Father Time

You cherish your downtime—those moments when you don't need to be anywhere or do anything. But if you're the average guy of the 1990s, getting this kind of time is as unlikely as finding a hockey player who has all his teeth.

And relaxation isn't something that you can afford to forgo. In fact, taking a few minutes each day to relax and let life's strains roll off isn't a luxury; it's a necessity if you want to stay vigorous, productive and healthy.

"There are three main things you can do to prolong your life. One is to exercise, one is to maintain proper nutrition, and the other is to relax. Relaxation can definitely help you age better. It's important for preventing a wide variety of disorders and for increasing your effectiveness and efficiency in life," says Frank J. McGuigan, Ph.D., director of the Institute for Stress Management at the United States International University in San Diego. "I don't think there's any question that relaxation can have a positive effect on phobias, depression, anxiety, high blood pressure, ulcers, colitis, headaches and lower back pain."

Slow Down, You Move Too Fast

For many of us, relaxing means shooting some hoops, whacking a golf ball or nailing a killer tennis serve.

But while those activities can be stress relieving, they can also trigger competition and frustration, two things that actually make it harder to relax, says Richard Friedman, Ph.D., associate professor of psychology at the State University of New York at Stony Brook.

"We know from carefully conducted experiments that most people don't really get into a relaxed physiological state when they're doing things that society generally considers relaxing, like reading a newspaper, playing sports or watching television," Dr. Friedman says. "The true way to get into a relaxed physiological state is essentially to let your mind go into neutral."

Popping your brain out of gear momentarily frees your mind, so you're not judging anything or pondering weighty decisions. For a few seconds or minutes, you're not thinking about what you could have done yesterday or what might happen tomorrow. Taking several of these mental rest stops each day lessens anxiety and helps you let go of stress and tension, Dr. Friedman says. This physiological state, called the relaxation response, has been shown to lower heart rate, metabolism, blood pressure and breath rate, slow brain waves and foster feelings of peace and tranquillity, says Herbert Benson, M.D., associate professor of medicine at Harvard Medical School and chief of the Behavioral Medicine Division at the New England Deaconess Hospital, both in Boston, and author of *The Relaxation Response*.

Sometimes relaxation or a feeling of ease and well-being arises naturally, like after a long, enjoyable run or a good laugh. But if you've ever had anyone tell you to relax when you felt stressed, besides becoming more frustrated or upset, you know how difficult it is to consciously allow yourself to regain a sense of stability and calm.

"To relax, you really can't try too hard. This is similar to trying to fall asleep. Often the effort involved in attempting to make yourself go to sleep will probably keep you awake all night," says Saki Santorelli, Ed.D., associate director of the Stress Reduction Clinic at the University of Massachusetts Medical Center in Worcester.

To truly unwind, Dr. Santorelli says, you actually need to concentrate or focus your attention on your breath or some other sensation that will allow your mind to settle into an inherent sense of stillness. There are plenty of ways to unwind, but before we talk about them, let's find out a bit more about the physical and psychological benefits of the relaxation.

Mellow Out for Better Health

When you're stuck in traffic, struggling to meet a deadline or facing any other stressful situation, your muscles tense, you breathe faster and deeper, your heart beats more rapidly, blood vessels constrict and blood pressure rises, the digestive tract shuts down, and perspiration increases. Over time, constant stress elevates blood pressure, total blood cholesterol and blood platelet counts, all of which can lead to atherosclerosis (hardening of the arteries) and heart attacks. Add to that other risk factors of a modern lifestyle—like a high-fat diet and too little exercise—and you're on course to an earlier demise.

In a study of monkeys, whose cardiovascular systems are similar to ours, researchers at Bowman Gray School of Medicine of Wake Forest University in Winston-Salem, North Carolina, found that emotional stress (caused by the disruption of the animals' social bonds) significantly increased coronary blockages. And these blockages occurred regardless of diet and blood cholesterol levels— two of the major risk factors for heart disease. When the monkeys were fed a typical high-fat diet, emotional stress magnified the process of atherosclerosis 30 times.

Stress is also linked to ulcers and colitis and can trigger backaches, headaches, leg pain, chronic fatigue, depression, anxiety and insomnia. It also can aggravate arthritis and diabetes, Dr. McGuigan says.

In fact, eight of ten people seen by primary care physicians have some stress-related symptoms, says Robert S. Eliot, M.D., director of the Institute of Stress Medicine in Jackson Hole, Wyoming, and author of *From Stress to Strength: How to Lighten Your Load and Save Your Life.*

Fortunately, practicing relaxation techniques can relieve or prevent almost all of the harmful effects of chronic stress, Dr. Benson says.

Relaxation training, for instance, is a core element in a successful program to clear clogged arteries and reverse heart disease without surgery pioneered by Dean Ornish, M.D., president and director of the Preventive Medicine Research Institute in Sausalito, California. While Dr. Ornish believes that all the components of his program are important—including regular exercise and a nearly fat-free vegetarian diet—he says that relaxation training is probably one of its most powerful components.

"We've shown, using PET scans and angiograms, that people who practice some form of relaxation, like yoga or meditation, and who meet regularly with a support group experience a greater degree of heart disease reversal than if they attack the problem only at the physical level, say with just diet or cholesterol-lowering drugs," Dr. Ornish says. A PET scan is positron emission tomography, a three-dimensional imaging technique that measures heart blood flow.

Studies by Dr. Benson and other researchers also have consistently shown that relaxation techniques significantly relieve high blood pressure, another risk factor for heart disease.

Practicing muscle relaxation techniques in addition to dietary and lifestyle changes, for example, helped a group of 32- to 55-year-old men with high blood pressure lower their systolic blood pressure (the upper number in blood pressure readings) an average of eight points in seven weeks. In contrast, a similar group of men who were encouraged to exercise, lose weight and limit their salt consumption showed virtually no change in their borderline high blood pressure.

Relaxation can also short-circuit lower back pain and headaches. Muscle relaxation, for example, helped 21 people whose severe chronic tension headaches weren't relieved by drugs reduce the number and severity of their headaches by 42 percent, according to researchers from the Center for Stress and Anxiety Disorders at State University of New York at Albany. Another group of people who simply tracked their headache activity showed no improvement at all.

Getting Down to Basics

If you ever used your older brother's prized T-shirt to wax your car, you know all about fight or flight, the two basic responses to stress. But Dr. Eliot suggests that we might be better off if we learned another approach.

"When you can't fight and you can't flee, then flow," he says.

While learning to be more relaxed and at ease takes time and attention, it can be done. "I look at relaxation as being comfortable in your own skin," Dr. Santorelli says. "That's tough for all of us at times, but it's possible to begin cultivating that capacity at any age."

Here are a few basics to help you mellow out.

Snuff out the smokes. "Our studies show that smoking causes blood vessels to clamp down and restrict blood flow," Dr. Eliot says. "That's like trying to drive with your foot pressed down on the brake. If there's a single thing that people can do to feel less stressed and more relaxed, it's kicking the habit."

Whittle your weight. "It's hard to feel relaxed if you're carrying around extra weight," Dr. Eliot says. "Your clothes don't feel comfortable, and your body image suffers." Being overweight also contributes to high blood pressure, heart disease and diabetes. Ask your doctor if losing weight could help you.

Team up with carbos. "Protein seems to raise energy levels and keep you alert," Dr. Eliot says. "So if you have a hamburger late at night, you'll probably be rehashing yesterday's sales meeting until dawn." Carbohydrates, on the other hand, trigger the release of hormones that will help relax you. So if you want to unwind after dinner, eat a plate of spaghetti, baked beans or other complex carbohydrates.

Write it down. Over a dozen studies have shown that if you write about your problems, you can help relieve stress, improve your immunity, make fewer visits to the doctor and have a more optimistic view of life, says James Pennebaker, Ph.D., professor of psychology at Southern Methodist University in Dallas. Spend 20 minutes a day writing about your deepest thoughts and feelings, Dr. Pennebaker suggests. Don't worry about grammar or style; just write how you feel about things that are really upsetting you. Then when you're done, throw the paper away. You may feel a sense of relief.

Keep time on your side. "Every time after you look at a clock or your watch during a day, take a deep breath while consciously raising and lowering your shoulders or dropping your jaw," Dr. Santorelli says. "That probably takes ten seconds and will serve as a reminder to you that you can be at ease while going about your daily schedule."

Laugh it off. Humor is a powerful relaxation technique, Dr. Eliot says. Laughter triggers the release of endorphins, chemicals in the brain that produce feelings of euphoria. It also suppresses the production of cortisol, a hormone released when you're under stress that indirectly raises blood pressure by causing the body to retain salt. So share a good laugh with a friend or keep a file of humorous anecdotes and drawings that you can quickly pull out.

Make time for others. "Take a moment to practice basic kindness," Dr. Santorelli says. "Smile and say hello to a co-worker, play with a pet or talk to a close friend. If you do, you might feel better and more relaxed and possibly be more productive."

Snooze away. Get plenty of uninterrupted rest, Dr. Eliot advises. If you get less sleep than you need, you might wake feeling tense and incapable of coping with life's basic hassles. Try to get at least six to eight hours of sleep each night. Avoid alcohol or sleeping pills. Although they can help put you to sleep, they can also interfere with your natural sleeping patterns and actually cause you to have a less restful night, Dr. Eliot says.

Going with the Flow

There are many methods available for the development of calmness and stability. The key is finding one that feels comfortable to you. "I feel that it is important to set aside a block of time each day to practice these methods and then incorporate them into your daily life. Often these can be so unobtrusive that most people won't know that you're doing anything special," says Dr. Santorelli. Here are some ideas.

Pay attention to your breath. Paying attention to your own breathing is a simple form of meditation that can be very calming, Dr. Santorelli says. Sit in a comfortable chair or on the floor so that your back, neck and head are straight but not rigid. Exhaling deeply, allow the inhalation to come naturally. Simply pay attention to the gentle rising and falling of your abdomen, the movement of your ribs or the sensation of the breath moving through your nostrils. There's no need to try "relaxing." Just focus your mind on your breathing. If your mind starts to wander, gently escort it back to your breathing.

As an alternative, lie on the floor, put a book on your abdomen and take several slow, deep breaths, Dr. Eliot suggests. Focus on the book moving up and down on your belly. As you breathe in, think to yourself "Cool, clear mind." Then as you blow out, think "Calm, relaxed body."

Take a slice of life. Another way of cultivating moment-to-moment awareness is to focus your attention on a food, Dr. Santorelli says. Take a single slice of orange or apple, an almond, a raisin or some other food you like. Look at it carefully. Roll it around in your fingers. Focus your mind on its color, texture or fragrance. Then after a few moments, consciously decide to take one small bite. Chew it slowly, paying attention to its taste and what happens to it in your mouth. Feel your tongue engulf it. Then slowly and consciously swallow it.

As an alternative, try focusing intently on an everyday activity, like showering or washing dishes. "Some people say that they feel much more at ease after practicing in this way," Dr. Santorelli says.

Climb every mountain. Visualizations and imagery can encourage the development of calmness and well-being, Dr. Santorelli says. Closing your eyes, once again become aware of your breath and bring to mind a favorite mountain in your life. It could be one you've climbed or yearned to visit. Allow your body to become the stable foundation, sloping sides and summit. Feel yourself steady, solid, grounded. As your sense of stability and steadiness grows, allow the weather to vary; some days the mountain will be awash in sunlight, other times covered with rain, snow, sleet or hail. Although the weather changes, notice that the mountain remains steady and dignified. "This image helps you realize that you can feel stable and secure and endure any storm that life has in store for you, like being stuck in a traffic jam, facing a deadline or living with the death of a loved one," Dr. Santorelli says.

Move that body. Exercise triggers the release of endorphins, but exercising the mind and body simultaneously may produce even better results, according to researchers at the University of Massachusetts Medical Center in Worcester. They asked 40 sedentary people to begin walking 35 to 40 minutes a day, three times a week, while listening to relaxation tapes. The tapes guided the walkers through a meditation that helped them focus on the one-two rhythm of their steps. The researchers concluded that this routine provoked more feelings of euphoria and reduced anxiety than in a matched group that exercised at the same intensity but didn't listen to the tapes.

"If you focus your mind on an unchanging, repetitive rhythm like exercise, the mind tends to go blank. That blankness is what you're shooting for," Dr. Friedman says. "It gives the brain a chance to restore itself and calm down."

To try it, pick an exercise (such as walking, running, swimming, climbing stairs or jumping rope) that has a natural rhythm. Focus your attention on that rhythm, even to the point of repeating the words "one, two" in your head in cadence with the exercise. Try to stay in that rhythm. As with breathing or other types of meditation, your mind may start to wander after a couple of minutes. If it does, refocus your attention on the repetitive movement of the exercise, Dr. Benson says.

Try doing this 20 minutes a day, three times a week, Dr. Benson suggests.

Unleash those muscles. There are about 1,030 skeletal muscles in the body. When you feel under stress, these muscles naturally contract and create tension, Dr. McGuigan says. One way to counteract that is progressive relaxation. By systematically flexing and releasing muscles, progressive relaxation can whisk that tension right out of your body.

"It's a good technique for beginners because it's practical and doesn't depend on imagination," says Martha Davis, Ph.D., a psychologist at Kaiser Permanente Medical Center in Santa Clara, California, and co-author of *The Relaxation and Stress Reduction Workbook*. "It works because it exaggerates the tension in the muscle so that you become more aware of what tension feels like. Secondly, you fatigue the muscle so that when you let go, the muscle is more than ready to relax."

Although there are many variations, Dr. Davis suggests this approach: Clench your right fist as tightly as you can. Keep it clenched for about ten seconds, then release. Feel the looseness in your right hand and notice how much more relaxed it feels than when you tensed it. Do the same thing with your left hand, then clench both fists at the same time. Bend your elbows and tense your arms. Release and let your arms hang at your sides. Continue this process by tensing, then relaxing, your shoulders and neck and wrinkling, then relaxing, your forehead and brows. Then squeeze your eyes and clench your jaw before moving on to tense, then relax, your stomach, lower back, thighs, buttocks, calves and feet. It should take about ten minutes to complete the entire sequence. Try to do these exercises twice a day.

Stretch them, too. Unlike progressive relaxation, which contracts muscles, gentle stretching allows muscles to stretch and relax. That's better for some people, particularly those with chronic muscle pain, says Charles R. Carlson, Ph.D., professor of psychology at the University of Kentucky in Lexington.

"If you tense a muscle that is already in pain, you'll likely just create more pain. That doesn't help you relax," Dr. Carlson says. "Gentle stretching does two things. First, if you gently stretch a muscle and release it, it will generally relax. But secondly, when you focus your attention on doing the stretch, it also helps the mind relax. Muscle stretching should always be done slowly and without pain. There should be no overstretching or bouncing of muscles."

As an example of stretch-based relaxation, begin by pushing up your eyebrows with your index fingers and pushing down on your cheeks with your thumbs. (While doing any of these stretching exercises, note what the tension feels like, so you'll learn to monitor your muscle tension, Dr. Carlson advises.) Hold that position for about ten seconds, then release and let the muscles around your eyes relax. After a minute of relaxing your muscles, let your head slowly sag toward your right shoulder for about ten seconds, then slowly sag your head toward the left shoulder for another ten seconds.

Next, at chest height, place your hands together as if you were praying. Then keeping your fingertips and palms together, spread your fingers as if you were creating a fan. Move your thumbs down along the midline of your body until you feel a light stretch in the lower arms. Hold that position for ten seconds. Then relax.

Next, interlock your fingers and raise your hands over your head. Straighten your elbows and rotate your palms outward. Let your arms fall back over your head until you feel resistance. Hold that position for ten seconds, then quickly release and let your arms rest at your sides for one minute.

Do these exercises at least once a day or whenever you feel tense.

RELIGION AND SPIRITUALITY

Power from Within
for the Long Haul

Whether you head for a familiar pew or take a nontraditional path, having a spiritual life can provide a powerful force for health. Faith not only fends off many forms of physical illness but also can take the emotional edge off aging.

If words like *faith*, *spirituality* or *religion* make you a little uncomfortable, you're not alone, says Mark Gerzon, author of *Coming into Our Own: Understanding the Adult Metamorphosis*. "Even talking about ways to bring spiritual dimensions into our lives makes some people nervous, because it may remind us of everything we didn't like as kids about church or morality." But you don't have to belong to an organized religion to benefit from a spiritual life as you age, he says.

Private and public expressions of spirituality—from meditation and prayer to attending religious services—increase emotional fulfillment while helping to relieve stress and depression. They also decrease your risk of heart disease and cancer. They may even help prevent alcoholism, drug use and suicide, researchers say.

Listening to Your Inner Voice

What is spirituality? According to *Webster's*, it means "relating to the spirit." If that seems a little vague, that's good, says Gerzon.

What matters most is to experience your own spirituality in your own way, Gerzon says. "The key thing about spirituality in the second half of life is that we've lived enough and seen enough people pass from this earth to feel an urgency," he says. "We begin to listen to our inner voices. And when we do, where they lead us is not predictable. They may lead us back to the church of our childhood, but they may also lead us to other places we never expected.

"So we need to broaden our view of what spiritual means. For some it could be tending flowers in the garden, and for others, saying Hail Marys at morning mass."

Perhaps your sense of the sacred has more to do with getting close to nature or to another human being than participating publicly in religious rites. Many people draw meaning and strength from this kind of private spirituality, says Gerzon.

One way of searching for a sense of wholeness is through meditation or prayer, which have been shown to decrease heart rate and blood pressure and to help you cope better with stress.

The Strength of Community

Most scientific conclusions about religion and health have been drawn from organized religion, because religious organizations provide researchers with measurable groups of subjects involved in specific behaviors, such as attending worship services or participating together in community service. But perhaps there is something about religious community itself—aside from a shared belief system—that makes you healthier.

When your beliefs encourage you to be involved in the community's social activities, you become part of a caring network that will be there for you when the chips are down, says Dave Larson, M.D., adjunct associate professor of psychiatry at Duke University Medical Center in Durham, North Carolina, president of the National Institute for Healthcare Research in Rockville, Maryland, and former senior research psychiatrist at the National Institutes of Health Office of Alternative Medicine.

In some ways, such as prolonging life, men benefit from the community aspects of religious life even more than women do, he says. Attendance is even more important for us, Dr. Larson says, because "women usually have a better network of support outside of their spiritual community than men do." Unlike men, women are encouraged from childhood to talk and build relationships and to work effectively together.

Erasing Stress through Spirituality

Raised to value independence, many men are just not very good at connecting with others on a deeper personal support level, Dr. Larson says. If a man stiff-upper-lips his way through most of the challenges he faces, this can easily lead to a deep sense of isolation. That isolation can become a major source of stress, he says.

Health experts have known for years that stress contributes to many phys-

Pray and Be Mellow

When you meditate or open your heart in prayer, you're calling on a powerful stress reducer, says Herbert Benson, M.D., associate professor of medicine at Harvard Medical School and chief of the Behavioral Medicine Division at the New England Deaconess Hospital, both in Boston, and author of *The Relaxation Response*.

Dr. Benson conducted some of the first scientific studies into the effects of prayer and faith on stress reduction. To help patients learn how to relax, he taught the simplest meditation method: Sit quietly in a comfortable position and silently repeat a word or phrase while passively disregarding other thoughts.

When patients were offered the choice of a word, sound or phrase to repeat, 80 percent of them chose a word or prayer from their faith. And that led to discovery, Dr. Benson says. People who used words from their own religion rather than neutral words (like "be calm" or "one") stuck with the program better. And their health improved as a result of the relaxation response, which is characterized by decreased heart rate and blood pressure and feelings of tranquillity.

The words may vary, Dr. Benson says, but the benefits don't. "In all the different religious contexts, there seems to be a similar potential for health-enhancing effects," he says. Here's how to bring those benefits into your life every day.

Choose a word or short phrase that's easy to pronounce and short enough to say silently as you exhale. When thoughts arise, as they inevitably will, gently return to the focus word. Practice this kind of meditation for 20 minutes twice a day, and you'll enjoy periods of stillness and quiet in your mind.

---

ical problems, including nausea, diarrhea, constipation, high blood pressure and heart rhythm abnormalities.

Studies have shown that strong religious beliefs go a long way to relieve stress, even if you simply hold your beliefs privately. But the stress-relieving effects of faith are most powerful, experts say, when you are regularly involved with a religious community.

Whether it's enjoying potluck suppers or affectionate hugs from the old woman who always calls you "Dear," activities at the center of a religious community also serve up sustenance of a different kind. The community can provide you with a sense of intimacy, almost like being part of a big extended family. And as a member, you participate in a reciprocal network of support, says Lawrence Calhoun, Ph.D., a psychologist at the University of North Carolina at Charlotte.

"When people in religious communities get sick, they visit each other, bringing food; they notify relatives and take each other to the doctor," Dr. Calhoun says. "When you're a meaningful part of a community like that, it can soften the sting of getting older."

Body and Soul

Psychologists Stanislav Kasl of Yale University in New Haven, Connecticut, and Ellen Idler of Rutgers University in New Brunswick, New Jersey, studied 2,812 elderly people in New Haven. They found that outwardly religious Catholics, Protestants and Jews were less likely to become medically disabled than those who considered attending church or synagogue unimportant. These people also remained more physically independent as they got older, largely because of their public religious involvement. But the researchers found, too, that men in poor health who did not participate publicly were strongly protected from serious depression by their private faith.

Even though holidays may have gotten a bad rap because of the commercialism that surrounds some of them, events like Hanukkah, Easter, Christmas and other religious holidays may mean even more to you as the years go by. The New Haven study found that very religious people are much less likely to die during the months before and after major religious holidays, when death rates among nonbelievers tend to rise.

Religion in your life can also be potent protection against cancer. This may be because some groups of believers, such as Mormons and Jehovah's Witnesses, encourage healthy lifestyle choices, like eating a vegetarian diet or avoiding smoking. Analysts from the University of Florida's Center for Health Policy Research in Gainesville reviewed data on cancer deaths across the United States and found that counties with the highest number of religious people also have the lowest rates of cancer.

Even faiths that do not recommend specific dietary or health habits still have a protective effect, the researchers believe, simply because they encourage moderation, cautioning their members against unhealthy excesses of any kind.

Strength for the Heart

When a man opens his heart to faith, he helps close it to heart disease, the leading cause of death for men.

A study of 454 men and 85 women in Jerusalem, Israel, showed that those who defined themselves as "secular" (nonreligious) had a greater risk of heart disease than those who followed the path of Orthodox Judaism. Even after the researchers accounted for smoking habits and cholesterol and blood pressure levels, a strong association between lowered heart disease risk and religious practice remained.

Although the researchers are unsure which aspects of belief are responsible, they speculate that the strong social support system of traditional Orthodox communities, like that of many other congregations, plays a heart-protecting role, perhaps by reducing stress and isolation.

In another study of religion and the heart, Dr. Larson and his colleagues studied data on blood pressure in more than 400 men in Evans County, Georgia. They found that either a personal belief in God or attendance at religious services (even without belief) tended to lower blood pressure, but people who both believed and attended had the lowest readings.

Soothing a Troubled Spirit

Men who are feeling alone in the world are much more vulnerable to depression and self-destructive behavior, psychologists say.

Dr. Larson and his research team reviewed more than 200 studies on religious commitment and mental health. They found that people who are religious have lower rates of depression, alcoholism, suicide and drug use than less religious people do. Young people who are religious do better in school and are less likely to be delinquent and sexually active. Married people who attend church regularly report greater marital happiness, are more satisfied with their sexual lives and experience lower rates of divorce.

The studies also showed that religious faith is directly connected to a higher sense of satisfaction with life in general and a greater ability to cope with life's stresses and problems, Dr. Larson says. The researchers examined specific "real life" behaviors, such as attending services, rather than attempting to measure attitudes or beliefs.

Kindling an Eternal Flame

It's common for men in midlife to feel a new interest in spiritual exploration, says Gerzon. Here are some ways to rekindle your spiritual flame.

Think it through. Before you recommit to the religion you were raised in or embrace another faith, examine it, says Alan Berger, Ph.D., director of Jewish studies in the Department of Religion at Syracuse University in Syracuse, New York. "Ask yourself 'What is it that my tradition teaches?' " he says. "Don't feel you have to accept it, but do know it."

Recognize that religion is more than rules. If religion seems only like a series of thou-shalt-nots, Dr. Berger says, "you need to un-skew your view. Go find yourself a better teacher, a new community. Read the texts yourself or with a partner and uncover the various levels of meaning. Understand that life is a fluid and dynamic experience that people need help with. Religion is the attempt to search for meaning in an otherwise chaotic universe."

Start right where you are. "It's fine to say 'I don't really know what I am spiritually,' " says Brother Guerric Plante, a monk at the Abbey of Gethsemane in New Haven, Kentucky. "Honesty has everything to do with spiritual growth." Once you're open with yourself about any confusion you feel, the way will become more clear.

Search with others. Read the religion and support group announcements in the newspaper to find a group or organization that may offer help for your spiritual search, Brother Plante says. "Faith can come through others—their example, their talk, their interest in others. Group therapy, religious services or even a 12-step group for addiction can rekindle a spiritual life if you're sincerely searching."

Learn from stillness. Clear time from your schedule to sit in quiet contemplation and listen to the stillness within you, says Gerzon. "If we derive meaning and purpose in life only from doing, we're in trouble," he says. "We need to find it from being, and meditation is a good way to start learning about how to simply be."

Stay open. Sometimes just encouraging your sense of curiosity and wondering about life will lead you to spiritual truths. When you ponder some of the age-old questions such as "Why am I here?" or "What is the meaning of life?" you encourage your spiritual insight to unfold, says Gerzon. "It's possible to find the spiritual dimension in answers, but we're more likely to find it in the questions themselves," he says. "When we're really moved by the spirit of life, it's because we're touching what we don't know, not what we know."

Find new spiritual challenges. You're more likely to grow spiritually if you seek out activities that are different from what you usually do all day, says John Buehrens, a minister for over 20 years and president of the Unitarian Universalist Association in Boston. If you spend your day in a corporate office, then serving a meal to the needy may be just what you need, he says. And a man who already serves others in his working life may benefit more from a discussion group instead.

Buehrens's own spiritual discipline? "I'm a pointy-headed, pear-shaped intellectual," he says. "So one of my spiritual disciplines is getting some regular exercise. It really is a time of meditation and prayer for me."

Think about somebody else. You need to get out of yourself to feel spiritually healthy, Buehrens says. "That's why community is so important to real spiritual growth, because we're drawn out of ourselves. We'll never find peace along religious, racial and ethnic lines unless we do this." His advice for the isolated? "Go help in a soup kitchen, go visit a nursing home and get your nose out of your navel," he says.

Keep a spiritual journal. Writing in a daily journal about your spiritual questions, doubts, beliefs and experiences can illuminate the meaning and value in your life, says Buehrens. "You may find that your unconscious is trying to get through to you with more life-enhancing and creatively responsible methods," he says.

Question authority. "All spiritual traditions try to teach an enhanced awareness of being, greater spiritual vitality and deeper compassion for other people," Buehrens says. But any spiritual community that doesn't respect questioning or the importance of your individual conscience may be an unhealthy one, he says. His advice? Follow your own conscience to the spiritual path that's right for you.

RESISTANCE TRAINING

Just the Lift You Need

Let's face it. You lift weights to look good.

Hold on. Let's be really honest. You do it to look big.

Make that BIGGER.

Make that BIGGEST.

So you make a weekly, if not daily, ritual of frequenting the weight room.

But did you know that all that effort may lead to more than just the ability to flex more brawn than the next guy? It may enable you to outlive him, too, because it helps maintain, if not improve, your quality of life.

Resistance training improves muscle strength and endurance, qualities that will enable you to do the activities you love well into old age. It can also help improve your cholesterol level, enhance your bone strength, maintain or lose weight and improve your body image and self-esteem.

"If people stay with it, continue to be active and continue to do activities that stress the muscles, they can fight off some of the effects of aging," says Alan Mikesky, Ph.D., an exercise physiologist and professor at Indiana University School of Physical Education in Indianapolis. "People can continue to do things they enjoy in life longer—and not only that but also maintain their performance in what they're doing."

Make It Your Strong Point

One of the major benefits of resistance training is its effect on muscle strength. Maintaining or increasing muscle strength is crucial to maintaining independence into old age, says Miriam Nelson, Ph.D., a research scientist and exercise physiologist in the Human Physiology Laboratory at the U.S. Department of Agriculture Human Nutrition Research Center on Aging at Tufts University in Boston. Adequate muscle strength is what enables you to do things like carry your own luggage, climb stairs and get in and out of bed.

Resistance training increases muscle strength by putting more strain on a muscle than it's used to. This increased load stimulates the growth of small proteins inside each muscle cell that play a central role in the ability to generate force. "When you lift weights, you stress or challenge the muscle cells, and they adapt by making more force-generating proteins," says Dr. Mikesky.

Weight training also helps improve muscle endurance, says Dr. Mikesky. So in addition to giving you the strength you need to lift a suitcase, it will give you the endurance you need to carry that suitcase for a longer period of time.

It doesn't take long to improve muscle strength, says Dr. Mikesky. "You can increase strength very quickly, in as little as 2 to 3 weeks," he says. Noticeable increases in muscle size take longer—about 6 to 8 weeks. Some studies have shown strength increases of 100 percent or more in 12 weeks, he says. The bad news is that you can lose strength gains just as quickly. "If you miss a week of workouts and go back and put the same weight on, it's harder," says Dr. Mikesky.

There are several different methods for resistance training, including free weights, weight machines, calisthenics and resistance tubing. Free weights involve the use of dumbbells and bars stacked with weight plates; the lifter is responsible for both lifting the weight and determining and controlling body position through the range of motion. Weight machines, on the other hand, allow you to lift plates, but the machine dictates the movement that you perform. Calisthenics, such as chin-ups, push-ups and sit-ups, utilize your own body weight as the resistance force. Resistance tubing involves the use of an elastic band that provides resistance to the active muscles. In one study conducted at Indiana University–Purdue University at Indianapolis, 62 older adults were put on a 12-week training program with elastic tubing. The participants showed an average increase in strength of 82 percent, as measured by the increase in the tubing's level of resistance.

"The difference between free weights and machines is that machines are more user-friendly," says physical therapist Mark V. Taranta, director of the Physical Therapy Practice in Philadelphia. Training with machines doesn't require a lot of skill or coordination. "With free weights, more balance is required, and there are more learning techniques required," he says.

There are different theories on what's the best type of resistance training program to follow. A lot of it depends on your individual goals. In general, lifting a heavy weight in three sets of 8 to 12 repetitions is the best way to build strength. And lifting a lighter weight for more repetitions helps build endurance and tone.

Heft for the Heart

Weight training can also give your cardiovascular health a lift, experts say. Studies of the effect of weight training on cholesterol profiles are controversial, says Dr. Mikesky, but some of them suggest an improvement in cholesterol levels similar to that brought about by endurance training.

In one study conducted at the West Virginia University Medical Center in Morgantown, resistance training helped increase levels of HDL (high-density lipoprotein) cholesterol, the good cholesterol, and decrease levels of LDL (low-density lipoprotein) cholesterol, the bad cholesterol. Twenty-five men lifted weights three times a week for eight weeks. HDL levels rose from 38.8 to 44.1, and LDL levels declined from 132 to 121. For men, the recommended level for HDL is at least 40 or above.

In another study, six men and eight women used resistance training three days a week for 45 to 60 minutes each session. Significant changes in cholesterol levels were observed. In men, the ratio of total cholesterol to HDL—a measurement that helps estimate how much LDL you have and serves as the best predictor of heart disease—was reduced by 21.6 percent. In the women, the ratio dropped by 14.3 percent.

Ideally, you want your ratio of total cholesterol to HDL to be low; a ratio of less than 3.5 is desirable. A ratio between 3.5 and 6.9 indicates moderate risk, and a ratio over 7.0 indicates high risk.

There's some indication that higher volume weight training—the kind that involves lifting a lighter weight for more repetitions—may have more of an effect on cholesterol levels than weight training that involves lifting heavier weights for fewer repetitions, says Janet Walberg-Rankin, Ph.D., associate professor in the Exercise Science Program in the Division of Health and Physical Education at Virginia Polytechnic Institute and State University in Blacksburg.

One study of ten men at Florida State University in Tallahassee found that men who performed high-volume weight training—sets of 8 to 12 repetitions performed with lighter weights and 60 seconds of rest in between—had lower cholesterol levels and higher HDL levels than men who did lower-volume training—sets of 1 to 5 repetitions with higher weights and three minutes of rest in between.

While researchers don't fully understand how weight training lowers cholesterol, one means might be its effect on body composition and weight, says Dr. Walberg-Rankin. Weight training sometimes leads to weight loss and the reduction of body fat, and that can cause cholesterol to drop, she says.

Resistance training can certainly have an effect on your body composition. Muscles burn more calories than fat, so by increasing muscle mass, you increase your metabolic rate and can burn calories and reduce fat tissue.

A Good Way to Bone Up

Resistance training puts stress on bone as well as muscle and thereby helps increase bone mineral mass and prevent osteoporosis, experts say. While aerobic weight-bearing exercise like walking and running helps maintain bone strength in the legs and hips, it's less effective on the spine and upper body. Resistance training helps maintain bone strength in those areas, says Dr. Walberg-Rankin.

One study of 46 young men conducted at the University of California, San Francisco, found that the bone density of men who lifted weights was higher than that of men who did not lift.

Boost Your Body Image

Resistance training is also a good way to feel better about the way you look. Researchers have found that resistance training is often superior to aerobic exercise for improving self-esteem and body image.

One reason weight training may be so effective in boosting self-esteem is that feedback is immediate. In addition to being able to see muscle growth and improved muscle tone, you can detect progress easily. "You know in two weeks when you can lift more weights on a machine," says Dr. Walberg-Rankin. That's a little easier to detect than an improvement in your aerobic fitness, she says.

How to Get to It

Why wait around when you can be lifting weights around? Here are some tips for getting started.

Check it out. Your physical health, that is. If you're planning to start a resistance-training program, see your doctor for a physical first, says Michael Kaplan, M.D., Ph.D., director of the Rehabilitation Team, a sports medicine and physical therapy clinic in Catonsville, Maryland. Your doctor will do a physical exam and take a health history. If you have a history of osteoporosis, heart disease or high blood pressure, be sure to mention it.

Don't go it alone. "If you don't have experience, get instruction from a reputable trainer or join a reputable health club," says John Skowron, physical therapist at Raleigh Community Sports Medicine and Physical Therapy in Raleigh, North Carolina.

Look for someone with a master's degree in exercise physiology or certification from the American College of Sports Medicine or the National Strength and Conditioning Association, he says. The trainer can help you decide on the best resistance training method for you and get you started on a program. If you are doing a home program with a gym machine or dumbbell weights, consult a video on proper weight-lifting techniques. If you're interested in using resistance tubing, consult a physical therapist or exercise physiologist.

Be sure to breathe. While you're lifting, do not hold your breath, says Dr. Walberg-Rankin. It doesn't really matter when you breathe in or out, she says; just be sure to do it throughout an exercise. Holding your breath can cause your blood pressure to skyrocket, which can be very dangerous.

Start out light. "Start with a minimum number of exercises and a very light weight," says Skowron. "This will minimize a lot of the soreness that may develop as a result of doing something new and different." Dr. Mikesky says to "start low and progress slowly." That means start with a lighter weight that you can lift 10 to 15 times and then progress slowly over the weeks to lifting heavier weights.

Keep at it. If you're persistent and consistent about lifting, your strength should gradually increase over a number of months. You may reach a point where you plateau, says Taranta, but it's important to keep lifting even at that plateau level to maintain strength.

Do lifts you like. There are many different exercises for each muscle group. "If you don't like an exercise, don't stay with it. Find one you like," says Dr. Mikesky.

Lower slowly. Focus on lowering the weight slowly. That half of the movement, called a negative, or eccentric, contraction, actually stimulates more muscle growth, says Dr. Nelson. One method is to take a longer time lowering the weight than raising it. Try lifting the weight to the count of three and lowering it to the count of four.

Get started. It's never too late to start weight training, says Dr. Mikesky. Muscle can adapt and increase in strength well into your older years, he says. Research at Tufts University in Medford, Massachusetts, has shown strength gains between 100 and 200 percent in individuals well into their nineties.

SEX

It Does a Body Good

Remember how much older and wiser you felt after your first time? Unlike your buddies, who were all brag, bravado and boyish bumbling, you suddenly felt like a man.

Now you are older and wiser, and the burdens of life often weigh heavily as a result. Guess what? Sex can relieve the pressure of those burdens, and it can do a lot of other good things, too. Medical researchers say sex eases stress, soothes chronic aches and pains, spurs creativity and revs up energy.

"Anything that makes you feel good, alive and physically excited will make you feel more youthful. All those things are associated with sex," says Lonnie Barbach, Ph.D., a sex therapist and psychologist in San Francisco and writer of the video *Sex after Fifty*.

It doesn't take a genius to figure out that the bliss you feel after sex is good for you. Scientists believe sex is a great tension reliever because it releases chemicals in the brain called endorphins. Endorphins are natural painkillers that calm you, create a sense of euphoria and temporarily melt down your stress, says Helen S. Kaplan, M.D., Ph.D., director of the Human Sexuality Teaching Program at New York Hospital–Cornell Medical Center in New York City.

Intimacy can also bolster your immune system and protect you against disease, says Dr. Kaplan.

Sex is a powerful tool that helps men cope with chronic diseases such as arthritis, says Sanford Roth, M.D., a rheumatologist and medical director of the Arthritis Center in Phoenix. Endorphins relieve the pain, but Dr. Roth believes sex also has a vital psychological impact.

"Many times when patients come to me, pain isn't their number one issue. They're more concerned about how the disease is affecting the quality of their lives, and sexuality is an important part of that," Dr. Roth says. "So maintaining sexual function in the face of disease helps people feel better about themselves and their lives."

It May Actually Cure That Headache

"Not tonight, dear, I have a headache" is an excuse older than the Dead Sea Scrolls, but it's not necessarily a valid one. While sex isn't a sure cure, researchers have found that it may relieve some headaches. In one small study, 47 percent of people with migraines said sex relieved their pain, says George H. Sands, M.D., assistant professor of neurology at the Mount Sinai School of Medicine in New York City. Researchers say one possible reason is that orgasms short-circuit the nervous system activity that's causing the pain. (On the other hand, sex can sometimes cause headaches. If it does, discuss it with your doctor.)

Sex can also be self-affirming. "Sex can help make you feel competent. It's a way of connecting with someone else. It can help you feel in charge of your own destiny," says Marty Klein, Ph.D., a licensed marriage counselor and sex therapist in Palo Alto, California, and author of *Ask Me Anything: A Sex Therapist Answers the Most Important Questions for the '90s*. "Sex is a place where you can go and not be bound by the ordinary rules of life."

"Sex often becomes more—not less—important as we age," Dr. Kaplan says. "It's one of the last processes to be affected by aging. First, the skin and your vision go, then you get arthritis and heart disease. So an older man doesn't remember things so well anymore. He can't climb mountains or play tennis. But he can still have sex. It's one of the enduring pleasures of life."

You probably were sexually aroused long before you were born—most baby boys get erections in the womb—and can remain sexually active until you die, says William Masters, M.D., of the Masters and Johnson Institute in St. Louis. Seven in ten men over 70 who have partners have sex at least once a week.

"Sex is a natural function throughout your life if you have an interesting partner and remain healthy. It's not going to go away," Dr. Kaplan says. "It's abnormal for sex to disappear. The normal person has sex until the end of his life."

Making Great Sex Better

You probably know the basics of terrific sex, including keeping your body in shape by avoiding fatty foods and not smoking, since those things can clog the arteries in your penis and make getting an erection difficult. But sometimes a few reminders are helpful. Here are some tips to add zing to your sex life.

Get physical. Aerobic exercise three times a week, 20 to 30 minutes a session, can improve your sex drive and performance, says Roger Crenshaw, M.D., a psychiatrist and sex therapist in private practice in La Jolla, California. Researchers at Bentley College in Waltham, Massachusetts, found, for example, that men in their forties who swam regularly had sex about seven times a month compared with only three times a month for their sedentary peers. In other words, the swimmers were as sexually active as men 10 to 20 years younger.

Put the squeeze on orgasms. Kegel exercises can help men sustain their erections and control orgasms, says Cynthia Mervis Watson, M.D., a family practitioner in Santa Monica, California, and author of *Love Potions*. Kegels strengthen the pubococcygeus (PC) muscles around the genital area. These are muscles that run from the pubic bone along the scrotum and back to the anus. To strengthen these muscles, sit with your legs apart. Practice tightening and relaxing these muscles. If you are unsure of where the muscles are, try to contract them to stop the flow of urine. Once you master the technique, squeeze those muscles, hold, then release for three seconds at a time. Work up to a set of 30. As these muscles become stronger, the scrotum will rise and fall as you tighten and relax them.

Talk it over. Talking with your partner helps both of you explain what you want sexually. If you don't tell her what you really want, then you can't expect her to please you, says Shirley Zussman, Ed.D., a sex and marital therapist and co-director of the Association for Male Sexual Dysfunction in New York City. After all, she can't read your mind. Avoid saying negative things like "That doesn't feel good" or "You know I don't like that." Instead, keep it positive: "I

What Women Really Want from Us

You tried being Mr. Sensitive, and women ignored you. Then you were Mr. Macho, and they abhorred you. Perplexed? So are most guys.

"The number one thing women want is to feel close to the man before they start making love," says Lonnie Barbach, Ph.D., a sex therapist and psychologist in San Francisco and writer of the video *Sex After Fifty*. "That means a woman wants to talk and be held and acknowledged as a person. Most women don't want you to suddenly throw them in bed and roll over on top of them. They want a relationship before the sex starts."

Women also don't want to feel rushed into sex or feel they have to respond to your advances in a particular way, Dr. Barbach says. In other words, guys, keep your expectations in check.

Women want sincerity and to be valued for their inner beauty, says Domeena Renshaw, M.D., director of the Sexual Dysfunction Clinic at Loyola University of Chicago Stritch School of Medicine in Maywood, Illinois. "If a woman is overweight, she's never going to believe her husband if he tells her he thinks she's glamorous," Dr. Renshaw says. "But if he says he remembers how much fun they had on their first date and how aroused he was to be with her, that will definitely arouse her."

What Celibacy Can Do

"Marriage has many pains, but celibacy has no pleasures," according to Samuel Johnson, an eighteenth-century wit. But that assessment is way off target, experts say. Many couples and more than a few single men find celibacy gratifying and say that it actually bolsters their relationships and self-esteem.

About one in ten married couples abstain from sex, according to Michael B. Broder, Ph.D., a clinical psychologist in Philadelphia and author of *The Art of Staying Together*. Some people are celibate because of religious convictions, medication side effects or chronic illnesses. But a growing number of couples are actually celibate because they want to strengthen their bond in other ways.

Singles choose abstinence to protect themselves from AIDS and other sexually transmitted diseases or even to finish their MBAs, says Shirley Zussman, Ed.D., a sex and marital therapist and co-director of the Association for Male Sexual Dysfunction in New York City. Some singles say that they are simply waiting for someone really special.

"One big advantage of choosing to be celibate for some period in your life is that it gives you an opportunity to fully understand the place of sex in your life or relationship," says Harrison Voigt, Ph.D., a clinical psychologist, sex therapist and professor at the California Institute of Integral Studies in San Francisco. "It offers you a chance to see how well you can really relate to others outside of the sexual sphere."

Here are some guidelines for choosing celibacy.

• Realize that you'll continue to have sexual urges but you don't have to act on them. In time, they might subside.
• Consider your celibacy a vacation—a time to rest or try new experiences. Instead of thinking of it as a deprivation, consider it a choice. See it as an opportunity to find deeper meaning in your life.
• Remember, it doesn't have to be forever. You can stop being celibate anytime you choose. When you do, sex may be even more exciting and rewarding than ever.

enjoy sex with you, but I have some ideas about making it even better."

Demonstrate. While talking helps, often showing your partner what pleases you is as useful. If she's rubbing your penis too hard, for example, take her hand and show her how you prefer to be stroked, Dr. Klein suggests.

Broaden your horizons. "Intercourse is overemphasized as a sexual ac-

Your Pal, the Condom

For most guys, wearing a condom is like having sex in a sandwich bag.

Yet the condom remains one of the most trustworthy methods of birth control and is indispensable in this age of AIDS and other sexually transmitted diseases (STDs).

Even the traditional story that condoms are uncomfortable and awkward is leakier than a cheap prophylactic, says Roger Crenshaw, M.D. a psychiatrist and sex therapist in private practice in La Jolla, California.

"If you don't feel comfortable in a condom, then perhaps you're not comfortable with sex itself or you are not with the right person," says Marty Klein, Ph.D., a licensed marriage counselor and sex therapist in Palo Alto, California, and author of *Ask Me Anything: A Sex Therapist Answers the Most Important Questions for the '90s.*

Sex in a condom shouldn't strangle your penis. Instead, it should unleash your inhibitions, since the chances of unwanted pregnancy and STDs are dramatically reduced, Dr. Klein says.

Always use a latex condom. The structure of latex is more tightly woven than that of lambskin and gives you far better protection against disease and unwanted pregnancy. Condoms containing spermicides are safer in the rare case of breakage.

Always put on the condom before any genital contact to prevent exposure to infectious fluids or sperm. After ejaculation, remove the condom before the erection fades, so semen doesn't escape. If a condom does break during ejaculation, immediately use a spermicide. Finally, never use a condom more than once.

---

tivity," Dr. Klein says. "Most couples would benefit from seeing sex as a much broader set of experiences." So simply take time to kiss, hug, caress, hold hands, talk or do other sexually pleasing activities, such as mutual masturbation, that make you feel close to your partner, he suggests.

Make time for whoopee. "I know it sounds comical, but some couples say they just don't have time for sex," says Carol Lassen, Ph.D., a psychologist and clinical professor of psychology at the University of Colorado School of Medicine in Denver. "Why? Everything else comes first. They can't have sex because they have to do the laundry or watch a football game or just get some sleep. They have very little time left for each other."

Rather than letting sex get lost in the daily grind, schedule time for it, says Michael Seiler, Ph.D., co-author of *Inhibited Sexual Desire* and assistant director of the Phoenix Institute in Chicago. "You'd make reservations in a fancy restaurant for 7:00 Saturday night. Why not say you'll meet in the bedroom at 9:00 P.M. Tuesday?" he says. "How do you know you'll be in the mood? You don't. But you don't know if you'll be hungry on Saturday night, either."

Check your hang-ups at the door. "Leave work, religion and your performance expectations outside the bedroom door," Dr. Barbach suggests. "Simply go into the bedroom with your body and your feelings. Focus on the emotional connection you have with your partner and the pleasure your body has in store."

Just do it. "Most men would benefit from not worrying whether they're doing it right," Dr. Klein says. "Instead of worrying about thrusting the right number of times or being in the right position, you'll have better sex if you simply focus on your own body and do what feels good."

Keep it fun. "Do you know what the Eskimos call sex? Laughing time,"

A Message from Your Dream Lovers

You dream that you walk into an elegant dinner party and discover that you and Sigmund Freud are the only men among a crowd of beautiful topless women.

What does it mean? Nothing except that you're probably an average guy.

"For men, sexual dreams are usually impersonal. We usually don't know who the woman is. She's just a gorgeous, willing female, like a *Playboy* centerfold," says Robert Van de Castle, Ph.D., professor emeritus of behavioral medicine at the University of Virginia Medical Center in Charlottesville and past president of the Association for the Study of Dreams.

Men who have sexual dreams probably have better sex lives than guys who don't dream about sex that much, he says. That's because men who are comfortable with their sexuality in the real world are more likely to dream about it.

If you have a sexual problem, it can show up symbolically in your dreams. A man who has problems with impotence may dream about a beautiful woman waiting for him in his bedroom, but he can't get to her because he can't unlock the door, Dr. Van de Castle says.

You can't even escape aging in your dreams. "Generally, we tend to dream about sexual partners who are our own age," Dr. Van de Castle says. "Occasionally, some older men still do dream about the young *Playboy* centerfold. But the vast majority of the people you see in your dreams are within 20 years of your own age."

Dr. Zussman says. "Sex can be fun, frivolous and relaxing. We are so far from that in our society. We feel like we have to have fantastic sex each and every time." Forget performance, she says. Concentrate on having a good time with your partner, and sex will be more like laughing time than working overtime.

See the light. If you want to delay your orgasm, focus on an imaginary light or candle, suggests Domeena Renshaw, M.D., director of the Sexual Dysfunction Clinic at Loyola University of Chicago Stritch School of Medicine in Maywood, Illinois. The light focus will momentarily divert your attention away from sex and extend your time to orgasm.

Get back to basics. "Couples stop doing the very things that brought them together in the first place," Dr. Seiler says. "They don't write each other little notes or send flowers. They don't give each other back rubs or go out on dates. You really have to work to keep the fun and play in the relationship. Without it, there won't be any fun and play in the bedroom."

So cook a romantic meal or have a warm bubble bath waiting for your lover when she gets home from work, Dr. Renshaw suggests. Pretend you are Anthony and Cleopatra. You might be pleased with where it leads.

Get inspiration. If your sex life has lost most of its fizz, try browsing through a few sex manuals or watching erotic videos together for new ideas, Dr. Renshaw says.

Keep an eye on her. "Sustained eye contact during sex breeds intimacy. Often it's more intimate than kissing or holding hands," says Harrison Voigt, Ph.D., a clinical psychologist, sex therapist and professor at the California Institute of Integral Studies in San Francisco. "It's a way to get people in touch with a powerful form of union that isn't physical."

Create a ritual. Lighting a candle, massaging each other's feet or collaborating on the exchange of some special intimacies can become a part of a unique ritual that can help some couples connect emotionally before sex, Dr. Voigt says. "A ritual is basically a mutual agreement that sex should be something unique for the couple. It doesn't have to be complex, but it should change the context of sex into something that is special rather than just rolling over in bed and saying 'Hey, let's do it.'"

Don't keep score. If you had sex four times last week but only once this week, don't push to keep pace. "Frequency isn't as important as truly enjoying the sex that you do have," Dr. Zussman says.

Don't take work to bed. Your bedroom should be a place where you and your partner can retreat for intimate interludes. If it's cluttered with computers, the television, a typewriter and filing cabinets, it's an office. "One man told me that when he gets home, his wife, who is a writer, sometimes has papers scattered all over the bed, and all interest in sex just drains from him," Dr. Zussman says.

SKIN CARE

Too Simple to Skip

Remember your first car? You tuned it up, changed the oil, laid on the car shampoo and polished that baby until the chrome screamed. You knew one of the first things your peers would check out was your wheels.

In the adult world, your wheels don't make the first impression—your face does. When your facial skin looks good, you look good. Healthy-looking, well-toned skin can knock years off the clock.

Not into face fussing? No problem. Good skin care doesn't have to be a fancy ritual. The basics can be quick and simple and give even better results than Turtle Wax on the hood of a 1968 'Vette.

Shaving the Edge off Your Years

For most men, skin care stops at the face, and men have a real advantage over women when it comes to facial aging. That's because when you shave every day, you remove the top layer of dead cells that can make your skin look dull. Shaving can give you a cleaner, younger appearance—but not if you leave your face looking like a war zone. These pointers will help.

Choose your weapon. Maybe you're sentimental over the memory of Dad's morning buzz or big brother's machete-like skill with a single-edge. The difference between an electric and any other kind of blade is just preference. It really doesn't matter which you choose. If you opt for an electric razor, though, shave your face before you shower or wash, says John F. Romano, M.D., a dermatologist at New York Hospital–Cornell Medical Center in New York City. The natural oils that accumulate on your skin overnight act as a protective barrier between your face and the shaver. And to be kind to your skin, prep with a powder-based preshave rather than one containing alcohol, which can dry the skin, he says. If the blade's your weapon, read on.

What's beneath the Beard?

While a well-kept, well-trimmed beard can give you a distinguished and somehow more credible look, it also adds years to your appearance. "Men look older with beards and mustaches," says Carol Walderman, a cosmetologist and esthetician in Baltimore who writes for skin magazines (we mean the skin care industry kind).

But there's a paradox. Beard and moustache hair also does a great job of protecting facial skin against sun damage—the primo cause of skin aging, Walderman says.

So what wins the toss? If you're happy with a distinguished look, enjoy your beard. But if you have worn one for years and want a youthful boost, shave it off. "You'll have really nice skin under there, and you'll look even younger than you expected," Walderman says.

Just be sure to protect your born-again face with sunscreen to keep that youthful edge.

Hydrate like mad. "Stand over the basin and splash a lot of lukewarm water on your skin first," says Seth L. Matarasso, M.D., assistant professor of dermatology at the University of California, San Francisco, School of Medicine. It will soften the hairs and make them easier to cut. A quick wetting of the skin isn't enough, he says.

Foam the runway. If razor burn is a problem, apply a layer of light lotion before you slap on your shaving cream, suggests Marina Valmy, a cosmetician at the Christine Valmy Skin Care School in New York City.

Let it stand. After you lather on shaving cream, find a way to kill two or three minutes, says Dr. Matarasso. The cream needs time to soften your whiskers.

Don't stretch. Don't stretch your skin taut while you shave, that is. It's just another of those little torments that can make your skin sag and lose its firm tone after a few years, says Dr. Romano.

Go with the grain. Shave in the direction your beard grows, says Dr. Matarasso. If you shave against the grain, you'll cut the whiskers so short they'll spring back below the surface of the skin. Then when they start to regrow, they can cause folliculitis—those sore red "razor bumps."

Plug the oops. If you slip and nick yourself, reach for the old standby styptic pencil. Its main ingredient—aluminum chloride—coagulates blood and stops bleeding, Dr. Matarasso says, and it won't harm your skin.

Bag the bracer. If you're terribly attached to your aftershave, at least dilute it with distilled water, says Carol Walderman, a cosmetologist and esthetician in Baltimore. Most skin bracers irritate and dehydrate the skin, she says. A better alternative? Swipe your wife's skin toner, or use witch hazel for that refreshing cheek smack.

Wash and Lube

Many guys hop in and out of the shower a few times a day, especially after a sweaty workout. But that much washing can be too much, says Albert M. Kligman, M.D., professor of dermatology at the University of Pennsylvania School of Medicine in Philadelphia. "We're too clean. Too much washing can be irritating." Once a day you can wash your face thoroughly, he says, but the rest of the time, unless your skin's really oily, a swift rinse will do the job. Here are a few additional tips on daily facial hygiene.

Use gentle suds. Wash with gentle cleansers like Cetaphil or mild soaps such as Neutrogena, Dove, Purpose or Basis, says Thomas Griffin, M.D., a dermatologist with Graduate Hospital of Philadelphia and clinical assistant professor of dermatology at the University of Pennsylvania School of Medicine. And don't scrub—it's your face, not a broiler pan.

Avoid extremes. Don't use very hot water to wash your face, says Leila Cohoon, a cosmetologist and esthetician and owner of Leila's Skin Care in Independence, Missouri. Use warm to very warm water to wash off your cleanser; cold water just sets it in a film on your skin, she says. You don't need icy cold water to "close your pores," either. Pores do not open and close as commonly thought.

Just say no to abrasives. Next time your girlfriend offers you her crushed-walnut-shell or apricot-seed scrub, turn her down, says Cohoon. You don't need to abrade your skin to get it clean, and these types of industrial-strength scrubs can scratch and irritate your skin.

Finish the job. A moisturizer is an important step in men's skin care that's often overlooked, says Dr. Matarasso. That may be because too many guys have tried applying lotion to bone-dry skin and hate the greasy feeling it leaves behind. The trick is to apply moisturizer to damp skin, says Dr. Matarasso. The water helps the moisturizer penetrate below the surface and into the pores, where it seals in water and temporarily smooths fine wrinkles. Moisturizers can be used anywhere you have dry skin, including the face, elbows and hands. Choose any moisturizer labeled "non-comedogenic," which means it won't clog pores and cause acne.

Protection for the Long Haul

Nothing can age your skin as much as a lifetime of sun exposure. If you want to keep away nasties such as age spots and wrinkles, add daily sunscreen to your routine. The easy way? Use sunscreen every morning, says Walderman. You can apply it in place of a moisturizer after you shave. Here's what else you need to know about sunscreen.

Aim for high-level protection. Your best bets are sunscreens with a sun protection factor (SPF) of 15 or higher, which protects you from burning 15 times longer than naked skin can, says Valmy. If you have sensitive skin, pick a PABA-free formula. (Many people are allergic to this ingredient; it also stains.) Or get a sunscreen made for babies' skin. It is light and has no strong fragrance, Valmy says.

Let it sink in before you head out. Be sure to apply your sunscreen at least 20 minutes before you go out in the sun, says Dr. Griffin. That will give it time to start working to protect your skin before you face the rays.

SLEEP

An Essential Part of Life

We all know a sleep-deprived man when we see one: droopy eyes with dark circles; a dazed, gloomy, spaced-out expression, poor posture; slow-walking; slow-talking. Not exactly the epitome of robust youth. Why are there so many of these zombies plodding about?

"Our society continues to spread the myth that the tougher you are, the less sleep you need," says Mark Mahowald, M.D., director of the Minnesota Regional Sleep Disorders Center at the Hennepin County Medical Center in Minneapolis. "You can't fool Mother Nature and get away with less sleep than you need without paying a price."

Suppose we take our somnolent sad sack and make him clean up his act and start exercising good sleep habits. Could he actually add some spark and vitality to his life? And could he actually reverse some of these signs of aging?

No question about it. "Sleep maximizes the quality of our lives," says Michael Vitiello, Ph.D., associate director of the Sleep and Aging Research Program at the University of Washington in Seattle. "When you sleep better, you feel better. You're more likely to perform at optimal levels and to maintain other healthy behaviors, like exercise and good diet. Combine sleep with these other behaviors, and all those things we associate with youth—appearance, energy and attitude—will ultimately improve."

Benefits to Body and Mind

Why is sleep so powerful? We know that the body releases its greatest concentration of growth hormone—the substance that helps strengthen our bodies and repairs damaged tissue—during sleep. Studies have also shown that there's a close connection between sleep and the immune system. Sleep-deprived individuals seem to experience a decrease in the activity of natural killer cells and other good guys that keep the body healthy and infection-free.

But most sleep specialists believe the mind, as well as the body, benefits from a good night's sleep. "Sleep seems to have a reactivating effect on the processes in the brain and the central nervous system," says Karl Doghramji, M.D., director of the Sleep Disorders Center at Thomas Jefferson University Hospital in Philadelphia. "Without sleep, neither functions at its maximum capacity. And it's possible that this could have a negative impact on our overall health."

Sleep, it turns out, is really a highly active state made up of a series of regular cycles. There are stages to each cycle: Stages one to three occur during light sleep, and stage four (also called delta sleep) represents our deepest sleep. A fifth stage of sleep (called rapid eye movement, or REM) occurs when we dream. Experts say that delta sleep and REM sleep are both essential for maintaining the brain's abilities to learn, memorize, create and reason.

Another very significant impact of sleep is how it affects our behavior, says Dr. Mahowald. "Sleep deprivation makes us moody and irritable."

Your Changing Sleep Patterns

Do you expect to run as fast or play tennis as well in your forties, fifties or sixties as you did in your teens, twenties and thirties? Of course not. But how about sleep? You probably think it will take no effort at all or even be easier. But for most of us, a good night's sleep could become harder to get.

Beginning in middle age and continuing into our golden years, it will take many of us longer to fall asleep. We'll experience frequent awakenings and spend less time in the valuable delta and REM stages. We'll spend less time sleeping, period.

"As we age, our internal clocks are much more easily disturbed," says Timothy Monk, Ph.D., director of the Human Chronobiology Research Program at the University of Pittsburgh School of Medicine. "The main effect can be that we don't sleep as well and we enter a state of malaise and depression—like a chronic case of jet lag."

Maximizing Your Zzzzs

How much sleep do you need? It depends on the individual. For most men, seven to eight hours will do the job. Some need more; some need less. There's no magic number, and every guy is different. "You should get as much sleep as you need to feel rested and able to function at your maximum the next day," says Dr. Mahowald.

How can you maximize the quality and quantity of your sleep? Here's help.

Keep a regular bedtime schedule. Going to bed and waking up at the same time every day (including weekends) helps maintain a consistent rhythm, says Dr. Monk. Establishing this regularity will help you fall asleep easier, sleep more soundly and wake feeling refreshed.

Eat three regular meals at regular times. "Our daily rhythms can become easily disrupted by external factors," says Dr. Monk. "You need certain external cues to keep your body clock running right. Keeping consistent meal times will help."

Get regular exercise. Contrary to popular belief, heavy exercise will not wear you out and make you sleepy, says Dr. Mahowald. But people who are physically fit and active will be better sleepers, so make exercise a part of your daily regimen. A mild walk before bedtime is okay if it relaxes you, but save your heavy workouts for earlier in the day; they can keep you awake for quite a while.

Take time to unwind. You can't expect to leap from the rat race directly into the sack, says Dr. Mahowald. Give yourself two hours prior to bedtime to relax and turn off the world by reading, watching television, listening to music—whatever helps you mellow out. Take care of business, bills and other stress makers during the day or early evening.

Establish bedtime rituals. Becoming a creature of habit may be all you need to conk out on cue, says Dr. Vitiello. Develop a pre-bedtime routine that has you doing the same things at the same time each night. For example: At

---

To Nap or Not to Nap?

Many individuals who don't get all the sleep they need at night benefit from a short siesta in the afternoon, says Timothy Monk, Ph.D., director of the Human Chronobiology Research Program at the University of Pittsburgh School of Medicine.

But not everyone has the time for a nap, and napping is not for everyone. "If you have insomnia, you may have a strong desire to nap in the afternoon, but that can worsen your sleeplessness at night," says Karl Doghramji, M.D., director of the Sleep Disorders Center at Thomas Jefferson University Hospital in Philadelphia. "In addition, many people are poor nappers. They actually feel worse after a nap due to what we call sleep inertia—the groggy feeling that can linger for hours."

What should you do? Drs. Monk and Doghramji say to experiment. If you feel tired and find a nap refreshing, if it doesn't interfere with your evening sleep and if your schedule permits it, by all means take a siesta. About 20 to 45 minutes just after lunch is usually best.

9:30 P.M., let the cat out; at 10:00 P.M., brush your teeth; at 10:30 P.M., catch up on your reading. Then cut the light.

If you can't sleep, don't. Don't stay in bed trying to make sleep happen, says Dr. Vitiello. You'll only condition yourself not to fall asleep while you're in bed. Instead, get up and read a book or do something constructive until you feel tired. And don't believe the myth about going to bed early if you have a big day ahead of you. Most people just spend that extra time in bed awake, only to have trouble falling asleep later.

Avoid late-night meals and munchies. A small snack before bed is okay, but don't eat a full meal, spicy foods or a Dagwood sandwich less than three hours before bedtime, says Dr. Doghramji. Your rumbling stomach can keep you up for hours and make sleep less refreshing.

Curtail your caffeine. Have your coffee, tea and colas in the morning or early afternoon, says Dr. Doghramji. Caffeine is a powerful sleep inhibitor that stays in the bloodstream for up to six hours.

Nix those nightcaps. Alcohol will help you fall asleep in no time, says Dr. Mahowald. But that sleep promises to be a restless one. Booze inhibits the quality of sleep by changing the REM and non-REM patterns. You may get plenty of shut-eye, but you'll feel like hell in the morning.

Limit late-night liquids. Frequent trips to the bathroom can keep you up all night.

Just say no to drugs. Sleeping pills, although often helpful, can upset your sleep patterns, too, says Dr. Doghramji. In addition, it's easy to get hooked on them, especially if you use them improperly. Your best bet is to try to fall asleep without any chemical assistance. If you must take sleeping pills, do so only under a doctor's watchful eye.

Limit your bedtime activities. Use your bedroom for sleep and sex only, says Dr. Vitiello. "If you introduce activities like paying bills, eating pizza and watching television, the mind and body get confused and may not want to go to sleep."

Go for a roll in the hay. Some guys find sex before sleep relaxing, says Dr. Mahowald. If making love knocks you out, go for it.

Get off the shift. "We were built to work during the day and sleep at night. That's why guys who work graveyard shifts often have trouble sleeping," says Dr. Monk. If this describes you, the tips given here should be of great help. If that's not enough, and you're still having problems, it might be time to start wrangling for a switch to day shift. Of course, it isn't always possible to make that switch, but it couldn't hurt to try.

STRETCHING

Loosen Up, Will Ya?

Okay, so you really dislike stretching. Make that hate stretching.

You've tried it, mostly when you were twentysomething and dating the woman of your dreams from down the street. She was into exercise, and your courtship involved meeting at a designated street corner to run.

But before taking off, she'd launch into this bend-over-stretch-back, pull-on-one-leg-now-the-other routine, and you had no option but to join in. You'd reach down to touch your toes, and—YOWEE!—your hamstrings would start screaming. It hurt like hell, but hey, you wanted to impress her.

Well, it wasn't long before that relationship went down the tubes, and with it, any semblance of stretching. It hurts too much, and besides, it takes precious time away from your weight-lifting workouts. And who needs it anyway?

You do.

A general warm-up followed by regular stretching raises the temperature within our muscles and enables us to move smoothly and with a full range of motion—like we did when we were younger. In addition to relieving stress and tension, stretching improves flexibility, enhances performance and helps prevent injuries.

Oh, Those Aging Muscles

As we age, our muscles and joints tend to become a bit tighter, says John Skowron, physical therapist at Raleigh Community Sports Medicine and Physical Therapy in Raleigh, North Carolina. That's because over time, connective muscle tissues shorten. That makes it harder to do the activities we're used to, whether on the playing field or around the house, because our muscles just aren't ready.

Advanced Placement Stretching

If you're a beginner, the type of stretching described in this chapter—static stretching—is probably the best way to get started. But if you're looking for other methods, here are some suggestions.

Passive stretching. A gentle force is applied by a partner to increase flexibility. For example, to stretch the hamstrings in your right leg, lie on your back with your left leg bent and the sole of your left foot flat on the floor. Raise your right leg, slightly bent, upward until you feel a stretch. Have your partner apply a gentle force to push the stretch a little farther.

PNF stretching. Proprioceptive neuromuscular facilitation, or PNF, stretching is a technique that stimulates certain reflex centers and nerves. It generally requires a partner, who provides resistance so that the muscle being stretched can be contracted against resistance before the stretch is continued. For example, begin the right hamstring stretch. While in the same position described above, have a partner raise your right leg until you feel a stretch. Then as a partner provides resistance against your push (he can do this by placing a shoulder against the back of your thigh), contract, or tighten, your hamstring without moving it and hold the contraction for 3 to 6 seconds. Then relax, have your partner move you into the stretch farther and hold it for another 20 to 30 seconds.

AI stretching. AI, or active isolated, stretching is a completely different approach advocated and practiced by Aaron Mattes, Ph.D., a kinesiologist in southern Florida and author of *Flexibility: Active and Assisted Stretching.* In contrast to static stretching, AI stretching involves performing each stretch for 1½ to 2 seconds, relaxing, then stretching again. It also involves contracting the muscle opposite the one you are stretching and using a rope or towel to move the limb to the point where the stretch is felt.

For example, to stretch your right hamstring, lie on your back with your left leg bent and foot flat on the floor. Then with a rope or towel wrapped around your right foot and your right leg extended, lift your right leg up, contracting your right quadriceps while you gently use the rope to assist the leg into the stretch. Hold the stretch for 1½ to 2 seconds, return your leg to the starting position, relax and repeat.

Here's what happens: Any time you do an activity, whether it's reaching up to paint a wall, carrying something down stairs or going for a run, your muscles move. Certain muscles contract, or shorten, with movement, while the opposing muscles relax, or lengthen. When the muscles and surrounding elastic tissue that need to lengthen are too tight, they can't move the way we want them to, and we lose what health experts call our full range of motion—that is, our movement becomes restricted.

This can cause all kinds of trouble. Sometimes it prohibits us from participating in activities at all. Other times we can participate, but our performance is compromised. Then there are the times when it leads to injury. When your body realizes it can't use a certain muscle group fully, it often tries to compensate by asking another muscle group to work harder than usual, a demand that may cause that part of the body to break down. And sometimes the muscles themselves become damaged—their tissues can tear, which is what happens when someone "pulls" a muscle.

Part of the reason we get tighter after age 30 has to do with our lifestyles, says Michael Kaplan, M.D., Ph.D., director of the Rehabilitation Team, a sports medicine and physical therapy clinic in Catonsville, Maryland. "Before they're 30, people tend not to have as many responsibilities. They often don't have the job that they have to do plus the house that they have to support, the kids they have to do things for," he says. Eventually, any of these responsibilities takes up most of their time; folks become less active and, as a result, less mobile and less flexible.

"There's no reason why people in their thirties and forties and even older can't have just as much flexibility as when they were younger—or even more flexibility," says Dr. Kaplan. "A 60-year-old can have more flexibility than a 20-year old," if he works at it and stretches, he says.

Improving Flexibility

Here's how it works. When you stretch a muscle, say the hamstring at the back of your leg, you place tension on it, and the muscle begins to lengthen. A stretch reflex inside the muscle tries to protect it from lengthening and asks the muscle to contract. But if the stretch is held long enough, a structure located where tendons adjoin to muscles, called the Golgi tendon organ, sends a message that triggers the muscle to relax farther, and lengthening continues.

That's what happens when you do the type of slow and steady stretching—called static stretching—that has generally been accepted as the right way to stretch these days. The idea is to move into the stretch slowly and gradually, hold it for 20 to 30 seconds, relax and repeat. Research conducted at the Institute for Sports Medicine at Lenox Hill Hospital in New York City showed that the majority of muscle relaxation occurs within 20 seconds of stretching.

How It Can Help

In addition to improving performance and helping to prevent injuries, stretching can help improve strength, says Mark V. Taranta, a physical therapist and director of the Physical Therapy Practice in Philadelphia. "People have to realize that strength will increase as flexibility increases," he says. "If you're flexible, you're able to generate more force," because the muscle is in a lengthened position.

And if you're feeling stressed out, stretching can provide some relief. "Stretching reduces tension," says William L. Cornelius, Ph.D., associate professor of physical education in the Department of Kinesiology, Health Promotion and Recreation at the University of North Texas in Denton. One way researchers have assessed this is by measuring the electrical activity elicited by muscles with a technique called electromyography, or EMG. Studies have shown that stretching helps reduce the amount of electrical activity passing through muscles, a sign that tension has been reduced, says Dr. Cornelius.

How to Do It Right

You can reap the benefits of stretching if you pay attention to your stretching technique. Here's what to keep in mind.

Warm up first. "You should warm up the muscle before you stretch it," says Lucille Smith, Ph.D., assistant professor at the Human Performance Laboratory at East Carolina University in Greenville, North Carolina. The general guideline is to warm up until you break a sweat. For activities involving the entire body, warm up with a brisk walk or light jog. If you're going to be exercising only one area of your body, concentrate on that area. Warming up raises the temperature of the muscle and makes it less susceptible to injury. "When the muscle is heated up, it's more pliable," says Taranta.

Go slow and steady. When you stretch, make it a slow and steady one, says Dr. Cornelius. Don't bounce. Move into each stretch gradually until you feel tension in the muscle and connective tissue, he says. Hold that position for 20 to 30 seconds, relax and do it again.

Be sure to breathe. "You really have to concentrate on your breathing," says Taranta. If you hold your breath, that can contribute to tensing of your muscles, whereas breathing helps relax them, he says.

Know every bit helps. You don't have to have 20 to 30 minutes to devote to stretching, says Dr. Kaplan. If you stretch your neck, shoulders, back, hips and legs for 2 minutes each at 30-second intervals, that makes for a 10-minute stretching workout.

Get into a routine. It's important to be consistent about stretching, says Taranta. If you don't stretch regularly, it won't have much effect, he says. Aim to stretch three times a week to start. Once you're in the habit, aim for every day.

Pay attention to the temperature. When it's cold out, you may need to spend a little extra time stretching to get your muscles warm; when it's hot, a little less, says Taranta.

Do more in the morning. If you exercise in the morning or have to do physical labor first thing, take the time to warm up and stretch a little longer than usual. "Core temperature and body temperature probably would be lower, and you'd probably be stiffer first thing in the morning versus later in the day, when you've already been moving around," says Dr. Smith.

Get in a group. Join or form a group of people interested in stretching together, says Dr. Kaplan. Yoga classes are one option. Or if you are part of a softball or volleyball team, make stretching together part of your practices and games, he says. "By yourself, you may lose incentive."

Go for the Basics

There are lots of stretching options. Here are a few basic stretches for each body area to get you started.

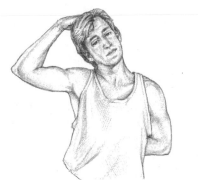

If your neck is feeling sore or tight, stretching can do wonders. While standing or sitting, hold your left arm behind your back. Then tilt your head as if you were trying to touch your right ear to your right shoulder. Use your right hand to pull gently on your head if you need more of a stretch. Hold the stretch for 10 to 20 seconds, relax and repeat. Try this three or four times for the left side of your neck, then reverse and do the same for the right side.

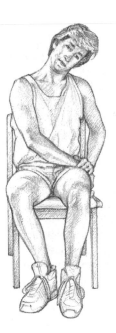

Here's another stretch to keep your neck from tightening up. Sit on a chair and cross your right arm across your body so that your right wrist rests on your left hip. Grasp your right wrist with your left hand. Tilt your head as if you were trying to touch your left ear to your left shoulder. At the same time, pull gently on your right arm with your left hand. You'll feel the stretch on the right side of your neck. Reverse the directions to do the same exercise for the left side of your neck.

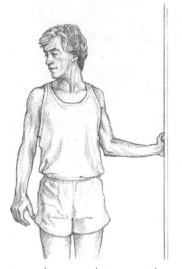

Standing in a doorway, let your right arm hang down by your side (above). Bend your left arm to 90 degrees and place the palm of your left hand against the door frame. Slowly turn your body to the right until you feel a gentle stretch in your left shoulder. Hold it for 20 to 30 seconds, relax and repeat. Reverse the instructions to stretch your right shoulder.

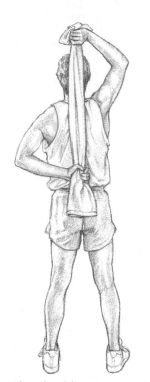

The shoulders are another area where stress and tension can take their toll. While standing with feet hip-width apart, grasp a towel in your right hand (above). Flip the towel up and over your head, as shown. Reach behind your back with your left hand and grasp the end of the towel. Stretch your left shoulder by pulling upward on the towel with your right hand. Hold the stretch for 20 to 30 seconds, relax and repeat several times. Reverse the instructions to stretch your right shoulder.

Standing with your feet hip-width apart, clasp your hands together in front of your body, keeping your arms straight (left). Raise your arms a couple of inches away from your body. Bend your head forward and gently pull your shoulder blades apart. Hold the stretch for 20 to 30 seconds, relax and repeat several times.

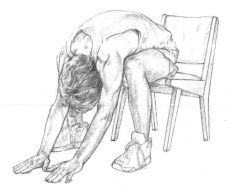

Sit on a chair with your knees apart. Bend forward and try to touch your hands to the floor (above). You should feel a gentle stretch in your lower back. Hold the stretch for 20 to 30 seconds, relax and repeat.

And then there's that achy-breaky back. To get some relief, try this stretch (above). Stand up straight with your feet hip-width apart. Place both hands on your hips and arch gently backward. Hold the stretch for 20 to 30 seconds, relax and repeat.

Lie on your stomach on the floor and place the palms of your hands on the floor by your chest. Press your upper body upward, keeping your hips on the floor (right). Remember to keep your lower back and buttocks relaxed. Hold the stretch for 20 to 30 seconds, relax and repeat several times.

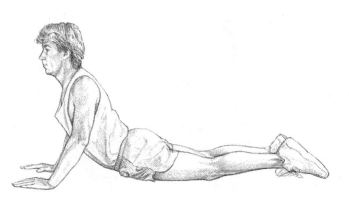

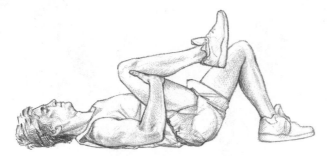

Lying on your back, bend both knees while keeping your feet flat on the floor. Then pull your right knee toward your chest, and grasping the back of your thigh, pull your knee toward your chest until you feel a gentle stretch in your lower back (above). Repeat with the opposite knee. You can also perform this stretch by pulling both knees toward your chest simultaneously (below).

Sit on the floor with both legs extended straight in front of you. Bend your right leg and cross it over your left leg so that the sole of your right foot is flat on the floor. Slowly twist your upper body to the right and place your left elbow over the outside of your right knee. Gently push on the bent knee with your elbow until you feel a stretch in your right buttock. Hold the stretch for 20 to 30 seconds, relax and repeat several times. Do the same for the opposite side.

To stretch your quadriceps, or thigh muscles, stand on your right leg, bend your left leg up behind you and grasp your left foot in your left hand. Pull your left heel toward your buttocks as far as is comfortable until you feel a stretch in the front of your thigh. Hold for 20 to 30 seconds, relax and repeat several times. Do the same for your right leg.

Here's a stretch for your hamstrings, the muscles at the back of your thigh. Lie on your back and bend both knees so that the soles of your feet are flat on the floor. Grasp the back of your left thigh with both hands. Holding your left thigh, slowly straighten your left leg until a gradual stretch is felt in your hamstrings. Hold the stretch for 20 to 30 seconds, relax and repeat several times. Then repeat the stretch for your right leg.

VEGETARIANISM

Hang On to Those Salad Days

Let's cut right to the meat of the matter here: If you're a typical American male, you're eating way too much fat. And you're getting most of it from your ol' barnyard buddies, Mr. Steer and Mr. Pig.

The result can be a nightmare of aging before your time. Diets heavy with fat can lead to elevated cholesterol levels, high blood pressure and digestive tract problems. And then there's that amorphous jiggle-bulge growing where your youthful waistline used to be.

If you're searching for a way to regain a little vigor, lose weight and help ward off serious health problems down the road, you might want to take a hard look at a meatless lifestyle.

"Very simply, vegetarians tend to be healthier people," says Reed Mangels, R.D., Ph.D., a nutrition adviser to the Vegetarian Resource Group in Baltimore. "You get much of your fat through animal products—and the fewer animal products you eat, the better you're probably going to feel."

Leaner, Lighter, Livelier

Study after scientific study shows that your average vegetarian is better off than his meat-eating brethren. Researchers in Germany, for instance, found that a group of 1,904 vegetarians had about half the overall mortality rate of meat eaters over an 11-year period.

The German study showed that vegetarian men suffered about 50 percent fewer cases of digestive tract cancer than people who ate normal diets. They also had less than half the expected rate of heart disease.

Other studies conducted on Buddhists, Seventh-Day Adventists, people in the developing world and Westerners show that vegetarians generally have lower blood pressure than meat eaters. Vegetarians may also have less risk of developing diabetes.

Vegetarians also report less trouble with constipation and gallstones. And people who switch to vegetarian diets say they just plain feel better—with more energy and vigor—after dropping meat from their diets.

What's behind all these magic results? For one thing, vegetarians tend to weigh less—partly because they eat less fat, Dr. Mangels says, and partly because they tend to lead more active lifestyles.

Vegetarians also smoke less. "Many of them have made a serious long-term commitment to their health," says Dr. Mangels. "It's reflected in their lifestyles, not just in the food they eat."

Most vegetarians eat diets that are much lower in fat—well below the 30 percent of total calories recommended by the American Heart Association and the National Cancer Institute. On average, Americans eat 40 percent of their calories in the form of fat.

Less fat, less weight, more exercise and fewer cigarettes can have a ripple effect on your health, according to Dr. Mangels. "It all goes hand-in-hand," she says. "You eat better, you feel better, your heart may be stronger, so you feel like doing more. The end result is better overall health."

There's even some evidence that vegetarian diets can help fight arthritis pain. Symptoms of the most common form of arthritis, osteoarthritis, may be relieved because people who weigh less don't put so much stress on joints like their knees, Dr. Mangels says.

And people with rheumatoid arthritis may get relief from vegetarian diets tailored to their needs, researchers in Norway report. They put 27 people with rheumatoid arthritis on a fast, then slowly introduced vegetarian foods to their diets, rejecting foods that resulted in pain flare-ups. After a year, those in the study said they had less tenderness in their joints, less morning stiffness and greater grip strength.

Steering Away from Red Meat

Sure, it all sounds good. But give up meat? What will they ask for next—Monday Night Football?

Hey, becoming a vegetarian isn't as hard as you might think. And you don't have to cut out meat entirely to reap most of the health benefits of vegetarianism. "If you can keep your meat intake to a small portion, like a side dish, you're probably all right," says Suzanne Havala, R.D., a nutrition adviser for the Vegetarian Resource Group and a dietitian who co-wrote the American Dietetic Association's position paper on vegetarianism.

Besides, Havala says, by the time you discover what variety vegetarian meals can offer, you may start missing meat less and less. "From my experience, people find vegetarian meals so delightful that they would just as soon forget about the meat altogether."

Here are some tips to get you started.

Lower the steaks. You don't have to eliminate red meat all at once, Havala says. "It's easier that way for some people. But lots of people like to taper off until they're not eating any meat after a few weeks or months," she says.

Try starting with one meatless day a week. How hard is that? As hard, Havala says, as eating cereal and a piece of fruit for breakfast, a peanut butter and jelly sandwich with a piece of fruit for lunch and pasta tossed with steamed veggies and a salad for supper.

Work your way up to two, then three or more meatless days per week. At that point, you can easily make the jump to full vegetarianism, if you want.

A World without Meat

When you were a kid, you learned all about the four basic food groups—meat, dairy, vegetables and bread.

As you grew up, you switched to new groups: beef, beer, chips and cheesecake.

It may be time to regroup.

"You don't need to eat meat to be healthy," says Suzanne Havala, R.D., a nutrition adviser for the Vegetarian Resource Group in Baltimore and a dietitian who co-wrote the American Dietetic Association's position paper on vegetarianism.

Here's a quick vegetarian primer, courtesy of Havala. And those new food groups are:

Breads, cereals and pastas. Eight or more servings a day. Examples of serving sizes include one slice of whole-grain bread; half of a bun or bagel; ½ cup cooked cereal, rice or pasta; and one ounce dry cereal.

Vegetables. Four or more servings a day. Serving sizes are ½ cup cooked vegetables and 1 cup raw. Be sure to include one raw serving that's rich in beta-carotene, such as carrots.

Legumes and meat substitutes. Two to three servings a day. Examples of serving sizes include ½ cup cooked beans, four ounces tofu and two tablespoons nuts or seeds.

Fruit. Three or more servings a day. Serving sizes are one piece of fresh fruit, ¾ cup juice and ½ cup cooked or canned fruit.

Dairy or alternatives. Optional, two to three servings a day. Serving sizes include one cup low-fat or skim milk, one cup low-fat or nonfat yogurt, 1½ ounces low-fat cheese and one cup calcium-fortified soy milk.

Eggs. Optional, three to four yolks a week. This includes eggs in baked foods. Note: Strict vegetarians, or vegans, do not eat eggs. Egg substitutes work fine in most recipes.

Fake it. Health food stores and some supermarkets sell stuff called meat analogs. You've probably heard of them—tofu burgers and meatless hot dogs are the most common. "Some people need to see something that looks like a meat dish at first," Dr. Mangels says. "Try them for a while. They might help you make the transition."

Don't fixate. People used to think that vegetarians had to plan their meals right down to the last gram to get adequate nutrition. "If you just make sure to get enough calories to meet your energy needs by eating a variety of fruits, vegetables, grains and legumes, you should be fine," says Havala.

Something to avoid: picking a favorite food and eating it five times a day. "Balance is the key," Dr. Mangels says. "Don't eat only grapefruit for two weeks straight, then switch to baked potatoes for half a month."

Be careful. Vegans—strict vegetarians who eat no animal products, including eggs or milk—must make sure they get enough B_{12}, a vitamin that aids in nervous system function. The vitamin is found mainly in animal products and in supplements. The Recommended Dietary Allowance is 2 micrograms.

If you drink low-fat milk, eat low-fat cheese or cook yourself an omelet, you're all set. But if you don't, try whole-grain breakfast cereal or soy milk.

Junk the junk. No diet, meatless or otherwise, needs to include lots of junk food. "To reap the most benefits from a vegetarian diet, limit or eliminate sugar and fat-filled foods," Havala says.

Ferret out the fat. Meat is loaded with fat. But it's not the only place you'll find that fiend. To lower your fat intake, Dr. Mangels suggests steaming foods, sautéing them in water, juice or wine and going easy on the cheese and mayo. "Low-fat salad dressings aren't a bad idea, either," she says.

Power up the proteins. Meat isn't the only food that's packed with protein. You'll get more than enough with a balanced vegetarian diet. "There is plenty of protein in grains, vegetables and legumes. Common meatless dishes such as bean burritos, vegetarian chili and stir-fried rice are packed with protein," Havala says.

C your way to enough iron. Again, a balanced vegetarian diet provides plenty of iron. But meat is still the best source of absorbable iron. You can increase the absorption of the iron found in vegetables by taking vitamin C. Havala suggests eating foods high in vitamin C at every meal. This includes tomatoes, broccoli, melons, peppers and citrus fruits and juices.

Don't have a cow over calcium. You'll get plenty of calcium in a balanced vegetarian diet, according to Dr. Mangels. If you drink milk and eat low-fat cheeses, you're in good shape. Calcium can also be found in collard greens, seeds and nuts, kale and broccoli.

Hit the road. "You don't have to be a stay-home eater just because you're a vegetarian," Dr. Mangels says. "You can eat out all you want. Just find a place with a good salad bar, and you're set." Most restaurants will give you a plate of steamed vegetables on request, too.

"Or try a Chinese restaurant. You can eat meal after meal there and never even think about missing meat," adds Dr. Mangels.

VITAMINS AND MINERALS

You Can't Live without 'Em

Breakfast? Oh, yeah. Coffee and a cold piece of toast. For lunch? Chips, cookies and soda. It's a candy bar for a jolt of late-afternoon energy. And suds and fries down at the tavern at the end of the day.

Is your daily diet providing the raw materials you need to function at your best? Not if you're eating like the guy we just told you about. He's not getting an adequate supply of vitamins and minerals, which means that the only thing keeping him going is cheap energy. And that won't last for long.

Vitamins and minerals, the building blocks of youth and vitality, keep you alive and kicking. While nutritionists are only just beginning to understand everything they can do, it's known that vitamins and minerals give you what you need to perform physically, mentally and emotionally. They rejuvenate and energize your cells. They make every single bodily process possible.

And bad things happen when a man doesn't get enough vitamins and minerals. For centuries, horrible deficiency diseases like scurvy, pellagra and rickets plagued mankind. These dreaded illnesses caused diseased teeth and gums, weak and brittle bones, unhealthy skin and hair; they even led to death.

The good news is that the modern American man follows a diet that has made most of these diseases extinct—thanks, in part, to the fact that many of the foods we eat, such as cereals, breads and grains, are fortified with vitamins and minerals. But it is still possible that you're not getting all the vitamins you need.

"As we age, our requirements for certain vitamins and minerals actually increase," says Jeffrey Blumberg, Ph.D., associate director of the U.S. Department of Agriculture Human Nutrition Research Center on Aging at Tufts University in Boston. "We tend to eat less food overall on a daily basis. So if your diet is already lacking a little in certain nutrients, as you get older, you stand a greater chance of widening that deficiency, and in some way your body will pay the price for it."

Growing evidence suggests that even a slight dip in vitamin and mineral intake may be to blame for a man's increased susceptibility to infection, slow healing, decreased mental capacity and chronic fatigue. The bottom line is this: To look, feel and perform at your best, you need to consume the right level of vitamins and minerals every day.

Vitamins Mean Vitality

How important are vitamins? Did you ever notice that the first four letters of the words *vitamin* and *vital* are the same? Coincidence or what?

Not at all. These organic chemical compounds facilitate and regulate every biochemical reaction and physiological process going on from head to toe. Each vitamin has a specific function, from helping bone growth to maintaining healthy skin to assisting the body in processing energy and so forth. Fall short in just one vitamin, and any number of vital functions can get out of whack.

Nutritionists divide the 13 essential vitamins into two groups based on their behavior in the body. Water-soluble vitamins—vitamin C and the eight B vitamins (thiamin, riboflavin, niacin, B_6, pantothenic acid, B_{12}, biotin and folate)—are fast-acting compounds that gravitate to the watery parts of body cells and assist the cells in chemical reactions and energy processing. They aren't stored for very long; the body quickly puts these vitamins to work and usually excretes any excess.

Fat-soluble vitamins—A, D, E and K—are found in the fatty parts of cells and regulate a wide variety of metabolic processes. They tend to be put in long-term storage and are then drawn upon as the body needs them.

While many studies have acknowledged vitamin intake as a factor in lowering the risk of chronic disease, several vitamins have been singled out for their unique ability to slow or even prevent the onset of age-related diseases like heart disease and cancer and to potentially slow the aging process itself. These vitamins—C, E and beta-carotene (a substance the body converts to vitamin A)—are known as antioxidants for their ability to neutralize destructive oxygen-derived particles believed to initiate many disease processes.

Minerals Mean Might

Millions of years ago, man first crawled out of the primordial sludge to assume his place on earth. So it seems only fitting that we have to draw from the soil from which we came to stay in good working order.

Like vitamins, minerals help keep the body functioning and facilitate biochemical reactions. But unlike vitamins, they are inorganic and not me-

(continued on page 558)

The 13 Essential Vitamins

Here's a handy table of vitamin requirements for men ages 25 to 50.

Vitamin	Daily Intake
Vitamin A	1,000 mcg. RE or 5,000 IU
B Vitamins	
Thiamin	1.5 mg.
Riboflavin	1.7 mg.
Niacin	19 mg.
Vitamin B$_6$	2 mg.
Folate	200 mcg.
Vitamin B$_{12}$	2 mcg.
Biotin	30–100 mcg.*
Pantothenic acid	4–7 mg.*
Vitamin C	60 mg.
Vitamin D	5 mcg. or 200 IU
Vitamin E	10 mg. alpha-TE or 15 IU
Vitamin K	80 mcg.

Daily intake values are Recommended Dietary Allowances (RDAs) unless otherwise noted.

Age-Erasing Benefit	Food Sources
Needed for normal vision in dim light; maintains normal structure and functions of mucous membranes; aids growth of bones, teeth and skin	Yellow-orange fruits and vegetables; dark green leafy vegetables; fortified milk; eggs
Carbohydrate metabolism; maintains healthy nervous system	Pork; whole- and enriched-grain products; beans; nuts
Fat, protein and carbohydrate metabolism; healthy skin	Dairy products; whole- and enriched-grain products
Fat, protein and carbohydrate metabolism; nervous system function; needed for oxygen use by cells	Meats; poultry; milk; eggs; whole- and enriched-grain products
Protein metabolism; needed for normal growth	Meats; poultry; fish; beans; grains; dark green leafy vegetables
Red blood cell development; tissue growth and repair	Green leafy vegetables; oranges; beans
Needed for new tissue growth, red blood cells, nervous system and skin	Meat; poultry; fish; dairy products
Fat, protein and carbohydrate metabolism	Found in small amounts in many foods
Fat, protein and carbohydrate metabolism	Whole- and enriched-grain products; vegetables; meats
Builds collagen; maintains healthy gums, teeth and blood vessels	Citrus fruits; peppers; cabbage; strawberries; tomatoes
Calcium absorption; bone and tooth growth	Sunlight; fortified milk; eggs; fish
Protects cells from damage	Vegetable oils; green leafy vegetables; wheat germ; whole-grain products
Clotting of blood	Cabbage; green leafy vegetables

*Value is the Estimated Safe and Adequate Daily Intake. There is no RDA for this vitamin.

The 15 Essential Minerals

Here's a handy table of the major and trace mineral requirements for men ages 25 to 50.

Mineral	Daily Intake
Calcium	800 mg.
Chloride	750 mg.*
Chromium	50–200 mcg.†
Copper	1.5–3.0 mg.†
Fluoride	1.5–4.0 mg.†
Iodine	150 mcg.
Iron	10 mg.
Magnesium	350 mg.
Manganese	2–5 mg.†
Molybdenum	75–250 mcg.†
Phosphorus	800 mg.
Potassium	2,000 mg.
Selenium	70 mcg.
Sodium	500 mg.
Zinc	15 mg.

Daily intake values are Recommended Dietary Allowances (RDAs) unless otherwise noted.

Age-Erasing Benefit	Food Sources
Strong bones and teeth; muscle and nerve function; blood clotting	Dairy products; green leafy vegetables; sardines with bones; tofu
Aids digestion; works with sodium to maintain fluid balance	Foods with salt
Carbohydrate metabolism	Vegetables; whole grains; brewer's yeast
Blood cell and connective tissue formation	Grains; legumes; shellfish
Strengthens tooth enamel	Fluoridated water; fish; tea
Maintains proper thyroid functioning	Beans; nuts; cocoa; grains; green vegetables
Carries oxygen in blood; energy metabolism	Red meats; fish; poultry; whole grains; dark green leafy vegetables; legumes
Aids nerve and muscle function; strong bones	Meats; poultry; fish; milk; beans
Bone and connective tissue formation; fat and carbohydrate metabolism	Spinach; nuts; pumpkin; tea; legumes
Nitrogen metabolism	Unprocessed grains and vegetables
Energy metabolism; teams up with calcium for strong bones and teeth	Milk; grains; iodized salt
Controls acid balance in the body; works with sodium to maintain fluid balance	Vegetables; fruits; meats; milk
Helps vitamin E protect cells and body tissue	Grains; meats; fish; poultry
Fluid balance; nervous system function	Salt; processed foods; soy sauce; seasonings
Wound healing; growth; appetite; sperm production	Seafood; meats; nuts; legumes

*Value is the Estimated Minimum Requirement. There is no RDA for this mineral.
†Value is the Estimated Safe and Adequate Daily Intake. There is no RDA for this mineral.

tabolized by the body. They provide structure to bones and teeth, are major components of blood, skin and tissue and keep the body's fluid levels balanced.

The 15 essential minerals are grouped into two categories. The major minerals—calcium, chloride, magnesium, phosphorus, potassium and sodium—are found in large quantities in the body and are abundant in our food sources. We require large amounts of these minerals.

The trace minerals—chromium, copper, fluoride, iodine, iron, manganese, molybdenum, selenium and zinc—are found in much smaller amounts in our bodies and in our food.

Once ingested, minerals make their way to every cell in the body. Some are stored, on reserve to replace those we lose in our urine and sweat. If we don't replenish our mineral stores as rapidly as they are being depleted, we run the risk of developing diseases such as iron deficiency anemia or osteoporosis.

A Man's Nutritional Needs

The most widely used guidelines for vitamin and mineral consumption are the Recommended Dietary Allowances (RDAs). These figures reflect the amount of a nutrient judged to be adequate for the average healthy person. "Because the levels exceed the actual needs of most people, you can actually be below the RDAs for a nutrient but still be well above the deficiency level," says Paul R. Thomas, R.D., Ed.D., staff scientist with the Food and Nutrition Board of the National Academy of Sciences in Washington, D.C. "Falling short of the RDAs usually isn't dangerous, but if your vitamin and mineral intake is routinely some 20 to 30 percent below the RDAs, deficiency problems could develop over time."

What about people who want to achieve superior health? "A growing body of evidence indicates a direct link between increased longevity and improved overall health when certain vitamin and mineral intakes exceed the RDAs," says Dr. Blumberg. "This suggests that perhaps the RDAs are inadequate for the changing needs of the aging adult."

But getting too much of some vitamins and minerals can be just as bad as not getting enough. "Taken in extremely high doses, many vitamins and minerals can be toxic," says Diane Grabowski, R.D., nutrition educator with the Pritikin Longevity Center in Santa Monica, California. "They can interfere with the functioning of vital organs like the heart, liver or kidneys. Or they can produce any number of harmless but aggravating side effects such as heartburn, nausea or frequent urination."

Research is in the works to determine the exact levels of each vitamin and mineral needed for optimal health. Until such results are found, doctors say that your minimum goal should be to reach 100 percent of the RDAs for every essential vitamin and mineral every day, especially if you lead an active life.

Food: Our Number One Nutrient Source

Meeting your nutrient needs is easier than you think. "A well-balanced diet consisting of a variety of nutrient-rich foods will easily supply all the vitamins and minerals you need—probably even more," says Grabowski.

Here are some tips for getting the maximum vitamin and mineral content from the foods you eat.

Stick with the basic five. "Concentrate on eating from the five basic food groups—fruits, vegetables, legumes and lean meats, grains and cereals and low-fat or nonfat dairy products," says Grabowski. "If you eat a lot of snacks that are nutritionally inferior or junk food, you're just giving your body empty calories that are devoid of vitamins and minerals."

Focus on fruits and veggies. "You should eat a minimum of five good-size servings of fruits and vegetables every day," says Grabowski. "In most cases, the darkest or most vibrantly colored fruits and vegetables have the richest vitamin and mineral content." This fruit and vegetable rainbow includes perennial favorites such as cantaloupe, oranges, peaches, tomatoes, spinach, yams and carrots. Ask your greengrocer to turn you on to some more exotic and unusual fruits and vegetables that are loaded with nutrients.

Eat 'em raw or just-cooked. Cooking food can draw out a lot of the vitamins and minerals, so whenever you can, try to eat fruits and vegetables in their natural raw or unprocessed state or minimally cooked. Try fresh fruits, raw or steamed vegetables and salads.

Don't boil. Boiling draws out more minerals and vitamins from foods than other cooking methods, says Grabowski. "The less time spent in the oven, on the stove or surrounded by hot water, the better." She recommends steaming or microwaving.

Store smartly. Exposure to air can rob food of vitamins and minerals. And light can penetrate glass bottles or cellophane wrap, destroying some vitamin content. Grabowski recommends using airtight containers as well as cartons or aluminum foil to keep light out. For long-term storage of foods or juices, try freezing. It keeps all the nutrients intact for a long time.

Be aware of medications. Certain drugs and over-the-counter medications can interfere with the body's vitamin and mineral stores. Aspirin, laxatives, diuretics, antibiotics, antidepressants and antacids can accelerate the excretion of some vitamins and minerals or impede their absorption. If you are taking any of these medications, consult your doctor before quitting or trying alternatives.

The Scoop on Supplements

Your diet should meet your nutritional needs. But many men don't eat a balanced diet and don't meet all the RDAs. If you think you need some nutritional help, seek out a health or nutrition professional who can evaluate your diet and suggest which nutrients you may need more of. Keep in mind, though, that supplements can't make up for all the damage done by poor eating habits.

Here are some guidelines for selecting and using supplements. Any supplementing at levels in excess of the RDAs should be done only in consultation with a physician.

Choose a good multivitamin. A safe and beneficial supplement would be a once-a-day type multivitamin with minerals, says Grabowski. Such a supplement should contain a mixture of all or most of the essential vitamins and minerals and contain close to 100 percent of the RDAs for each.

Be wary of single-nutrient supplements. In most cases, you probably don't need to have bottle after bottle of individual vitamins or minerals if you are taking a multivitamin and eating right. Exceptions would be if you are under a doctor's treatment for a specific deficiency or if you are seeking antioxidant protection by taking extra vitamin C, vitamin E and beta-carotene. Otherwise, avoid single supplements—especially vitamin A, vitamin D and iron, says Dr. Thomas. High doses can be toxic, producing nasty side effects such as vomiting, hair loss, bone abnormalities, anemia and renal, liver and cardiovascular damage.

Let content be your guide. Generic and store brands are typically comparable in quality to big-name brands, says Dr. Thomas. In fact, generics are often produced by manufacturers of the big-name brands but cost a lot less. Your pharmacist should be able to tell you if a generic is worthwhile.

Stay away from "super-supplements." You may see some supplements labeled "high potency" or "extra strength." These products typically contain levels of vitamins and minerals that greatly exceed the RDAs and may be hazardous, says Dr. Thomas. Or you may just end up excreting the excess, in which case you're wasting your money.

Forget the gimmicks. Phrases like "anti-stress formula" are bogus, says Dr. Thomas, and although "time-released" and "effervescent" are legitimate descriptors, in some supplements those qualities may not matter. For example, effervescence in calcium may be helpful, but it is not needed in vitamin C.

Don't go natural. Also, ignore claims about natural or organic ingredients, says Dr. Thomas. There is no standard definition of *natural*. Some "natural" supplements, in fact, may contain mostly synthetic nutrients.

Avoid multiple dosages. If the label tells you to take more than one a day, check the total amount to see how it compares with the RDA. If it's way over, this may be a ploy to get you to shell out more money, Dr. Thomas says.

Take 'em with your food. As a general rule, vitamin and mineral tablets will be absorbed more efficiently by the body if they are taken during a meal rather than on an empty stomach, says Dr. Thomas. They will also break down better if they're taken with water or some other beverage.

Check the expiration date. When shopping for supplements, make sure an expiration date is on the label. If the date has passed or is just around the corner, find a bottle with a longer shelf life.

Store in a cool, dry place. Supplements can lose their potency if exposed to light, heat or moisture. Because of this, a kitchen cabinet, away from the heat of the stove, may be a better place to keep your supplements than a windowsill or a bathroom medicine chest. The refrigerator is a good place, too. Try to use a non-transparent container. And always secure the cap tightly.

YOGA

Relaxation for Real Men

Yoga suffers from this unfortunate public relations problem. Mention it to most guys, and they picture some serious-looking mystic twisting himself into horrible little body knots. That may be his idea of stress reduction, but it sure doesn't sound like yours.

Well, try to keep an open mind. Because if you're looking for a top-shelf age eraser, something that will leave you feeling limber, relaxed, focused and downright youthful, you really ought to consider yoga.

"So many things you do in life are energy users," says Alice Christensen, founder and executive director of the American Yoga Association in Sarasota, Florida. "But yoga provides a constant source of energy. When you practice yoga, you actually have more vitality and vigor. In that way, I really think it can help to make you feel younger."

New Health from an Ancient Art

Yoga has been around for thousands of years. Literally translated, it means "union." Yoga advocates believe that mind, spirit and body are inseparable. And they believe that exercises called asanas, or poses, can aid in flexibility, relaxation, increased strength and inner peace.

Though there are as many as eight different branches of yoga, most Westerners focus on hatha yoga. This type of yoga stresses relaxation through asanas and breathing techniques and is often taught in classes at local YMCAs or fitness clubs.

Hatha yoga is not aerobic exercise. But studies show it can help soothe your body and mind in a number of ways.

The most obvious benefits appear to come in stress reduction and mood enhancement. A study of 170 college students showed that those taking beginner yoga classes had less tension, depression, anger, fatigue and confusion

Scan Away Your Stress

Some days you stagger home from work wearing a 50-pound suit of worries. Tension at the office has left kinks in your neck, throbs in your head and knots on the soles of your feet.

But a yoga-like exercise called the body scan can help you focus on those aches and slowly work them out of your body. Taught to patients at the University of Massachusetts Medical Center in Worchester, the body scan is a great way to identify and beat your own stress hot spots.

Here's how to do it.

Lie on your back, close your eyes and simply breathe. After a few minutes start concentrating on the toes of your left foot. Note the sensations: Are they warm, cold, tired or cramped? After a minute or so, imagine releasing the weight of your toes, feeling them melt right into the floor.

Now concentrate on your left leg, practicing the same routine on your foot, ankle, calf, knee, thigh and hip. Then do the same for your right leg. Move up your torso, pausing at your pelvis, lower back, belly, upper back, chest and shoulders. On your arms, move on to the fingers of both hands, the back of the hands, the palms, the wrists, the forearms, the elbows, the upper arms and the shoulders. Finally, move on to your neck, then into your head, paying attention to your chin, mouth, nose, eyes and eyebrows, forehead, ears and scalp.

The American Yoga Association, in Sarasota, Florida, advocates a similar complete relaxation exercise that is introduced just before meditation, though its plan works from the head down and then up the back of your body.

"The subtle benefit of practicing this type of exercise is that you'll become more aware of your body on a daily basis," says Alice Christensen, founder and executive director of the American Yoga Association. "Then even when you're sitting at your desk at work, you'll notice 'Oh, my stomach's tense' or 'I'm clenching my teeth.'

"The simple act of bringing awareness to the tense area will help you to release the tension."

after class than they did before. The students' reported feelings were similar to those of others who had started more strenuous activities like swimming. The study reported that the students began to notice stress reduction after taking their first class.

Yogic breathing techniques may also help people with asthma. A British study of 18 patients showed yoga breathing could reduce symptoms of asthma, though it did not eliminate them. Some doctors are now prescribing yoga as part of therapy to help their asthma patients gain more self-control over their breathing difficulties.

Christensen says yoga can also be tremendously helpful to people with back pain, as long as they follow the yoga principles of stretching slowly and only as far as the body wants to go. And she says it may help people with arthritis as well. Though there are few studies linking yoga and arthritis, Christensen says many of her students with common age-related arthritis report feeling more flexible and in less pain after starting a yoga class. Christensen warns, though, that people with bone-crippling rheumatoid arthritis should not attempt yoga exercise when their joints are swollen and painful.

In addition to the physical advantages of yoga, there's a meditative side that's impossible to measure with a stethoscope. "Yoga quiets the constant talk that's in your mind," Christensen says. "You deal constantly with scattered thoughts, other people's voices, emotions, desires. And you don't even notice it after a while."

Yoga can help clear that from your mind. "It helps improve your concentration and allows you to become more observant of your thoughts, feelings and reactions," says Christensen. "Much of the time we move through the world like the steel ball in a pinball machine, bouncing off one thing after another. Yoga meditation increases awareness, so you can make more conscious choices in your life."

How to Get Started

If you'd like to enjoy some of yoga's healthy benefits, here are some tips to help get you started.

Take a deep breath. Yoga begins with breathing, something we Westerners rarely think about. Most of us inhale from our chests, taking quick, shallow breaths. Yoga practitioners, however, breathe from their diaphragms, the large, dome-shaped muscle that arches across the base of the lungs. When a person inhales deeply, the diaphragm expands, allowing more air into the lungs' lower lobes.

To get started, sit comfortably on the floor, supporting your hips by sitting on a firm cushion. Or you can sit on the edge of a chair. Place your hands on your belly, a little below your navel. This is the area—not your chest—that should expand when you inhale. Remember to always breathe in and out through your nose. When you inhale, feel your hands rise. When you exhale, contract your belly. Breathe smoothly and evenly. After a few breaths, place your hands on your legs and continue breathing with your eyes closed, concentrating on the sound of the breath.

Ideally, you should breathe from your diaphragm all the time—at work, at

If It's Good Enough for Kareem...

Kareem Abdul-Jabbar played a young man's game for 20 years. And he played it better than anyone. At his retirement, he had scored more points than any other man in the history of professional basketball.

Sure, he was seven-foot-two. Sure, he had the sky hook, the most unstoppable shot ever. But he had another secret weapon that he says kept him in the game well into his forties, an age when many athletes are already burned out.

"There is no way I could have played as long as I did without yoga," Jabbar says. "My friends and teammates think I made a deal with the devil. But it was yoga that made my training complete."

Jabbar discovered yoga in 1961 when he was 14 years old. He started practicing on a regular basis in the 1970s. And a decade later, in his early forties, Jabbar was still running the floor with younger players and winning championships left and right.

Even in retirement, Jabbar remains convinced that yoga was a key to his phenomenal success. And he says any weekend warrior can get many of the same benefits.

"Once I started practicing it, I had no muscle injuries during my career," Jabbar says. "Yoga can help any athlete with hip joints, muscles, tendons and knees. Plus it keeps you in touch with your body."

home, in the car, wherever. Christensen says this helps you get more oxygen into your system, making you more alert. You'll also find yourself breathing at a more relaxing pace of maybe 10 to 14 times per minute instead of the typical 16 to 18 times. Remember, always breathe through your nose.

Find a good class. Lots of places offer yoga classes, but not every class is the same. Christensen suggests looking for a teacher who practices yoga every day and sees his own yoga teacher on a regular basis. Ask the teacher for references. Take a trial class before you invest long-term time or money. And if you have specific problems, like a bad back or arthritis, make sure you find a teacher who will individualize instruction for you.

Fly solo. If you're having problems locating a class, the American Yoga Association has a correspondence course. The course packet includes an instruction book (*The American Yoga Association Beginner's Manual*) and an audiocassette on relaxation and meditation. The course can be helpful when you're practicing at home, even if you're enrolled in a class. The association also offers a videotape and other instructional materials. A catalog is available on request. For more information write to the American Yoga Association, 513 South Orange Avenue, Sarasota, FL 34236.

Go at your own pace. Yoga isn't football. You're not there to out-stretch or out-meditate or out-breathe your friends who practice yoga or the other people in the class.

"At the very least, you need to know that you should not compete," says Martin Pierce, director of the Pierce Program, a yoga studio in Atlanta. "If you are looking around at others thinking you must do as well as they do, you are going to create more stress for yourself." Direct your attention inward, Christensen says. "Pay attention to your own experiences, and you will achieve the most lasting results."

Strike that pose. Christensen says many yoga stretches, or asanas, are easy for beginners. But whatever your level of expertise, remember: Don't push your body. Stretch slowly and evenly. Don't bounce. And push only as far as your body lets you. "Going too far will injure you. Be a friend to your body," Christensen says.

Always check with your doctor before you start practicing yoga or any exercise program. See the illustrations for examples of asanas you can try at home.

Stick with it. You may start feeling better about yourself after just one yoga session, but don't stop there. "People can't expect to benefit greatly from yoga without making a commitment to it," says Jon Kabat-Zinn, Ph.D., director of the Stress Reduction Clinic at the University of Massachusetts Medical Center in Worcester.

"Yoga practice should be regular—daily, if possible," Christensen says. "At the very least, if you want results, it demands three exercises and a few minutes of breathing and meditation. This can take as little as 15 minutes. If you find yourself wanting to practice more, an hour a day is plenty. The important thing is to enjoy what you do."

Keep working out. Beginner yoga is not aerobic exercise. Christensen recommends that you continue with bicycling, walking, running or some other activity that gives your heart a workout. "Think of yoga as an added dimension to your fitness program," she says. "It is never boring, because besides offering the physical benefits of limberness, health and strength, it adds meaning to life."

Yoga for Beginners

If you're interested in trying yoga, these four poses are a good place to start. Remember: Don't stretch past the point of comfort.

The tree pose. This is a balance pose that improves poise, posture and concentration. Stand with your feet parallel. Shift weight to your right leg and place the heel of your left foot against your right ankle. Hold on to a wall or chair for support if you need to. Slowly raise the left foot higher, assisting with your free hand, until the foot reaches your right inner thigh. Place your arms at your sides. Then slowly bring them over your head as straight as possible with your palms together. Relax your stomach and your breath. Stare at one spot for balance. Hold for several seconds or as long as you can comfortably. Then slowly lower and repeat on the opposite side.

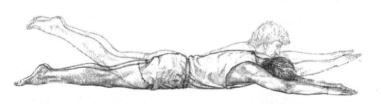

The boat pose. This is an excellent exercise to strengthen the back and improve posture. Lie on your stomach with your arms outstretched in front and your forehead on the floor. Breathe out completely, then breathe in as you raise your legs, arms and head all at once, looking up. Breathe out and lower. Repeat twice more.

(continued)

Yoga for Beginners—Continued

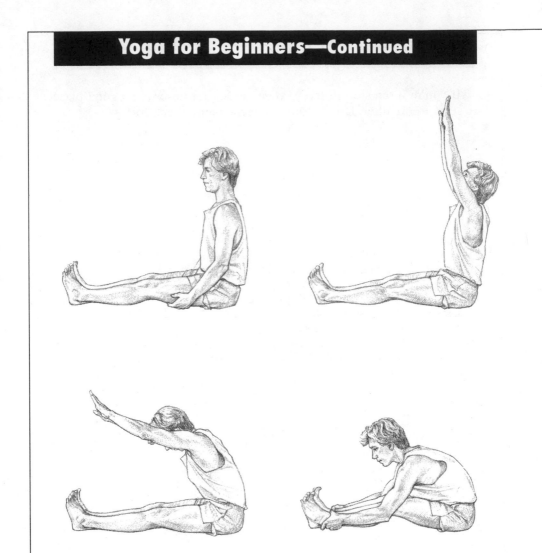

Seated sun pose. This exercise limbers the back and legs, massages the internal organs and improves circulation. Sit on the floor with your legs outstretched and your toes pulled back toward your face (upper left). Breathe in and raise your arms to the sides and over-head (upper right). Stretch and look up. Then tuck your head, start to breathe out and slowly bend forward as far as you can without straining (lower left). Get a good grip on your legs wherever you can reach, bend your elbows and gently pull your upper body down toward your legs (lower right). Use your arms to pull, not your back muscles. Hold for a few seconds. Breathe in and raise your arms back up overhead. Then breathe out and lower your arms to your sides. Repeat twice more.

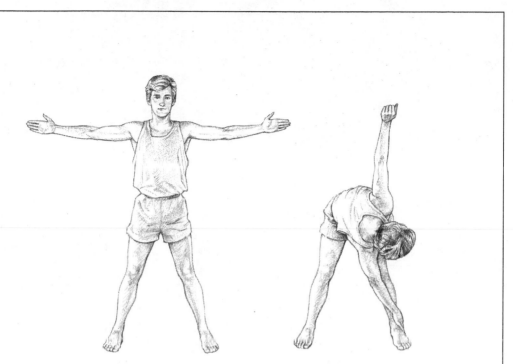

The twisting triangle. This exercise limbers the back, hips and legs and may help relieve depression. Stand with your feet pointed straight ahead, as wide apart as you can stand comfortably (left). Breathe in and raise your arms out to the sides, then breathe out and twist to the left (right). Grasp the outside of your left ankle with your right hand, extend your left arm straight up with fingers slightly curled and look up at your left thumb. Hold for just a moment, then breathe in and return to a standing position with your arms outstretched. Breathe out and repeat to the right leg. Stretch three times to each leg.

Sources and Credits

"Are You Burning Out?" on page 58 is adapted from *Burnout: The High Cost of High Achievement* by Herbert J. Freudenberger. Copyright © 1980 by Herbert J. Freudenberger and Geraldine Richelson. Used by permission of Doubleday, a division of Bantam Doubleday Dell Publishing Group, Inc.

"Is Alcohol Controlling Your Life?" on page 118 is adapted from the *American Journal of Psychiatry*, vol. 127, no. 12, 1655, June 1971. Copyright © 1971 the American Psychiatric Association. Reprinted by permission.

The table in "What's a Healthy Weight, Anyway?" on page 223 is from the U.S. Department of Agriculture and U.S. Department of Health and Human Services.

"Chart Your Flow" on page 230 is a test courtesy of the Male Health Center, Dallas, Texas.

"Is Tension Adding Up?" on page 289 is adapted from *Is It Worth Dying For?* by Robert S. Eliot, M.D., and Dennis L. Breo. Copyright © 1984 by Robert S. Eliot, M.D., and Dennis L. Breo. Used by permission of Bantam Books, a division of Bantam Doubleday Dell Publishing Group, Inc.

"Is Work Wearing You Out?" on page 290 is from the American Institute of Stress. For more information, write to 124 Park Avenue, Yonkers, NY 10703.

"A Swift Solution" on page 293 is reprinted by permission of the Putnam Berkley Group from *The 15-Minute Executive Stress Relief Program* by Greg Herzog and Craig Masback. Copyright © 1992 by Herzog Body Tech, Inc.